YOUR ORTHOMOLECULAR GUIDE FOR
HEALTHY BABIES AND HAPPY MOMS

Vitamins&
Pregnancy
The real story

Helen Saul Case

Basic
Health
PUBLICATIONS, INC.

Basic Health Publications, Inc.
an imprint of
Turner Publishing Company
424 Church Street • Suite 2240 • Nashville, Tennessee 37219
445 Park Avenue • 9th Floor • New York, New York 10022
www.turnerpublishing.com

Vitamins & Pregnancy, The Real Story:
Your Orthomolecular Guide for Healthy Babies and Happy Moms

Library of Congress Cataloging-in-Publication Data is available
through the Library of Congress

Editor: Karen Anspach
Typesetting/Book design: Gary A. Rosenberg
Cover design: Kimberly Richey

Printed in the United States of America
10 9 8 7 6 5 4 3 2 1

Contents

Acknowledgments

Thanks to my wonderful husband for his constant love and support.

Thanks to the editorial board and contributors to the *Orthomolecular Medicine News Service*.

Thanks to Steven Carter, Executive Director of International Schizophrenia Foundation. Thanks also to the editors of the *Journal of Orthomolecular Medicine* and the International Society for Orthomolecular Medicine.

Thanks to Ralph K. Campbell; Jack Challem, "The Nutrition Reporter"; Thomas E. Levy; W. Todd Penberthy; William B. Grant; Barbara Smith; Steve Hickey; and Robert G. Smith.

Special thanks to my mom, who by her own example demonstrated the value of orthomolecular medicine during her pregnancies.

Special thanks to my dad, who has dedicated his life to helping improve the lives of others.

And finally, thank you to my children, who are walkin' talkin' proof that this stuff works.

Foreword

by Ralph Campbell, MD

I am a father and I am a pediatrician. Both of "us" realize that with experience, we do things better. If only we could make our care for our firstborn retroactive, especially in terms of applying what we have subsequently learned about good nutrition! Well, here is your chance to do it right straight away. An ounce of prevention is worth a ton of cure. Helen Saul Case gets right to the heart of the matter by beginning at the beginning—an oft-neglected practice—with a discussion of nutritional supplements when you are just considering pregnancy. She continues with what is to be done after pregnancy is confirmed. Thinking ahead is the epitome of true motherhood and demonstrates a keen desire to do everything possible for the good of her offspring. At the same time, the mother-to-be can help herself to better personal health, which translates to having more energy and a better outlook on life, all of which benefits her baby.

Why do we need this book? Because doctors do not receive much, if any, useful training in nutrition. I had zero nutrition courses when I was in medical school. Afterward, the pharmaceutical companies provided precious little information of value about vitamins. Their attempts at formulating "prenatal vitamins" have been, at best, a cruel joke. Quantities are too low. Ferrous sulfate makes pregnant women nauseous. Artificial color in the tablet helps no one. The vitamin or mineral du jour—the rare nutrient that "modern medicine" currently accepts—is introduced and touted in a new formula. Well, that is better than nothing, but only just. Folic acid to prevent spina bifida; calcium "for healthy bones and teeth"; all given in the dose that meets the so-called "safe" (that is, pitifully inadequate) standard of the times. Preparing mothers with what they really need for optimal health means giving optimum quantities of nutrients to do the job. Orthomolecular medicine recommends more for good reasons. This book is full of good reasons that will enable women to tactfully negotiate the issue with their obstetricians. My experience has been that most doctors give little thought to the subject, and simply automatically issue their favorite brand of a designated daily, prenatal vitamin-mineral. That is cookie-cutter medicine, and it isn't good enough. The United States has a poor world standing as far as infant mortality goes. That is sad, and that can be improved immediately. This book will fill a void that has been present for decades.

Helen Saul Case is the daughter of orthomolecular medical writer Andrew W. Saul. He has reason to be proud. Our children who have picked up our message have certainly benefited and are able to pass it on. Mrs. Case shares information with you in a readable, nontechnical, but solid, scientifically grounded manner. I am impressed that she has foreseen almost every instance that would prompt questions and has provided clear, appropriate answers for everything from breastfeeding to postpartum depression. I hope that this book will be widely read, digested, and acted upon. It is very much needed.

Preface

I want to write this book for one simple reason: I wish I'd had one like this when I was pregnant. Having been born and raised with nutritional medicine, I have always felt comfortable with the use of vitamins and confident in both their safety and efficacy. When I found out that I was expecting a child, I felt I should have been able to seamlessly transfer this knowledge and apply it to care for my "new" pregnant body. But now, even *I* was nervous about taking nutritional supplements. It was one thing to be secure about my own choice to take vitamins. It was yet another to make this decision for a life I hadn't even met. I started questioning what I knew. I started looking for clarification. Nothing motivates a person to learn quite like the responsibility of having a child. I wanted to make sure I was doing the right thing.

I didn't just want to be sure. I wanted to be *really* sure. Was I taking enough of the vitamins my baby needed? How could I make certain I was getting the most beneficial dose? (An amount I suspected differed from your standard prenatal vitamin.) I knew I had a lot to learn, but by golly, I was going to learn it.

I believe the information we get from our doctors about vitamins is extremely insufficient. Pregnant women will simply be told about the standard government recommendations, provided there is even time for this discussion. I spent far more time in the waiting room than I ever did in an appointment with my obstetrician. There was little opportunity to ask detailed questions and get thoughtful, thorough responses. I doubt the word "orthomolecular" would have been in any of the answers anyway.

We need to have access to all the information out there, not just some of it. Many women and their babies would benefit from getting an abundance of nutrients during pregnancy, especially if there are health concerns, but the word "orthomolecular" is also conspicuously absent from most pregnancy health guides and parenting books.

I strongly believe that natural, alternative, drugless solutions are of great value during pregnancy. Upon investigation, you will find that many doctors and researchers agree. We need to know as much as we can about all of our options so we can make the best decisions for ourselves and for our babies.

This book was written and edited throughout my own pregnancy, from the day I found out I was going to have my second child and into the first two years of my new baby's life. I'll share with you what I have experienced with both of my children and what I have learned about the value of optimal doses of vitamins during pregnancy.

Vitamins & Pregnancy: The Real Story isn't just another pregnancy health book. This one is different. Typically, other pregnancy guides flatly discourage the use of vitamins at even the slightest increase over government recommendations. None of them really address the role of high doses of vitamins for a safe and healthy pregnancy. It is time for a change. Instead of searching through facts and myths about vitamins and preg-

PROCEED WITH CAUTION

If you are looking for a book about the miracles of modern medicine and pregnancy, read something else.

If you want to know how nutrition and vitamins can make life before, during, and after pregnancy a whole lot easier, remarkably healthier, and a lot less scary for both you and your baby, read on. An orthomolecular pregnancy is a healthy pregnancy. I have seen it work up close and personal. So, too, did my mother.

When you need information, it's nice to know where to find it. This book is for first-time moms and repeat moms alike. It is for parents about to begin this incredible journey and parents who have been down this road before. In fact, this book is for everyone who has suspected there is more to the story about vitamins and pregnancy than they may have heard. If you are ready for the real story, then you have come to the right place.

nancy, this book is intended to make your life just a little easier by putting a collection of this valuable vitamin information conveniently into your hands.

We know all too well what an immense personal responsibility we have when we bring life into this world. The best decisions are those we make when we come armed with information. Since we only get part of the story about vitamins at the doctor's office, I'd like you to hear about the rest of the story here.

You will notice that I quote extensively from the *Orthomolecular Medicine News Service* in this book. This is intentional. You can subscribe, free of charge, to *Orthomolecular Medicine News Service* articles at http://orthomolecular.org/subscribe.html and access the article archive at http://orthomolecular.org/resources/omns/index.shtml. This noncommercial, peer-reviewed publication contains research, clinical experience, and analysis from over twenty-five natural healing physicians and experts.

You'll also notice that I often quote my father, Andrew W. Saul. This is also intentional. I think that if you are going to quote someone, you may as well pick the person who you think can say it best. After all, my father has been teaching others (that includes me) about vitamins and natural healing for over thirty years, and I happen to like his delivery. We are a father-daughter orthomolecular team. It seems only natural to me to quote the most influential person of my professional career.

CHAPTER 1

Preg Trek

"A grand adventure is about to begin."
—WINNIE THE POOH

Pregnancy is hard. Parenthood is harder. It is tough, tiring, and terrifying to bring new life into this world and then try to keep it healthy and out of prison.

It is decided. You are going to have a baby. Life is about to throw you a million hardballs all at once (not counting the ones that got you into this position) and you left your helmet at home. So grab the nearest object, sister, and start swinging.

We are going to put words on these pages that you can use to help you get through what may be one of the toughest times in your life. Let's tell it how it *really* is, and then let's make it *better*.

DESPITE OUR BETTER JUDGMENT, WE ARE PREGNANT

"If you want to know what it's like to have a fourth child,
imagine you are drowning and someone hands you a baby."
—JIM GAFFIGAN

The experience of being a mom is disconnected from the love we feel for our kids. It is separate. It is "other." Motherhood is hard, messy, unrelenting, and physically exhausting. We are going to feel crappy once in a while. We are going to be drained dry. It is insanely hard to be pregnant. To give birth. To be a parent. Feel free to take a moment and mentally curse the carefree families in their unstained clothes in the "if you place presliced cookies on a baking tray with your kids, they will love you more" commercials. Take a moment to roll your eyes at the "happy family on vacation" advertisements. Where *are* all the screaming children in the Disneyland commercials? Scratch that—where are all the screaming *parents*?

Truly, I'm not here to depress you. We are going to keep it real, is all. This is no time to sugarcoat the truth.

I love my children dearly. I would do anything for them. But this book is not about our emotional capacity to love another human, in or out of the womb. We are here to dive headfirst into what can plague us during pregnancy and after, and how vitamins and nutrition can help.

One thing is for sure: pregnancy and motherhood is drastically harder when it is compounded with health issues. Let's try to make them never happen. If you've got them, let's work to make them go away.

Good Health and Real Choice

I don't know what I would have done without vitamins. On top of all that motherhood gifted me in a big basket—with a card that said "Ha ha!"—there is no way I could have handled the inevitable stress and health issues that come with pregnancy and being a mother of two without them.

Vitamins gave me options. I did not have to rely solely on a medical system filled with doctors who study standardized medicine and dole out medications, nor did my children.

Vitamins gave me choice. I was not reliant on drugs: over-the-counter, prescription, or illicit.

Vitamins gave me comfort. I did not fear side effects, complications, dosage errors, or death.

Vitamins gave me a safe way to prevent and treat illness. We all get sick. How we get *better* is where we differ.

WAITING FOR BABY

> "By far the most common craving of pregnant women
> is not to be pregnant."
> —PHYLLIS DILLER

It seems there is a lot of time to think and reflect while pregnant. In fact, it seems like there is little else to do. This was especially true while I was pregnant with my first child.

With my first, my daughter, I spent my days thinking "I'm *pregnant*. I'm *pregnant*. I'm *PREGNANT*. I'm going to have to give *BIRTH*," in unceasing loops. I had plenty of time to obsess. What is one to do with all those moments we have to think each day? Worry, that's what. And worry I did. About everything and anything. To get some answers, I signed up to baby newsletters and chat rooms and blogs. E-mails arrived weekly that kept me up-to-date about the current size of my baby (comparing her to some fruit or vegetable) and also kept me terrified with endless lists of seemingly crucial "do's and don'ts" that had me convinced that eating a smidgen of soft cheese or changing my kitties' litter box was going to do me or my baby permanent harm. There was no end to the things I could work up a panic about: Crib safety. Car seat safety. Proper infant car seat installation. Paint fumes. Microwaves. Logos on baby clothing that made her a walking advertisement. Pink clothes are not okay. Pink clothes are okay. No raw fish sushi, darn it anyway. What vitamins to take. Giving birth. I don't have enough baby clothes. I don't have the *right* baby clothes. Must buy more blankets. Baby will suffocate. Must get rid of all blankets. And so on. Endless, torturous, emotionally draining internal dialogues debating all the things that might go wrong, all of the things I don't even know I might be doing wrong, all of the things that I must buy because I Have To Have Them Before I Have A Baby . . .

And then here come all those well-meaning folks, with their hands on your belly threatening to sugar you up with orange juice so the baby will kick. I kept hearing people tell me that time was flying by. For whom? Them? I spent each day of nine months in feverish anticipation. They smile and want to know how everything is going. I was exhausted. I was puking. I was scared stiff. Instead of sugar-coating my answer with a polite, "Oh, just fine thank you," I found myself telling *the truth*. As they got a little paler, I felt a little better. We can't be Little Miss Sunshine all the time.

Shower Power

This is the true genius of the baby shower. In years BC, or "before child," I used to think such an event was tedious and unnecessary. More to the point, I thought baby showers were positively awful. Must we send *each* tiny outfit slowly around this great circle of cooing females to be meticulously admired for each ridiculous and pointless detail before the guest of honor opens another damn present? Does everyone have to bring all their hyperactive children and let them eat every sugar-encrusted morsel in the place and scream over every conversation just to show the poor new mother what she's in for? Must we all touch her protruding stomach? Must we play juvenile pregnancy games? Maybe it's not polite to measure how large around the middle she's become. Even a good friend, who became a mother years before me, didn't invite me to her shower, knowing full well she was doing me a great kindness.

My own pregnancy did not change my mind. A few months along and in a fit of hormonal rage, I vowed I would never have a baby shower. Ever.

Okay. I had sex. I got pregnant. This has happened billions of times on this planet. This isn't exactly rocket science. My children were *planned*, for goodness' sake. Why do I deserve "congratulations"? I called my mother and I declared I didn't need a shower and I didn't, and I quote, "want people to go out and buy a bunch of pink and blue sh*t." Patiently, my mother listened. And bless her heart, she said nothing and waited.

With time comes clarity, and thankfully I have not been spared.

First, I considered that maybe the baby shower really wasn't for *me*, it was for the baby. I relaxed my stance a bit and I resigned to have one. There had to be something I could put on the shower page of the baby book. Of course, I had a few rules. We would serve liquor—to make the party less boring for everyone else–and ban all big-belly games. I, of course, would not drink.

I have heard women declare that being pregnant was the best time of their lives. "I loved being pregnant," they would say. I would try to understand, but I never really got it. I did not "enjoy" pregnancy. I found it to be a daily challenge of aches and pains and new bodily symptoms I couldn't have dreamed up if I tried. Pregnancy books left out a whole lot on those pages. (I confirmed this after my first baby was delivered.) The giggly woman who taught the child-birthing classes at our hospital was irritatingly upbeat as she explained things so simply to us, as if *we* were the babies, that we learned nothing new at all. As much as I read, nothing could have prepared me, truly, for the experience of pregnancy and new motherhood.

In the end, it was each pregnant woman for herself. And no matter how supportive my husband was, I felt alone. Suddenly, I found this intense irrational need to be around a bunch of women who were going to do nothing but be positive and uplifting and excited and congratulatory. I wanted the fantasy of the carefree pregnancy so often pictured in magazines and on TV. I wanted to pretend, for a couple of hours, that motherhood was the classical music and soft focus pastel image we see in a Johnson's baby shampoo commercial.

I wanted a baby shower.

I called my mom and told her, who was going to make sure I had one anyway. I actually began to look forward to the event, and I planned an outfit accordingly.

Most days, my husband's joy and anticipation carried me through my pregnancy. But that one day, just that one, when a whole gaggle of women were excited for me and for baby, changed who I was. I didn't care that it was all temporary. It didn't matter that the few hours of escapist bliss in no way represented motherhood and the trials and tribulations yet to come, save those transcendent moments when a child smiles at you for the first time or runs through your yard with the wind in her hair.

It was the best day of my whole pregnancy.

I vowed, from this point on, I would attend all future baby showers with bells on. I would coo, congratulate, and pass every precious puffy little outfit around the room and be genuinely excited to do so. I would stay to the bitter end with a big smile on my face. A whole roomful of people helpful and supportive of you? Bring it on. For goodness' sake, we don't get enough of these moments when we are a mom.

Then I realized—the shower isn't for the new baby on the way. It's for the mother who needs, very much, at this moment, a temporary feeling of complete and resounding love and support. Looking back, I wish the shower had happened months sooner. The whole day was so special, I found myself wishing I had had its energy with me for a greater part of the pregnancy experience.

Planning for Baby

With my first baby, I spent my entire pregnancy planning how *I* wanted things to be: now, during birth, and after. This is because first time moms' minds need distraction. They need stuff to do. We have our jobs to keep us busy, but before children take over the house, there are still plenty of hours in the day to plan, to dream, and to obsess. Thoughts have all day to flow in and out and between all those other tasks we attend to. This is why there are so many pregnancy books: there is still time to read and think, especially before your first child. And then you will probably never read them again (except for this one, of course). With my free hours I made mental lists, made demands, bought supplies, cleaned house, cooked (not nearly enough) meals to put in the freezer, and loaded my iPod with hours of Ayurvedic pan flute and sitar music to soothe me during labor. I bought breath mints for the hospital, packed my emergency duffle, and put it by the front door, inclusive of a neatly typed and color-coded list of important phone numbers to hand to a nurse to notify folks of the birth, just in case my cell phone was dead or I couldn't speak or my husband went missing. I even carried a towel in my car and an extra pair of pants. (My husband's response to my fear of water breakage in public simply was, and without jest, "You could always wear Depends." You may wonder *why* he didn't suddenly go missing.)

I never did need that package of breath mints. Correction, I probably *needed* them, but there was a heck of a lot more I cared about than my breath at that particular time, and no one dared suggest otherwise. I found most labor-preparedness activities are distracting at best; some were ultimately useless. I had an overnight bag full of things I never touched. I had a birth plan I didn't even look at. The house didn't stay clean for long.

And yet after all of it, we had a beautiful healthy baby and nothing else mattered.

There is much we cannot control during our pregnancy, and I'm not about to pretend I have all the answers. But what I do know is that there is a great amount of valuable vitamin research out there that can help make our pregnancies as successful, comfortable, and stress-free as possible. The old saying is that life is a journey, not a destination, but in this case we *are* waiting expectantly for a "destination"—a baby in our arms. Let's make the journey to get there as good as it can be.

Reality Strikes

It figures, too, after all of that worrying, nothing could have prepared me for the real time, real life, engrossing and passionate, visceral experience of motherhood. After I gave birth, all that stuff I worried about, like, um, childbirth, was far more intense than I had ever anticipated. It looked like I had the *right* to feel the way I had all of these months.

At three in the morning, moments after her birth, my husband stared down at her, this beautiful, vibrant little girl, and with tears in his eyes.

"No wonder why people have so many of these."

I paused, I blinked, and I looked down below my waist. I was still laid out on the table, knee-deep in the results of biology, with doctors working carefully for well over half an hour on the final checklist of details to attend to after any baby is born. Nurses worked to clean me and the surrounding fifteen feet. Originally, when I walked into the delivery room, I scoffed at dust and hairs on the floor, vowing to not touch the tile with my bare feet. Now, I marveled how it was possible that the room could have been as clean as it was, given what I just witnessed had happened here, and happened on a daily basis.

I looked back to my husband, still very much in the moment with his new baby and I said, "*I can't.*"

And I couldn't. After everything I had gone through, from day one of being consciously aware of my pregnancy until now (and I still did not know how hard the days ahead would be), I could not for the life of me figure out why people ever had more than one child. They must be out of their minds.

For those of you that are already parents, and those of you that are parents of more than one child, you already know why. Now, I do, too.

The Second Child

June 6th, 2012

Yesterday, I found out I was pregnant. This will be our second child, and my husband is thrilled.

Having done this before, I am all too well aware of what is in store for me over the next nine months and beyond.

I, too, am excited to have another baby. I'm not as excited about all it takes to get there.

Sometimes it seems as if there is no place for women to express feelings like this, save the numerous online pregnancy posts and the underground market of tell-all motherhood books. With so many families out there longing for children that they might never be able to have, for families who have suffered miscarriages, still-births, and any number of the other issues that come with making and having a child, it can sound downright ungrateful when those of us with the good fortune to be pregnant, carry to full term, and deliver healthy babies come around and start complaining. We may feel pressure to hush up about how we really view motherhood. Sure, we are excited. That anxious, feverish, twitchy kind of excited. We may also be terrified.

Looking for comfort? Good luck. You'll be scared silly by all the don'ts, nevers, stay aways, and better nots plastered in prenatal pamphlets, posters, and popular parenting magazines. You can't sit in the waiting room of the doctor's office without ample access to issues of "Fretful Mother" (as Marge is seen leafing through on an episode of *The Simpsons*), the pages of which will have you second-guessing absolutely everything you do before, during, and after baby is born.

After already having had one child, no one can accuse me of not knowing any better. Those of you choosing to go around again know this, too. So why *do* we do this?

It's because babies are awesome. And if you want to have a baby of your own, there are specific procedures you must follow to get there. While there is nothing easy about choosing a surrogate or the adoption process, I feel that those of us who are biologically staged and ready to bring life into this world have a tough job on our hands, and we need more than just a bit of understanding and sympathy.

With my son on the way, kicking merrily in my womb as I write, I am pleased to report to having a much more "present" pregnancy. I don't spend my time worrying, obsessing, purchasing, or fretting. I spend my time chasing after my daughter, identifying every object known to man that she points to, giggling at silly faces we make, coming up with creative ways to make sure she gets plenty of vegetables, rediscovering everything in the world through the eyes of a person who's never seen any of it before, and simply playing the day away.

My daughter has brought me into the present moment: *this* moment. There is just no escape. Kids don't really give you a chance to reflect for long on what has already happened, or dwell on what the future holds. Sure, you can spend time cycling through those thoughts once they have gone to bed, but while they are up, they demand your constant attention one way or another with the necessities of the day: clean diapers, meals, and teaching them how to be human. Kids force you to be here now, and

I can only imagine that as the number of children in one's house increases, so decreases the opportunity to live anywhere but right here, right now.

As I prepare for baby number two (if you want to call it "preparation"), so much has become less important, as *he* has become more important. The color of the nursery isn't particularly significant. Matching furniture isn't exactly obligatory. A diaper stacker may not be the "essential convenience" it is advertised to be.[1] What he will wear doesn't really bother me either. Yeah, I've purchased boy outfits, but only a few. My self-restraint didn't exist when my previously pregnant self shopped for girl clothes. (Everything is just *so* darn cute.) But now, instead of buying one of everything in every color and every future size, maybe if he ends up in a pink-flowered onesie his sister used to wear because he's accidentally defiled the rest, and laundry just hasn't made into the machine that day, that's okay. No one but my husband and I will see him adorned in daisies, and who knows, maybe he'll grow up to be an ecologist.

With my daughter there were so many things I thought I *had* to have. The hours I spent in the ob-gyn office scanning through parenting magazines (far longer than I ever spent with a fetal Doppler pressed to my abdomen or a tape measure across my belly) certainly didn't help ease my hunger to own all-things-baby. Gosh, it was so expensive to have a child—but look at all of these things I can't possibly do without! I would read over the ten top-rated jogging strollers, and would be in awe that some cost $700 or more. What about The Perfect Nursery? This had to be something to dwell upon, and I was happy to do so. I have to be a great mother. I mustn't compromise. I would scribble down frantic little lists and stuff the oddly ripped pieces of paper into my purse. Baby swings. Baby carriers. Play yards. Linens. Maternity clothes . . . my, that's a cute dress! (Online later, I'd find not a single thing in that store magazine advertisement that would cover my rear end for less than $300 bucks. Forget that!) Sweating and hyperventilating, I'd be called back to the examination room, always surprised that my blood pressure hadn't shot straight up.

I prepared the house from roof to floorboards. I cleaned, disinfected, re-cleaned, redecorated, and reorganized. Furniture, bedding sets, baby changing and bath time supplies, infant toys, and clothing were purchased.

But when all was said and done, many of these absolutely critical, positively indispensable, incredibly necessary-to-have baby items remained untouched, still wrapped in factory packaging, now waiting to be donated.

What have I bought so far for baby number two? An extra car seat and a crib. Done.

It is immensely liberating to face the coming of the new baby with the experience of already being a mom. Plenty of folks will judge my parenting, but that's inevitable. The difference is whether or not I care about their opinion. Before, I could be likened to the incredibly self-aware, self-conscious middle schooler who is convinced that all eyes are on her at all times scrutinizing her appearance. Do I fit in? Are my jeans cool? Do I look enough like the others? Now in my thirties, I have a more casual, carefree demeanor. For example, "I don't care if I'm seen in this, I'm just going to Walmart" and other I'm-a-mother-now wardrobe decisions come easy. Such decisions also come with the wonderful side benefit of not giving a damn about what other people think. My baby girl manages this relaxed attitude without even knowing it. She is often dressed in a cozy gray hoodie and is, of course, mistaken for a boy. She smiles. I smile. Neither of us bother to correct them. It's just not a big deal.

We can probably imagine a crazed bride scanning the pages of *Vogue* for the perfect dress and accessories, and venue, and decorations, and body, and groom—only to find herself feeling diminished. There is much that is out of reach if you are a bride to be, or a new mother to be. There is plenty to want, if you want it. And for those who do want it, it can cost a small fortune. A bride may end up mortgaging her future for that $20,000 Vera Wang dress, the perfect favors (which nobody keeps anyway), a delectable catered meal, the hippest DJ in town . . . all for Just. One. Day.

I think of the brides or grooms that spent so much time planning their weddings, they forgot to fully consider the person they are about to marry. We have all been to those events where the wedding itself was dreamlike and amazing, except for the fact that you can tell the couple isn't going to make it past year two. It's pretty sad, really, but the planning of a marriage, or a baby, can sometimes cloud the reality of the situation.

Know in your soul the partner you are about to spend the rest of your life with is the right one. Know in your soul that when you are going to have a baby, having a healthy, happy child is the only things that matters.

During my first pregnancy, I was perfectly willing to be drowned in the social expectation of motherhood. Fussing over all the products I thought I needed to purchase was a welcome diversion from my physical concerns.

"The baby is going to fit through where?!"

I spent my nights fretting. During my second pregnancy, I set aside all judgment, including my own of myself. I avoided baby newsletters, sensationalist advertising, and parenting magazines. I focused on the wonderful child I already had, and considered how even more wonderful it would be to have two. I took care of my baby, and consequently, I took better care of myself by focusing on what was in front of me and nothing else. There is so little we truly can "control" during pregnancy. I decided to spend more time centered on what I could influence. My health was one. The way I spent my time was another.

I have yet to meet my son-to-be, but he has already taught me so much. I know I will love him for a million reasons, but at the moment I love him because he gave me a second chance to be pregnant—this time more happily so—and for that, I thank him.

My baby girl is waking up from her nap, so I'll let my keyboard cool down for a bit. It's time to play.

The Care and Feeding of the Stork

When I was six and a half months pregnant, I went to my ob-gyn for the standard spend-at-least-a-half-an-hour-waiting-and-probably-more-for-a-two-minute-pregnancy-checkup appointment.

Things were moving rather quickly that day, which is always nice. It wasn't so much the waiting that would get to me, but the *heat*. Those little exam rooms are stifling. I'm confident they are kept at a balmy ninety-five degrees Fahrenheit year round. Once while waiting and sweating right through my shirt, I tried to crack the door open, hoping some cooler air would drift in from the hallway. I was politely asked to keep it shut; otherwise the doctor wouldn't know I was ready to be seen.

Note to self: Wear absolutely nothing but a classy spaghetti string tank top and shorts to my next pregnancy checkup even in the dead of winter. Yes, underwear optional.

Properly dressed today, I was comfortable as could be. As she checked my blood pressure, the nurse asked how I was feeling.

I said, "Great!"

She replied, "No complaints, then?"

"Nope."

"Most people have a very long list," she said. (I guess she would know, right?) "But it is great that you are doing so well."

And I was. Aside from the growing pains of mommyhood and pregnancy —my shoulders getting tight from carrying my one-and-a-half-year-old around, and my back lower back getting sore from time to time from the weight of a blooming belly—I really had nothing to complain about. Really.

This was my second pregnancy. My first had been more physically challenging as my body adjusted to the new experience of growing a human being. (When those hips expand . . . !) I had my share of nausea and exhaustion, especially early on, but no medical issues whatsoever. This pregnancy was going even more smoothly. I was less nauseous this time around, too, though still tired and in need of the occasional nap. Once again, I was free of *any* medical issues.

My doctor entered the room. He measured my pregnant belly, told me my glucose tests were great, and, since I had no questions for him, he sent me on my way. I think our face-to-face time was a minute and a half, tops. On his way out he said, "You are making my job easy, Helen!"

Now it is possible these folks are just being polite. Or perhaps I'm an anomaly. I have yet to meet anyone who was raised like me, from the womb into adulthood: where vitamins and nutrition were routinely used for the successful treatment of our illnesses and, equally important, the prevention of illness. My brother and I never met our pediatrician. It's true. We had one; we just never needed to go. My parents didn't even know exactly where the office was until one day they drove by it simply by chance. My mom said, "Hey, isn't that it?"

Lest my parents appear to look recklessly irresponsible, consider this: the secret of good health is not about avoiding doctors, but about not needing to go. I saw it as a child, I saw it as a college student, I saw it as an adult, and now I see it as a mother.

Of course, when you are pregnant, it is prudent that you visit your doctor or midwife. I sure appreciated my doctor's help, and he liked that I was healthy.

Good diet and vitamins have always served me well. And now, my baby was benefiting. This book will help your baby share in these benefits, too.

Rock-a-bye baby
Inside my tum,
Soon your nine months
Will be done.

Out will come baby,
In our arms you'll go,
And we will love you
Forever more.

—My version of the song I used to sing
to my unborn children

CHAPTER 2

Vitamins and Pregnancy: Fact versus Fiction

It is rare that anyone addresses the most important question:
"What works best?"

—W. TODD PENBERTHY, PhD, Research Professor,
University of Central Florida

There are literally hundreds of prescription and over-the-counter prenatal vitamins on the market. They are essential for healthy pregnancies, but they may not meet the needs of all women and all babies.

In optimal quantities, vitamins help ensure healthy, full-term babies and healthy moms. But what is "optimal?" With so much conflicting information out there, it's time to look into what nutritionally-oriented physicians have found beneficial. It's also time to look at research that has been largely ignored.

In a healthcare system dominated by modern pharmaceutical medicine, orthomolecular (nutritional) medicine tends to linger quietly in the shadows. It's only fair that we take the time to level the playing field a bit. In all fairness, medical doctors aren't trained to utilize vitamin therapy. If there is a problem during pregnancy, doctors reach for drugs, not nutrients. But we have options. We have access to safe, natural, drugless solutions. We can avoid prescription drugs and use vitamins and nutrition to tackle pregnancy problems instead.

"Drugs are not the answer, unless you are a drug company."
—*Orthomolecular Medicine News Service,*
Vol. 4, No. 8, Aug 2008

We're going to debunk the myths that say vitamins are harmful and bring forward the evidence showing that vitamin supplements are helpful in pregnancy, even at dosages above our government recommendations. In the following chapters, we'll look at each vitamin and its benefits and its safety, one by one.

I don't believe in scare tactics that discourage moms from taking therapeutic doses of vitamins. I believe in what orthomolecular doctors have found to be true in practice, I believe in evidence, and I believe in what I have experienced through two healthy pregnancies.

Be as informed as you can be. You will decide for yourself if nutritional medicine is right for you. Talk to your doctor or midwife. Look into the research. Do not believe, even for a second, that what is fed to you in the mass media is the whole story. (Does *anybody* still believe everything they see on TV is true?) Keep reading; keep researching. As you may well know, it is a liberating experience to be in charge of your own health.

WHAT DOES THE WORD "ORTHOMOLECULAR" MEAN?

"Nutritional Medicine is Orthomolecular Medicine."
—*Orthomolecular Medicine News Service*

By definition, "ortho" means "right." Orthomolecular medicine is nutritional medicine: it is the practice of using nutrients that are normal and familiar to the body to prevent and cure disease. Two-time Nobel prize winner Linus Pauling came up with the name "orthomolecular" to describe using the "right" molecules to heal the body and to keep it healthy in the first place. It doesn't have to be complex; it basically means we should eat right and take our vitamins. "Anyone who wishes to become familiar with orthomolecular medicine may do so by simply beginning with a wholefoods, sugar-free diet, and a few vitamins," says orthomolecular medicine pioneer Abram Hoffer, MD.[1] This is something many of us are trying to do anyway during pregnancy.

"Orthomolecular" describes a way of living that promotes health and discourages disease. It encompasses a way of feeding the body with the very substances it requires to live. We depend on nutrients to survive. So does our baby. We depend on getting the right amounts of these nutrients to be healthy. It's true that some people require more nutrients than others.[2]

Sure, "orthomolecular" is a fancy word. But you do not need to use the word—rather, the goal is to *do* this word.

Orthomolecular medicine is twofold: prevention and treatment. Both are of value during pregnancy. Our goal is to achieve the best possible health for ourselves and for our baby by obtaining effective doses of nutrients. If there are health issues present during pregnancy, nutritional therapy is all the more important. Pregnancy is no time to "test" medications. Instead, you can choose to address illness by providing your body with the right nutrients to help it heal and do so safely. For those of us entrenched in a medical perspective, it may still be hard to believe: nutritional treatment is effective, cheap, and free of side effects.[3] It is safer for us and far safer for our baby. I know it works, and I have two healthy kids to prove it. My mom would say the same about us; she proved it a generation before me.

> *"Anyone who wishes to become familiar with orthomolecular medicine may do so by simply beginning with a whole-foods, sugar-free diet, and a few vitamins."*
> —ABRAM HOFFER, MD

PRE-PREGNANCY NUTRITION

All women of childbearing age should take a multivitamin *at the very least*. Here's why. Half of all pregnancies in the United States are unplanned.[4] *Half.* While there is never a bad time to start paying attention to good nutrition, taking care of your health *before* you get pregnant is ideal. We aren't eating enough fruits and vegetables every day.[5] In fact, only a sorry 11 percent of Americans get the recommended amounts of fruits *and* vegetables in their diet.[6] The advice is simple: make half of each plate fruits and vegetables.[7] Better yet, make them organic fruits and veggies. All you have to do is take a look at what's on the average checkout line at the grocery store or the dinner table to know this is not happening. There is no substitute for a diet rich in fruits and vegetables. Could we at least manage to take a vitamin tablet?

A little of a vitamin may be enough to prevent deficiency. More often, dosages of vitamins in amounts much higher than government-recommended dietary allowances are required for ideal health. Dosages will depend on the individual and the need. A dry sponge holds more liquid; sick or

MULTIVITAMINS PROTECT AGAINST HEART DEFECTS

Maternal multivitamin intake is significantly beneficial to a growing baby and her mother. The *Journal of Obstetrics and Gynaecology Canada* states, "Promoting the use of folic acid and a multivitamin supplement among women of reproductive age will reduce the incidence of birth defects."[8] A study in the *American Journal of Epidemiology* found taking multivitamins during pregnancy could prevent heart defects. In their discussion the authors state, "We found that women who reported using multivitamin supplements in the periconceptual period were at significantly lower risk of having babies with congenital heart defects than were women who reported not using multivitamins."[9]

stressed body requires more vitamins.[10] So, too, does a pregnant gal. This is why doctors recommend taking prenatal vitamins, and with good reason. Will your prenatal vitamin be sufficient? It might. You and your baby may also benefit from individualized doses of nutrients best suited to you and your needs.

Good nutrition can help you get pregnant and stay pregnant. Already had a baby? Good nutrition helps your body prepare for the next one and heal from the last one. Have you used hormonal birth control in the past? Among many other side effects, the pill depletes your body of vitamin B_2, vitamin B_6, vitamin B_{12}, folic acid, vitamin C, magnesium, and zinc.[11] It would be wise for any woman who has used hormonal birth control to address nutrient insufficiency before she becomes pregnant.

It's Time to Say "No" to Drugs

The media spends so much time telling you what vitamins *not* to take that many women have been scared off beneficial supplements, even multivitamins.[12] What is more concerning is the sheer number of people taking pharmaceuticals: 70 percent of Americans (seventy!) take at least one prescription drug,[13] and so does their dog.[14] More than half of Americans take two medications,[15] very many of which, such as antidepressants, can be harmful to a developing baby. To top it off, women are more likely to take medication than men. "Women receive more prescriptions than men across several drug groups, especially antidepressants," reports Mayo Clinic.[16] This means many unplanned pregnancies could also come with many unwanted drug-induced birth defects. Since half of pregnancies are unplanned, there is no "good" time for a woman of reproductive age to be on prescription drugs. Those first few months—and before—are especially crucial for the development of a normal, healthy baby. This is no time to be taking prescription drugs that could harm an infant. And yet, many women will and do. Others may stop taking medications too late. Some will be advised to continue taking their prescription anyway.

Many drugs come with warnings on the label of the little orange container that caution not to take the medication while pregnant or nursing or if you intend to become pregnant. Others have that information crammed onto a tissue-thin insert. I read one that said, "Do not take this drug if you become pregnant." Well, if you *know* you are pregnant, maybe that means something to you. Unplanned pregnancies and the simple fact that we may not know we are pregnant until we miss a period means our baby may be exposed to a medication that specifically warns against use during pregnancy at the earliest stages of development.

"Just say no to drugs" is still very good advice. We know to say no to alcohol and tobacco while we are pregnant. We can say no to pharmaceuticals, too. Think about it: if it isn't good for a developing baby, how can it really be good for us? I imagine that many women who take pharmaceuticals for their health issues must feel they have no other choice; perhaps the medication feels like (or has been presented as) the only option.

"Well, I only took the medication for a few weeks. Hopefully the baby will be fine," we may tell ourselves.

Maybe our baby will be fine. Maybe she won't. In and of itself, the word "maybe" is not one we want to use to describe whether or not our child is healthy and developing normally. What an awful feeling that must be. It's time to lift this burden—we do not have to be on drugs to be well. There is another way.

Many of us already know this. As Abraham Lincoln said, "You cannot fool all the people all the time." We are getting smarter. We are figuring it out. People who have taken pharmaceuticals and have failed to get better know full well that drugs do not have all the answers. People who have suffered devastating consequences of prescription medication side effects, or have children who have suffered, aren't going to accept it anymore. Many people have witnessed this broken system, and find this reason enough to seek healthier, natural alternatives. No, we will not be fooled. There is a safer way. There is a better way.

When 75 percent or more of doctor office visits and hospital visits involve prescription drug therapy,[17] we cannot count on our doctors, or the media, to recommend vitamins instead of medicines. We must choose to protect our own health and that of our unborn children. We must look into nutrition for ourselves. Nutrients will always be safer than drugs. Period.

THE IDEAL PREGNANCY

What would a perfect pregnancy look like? Feel like? How would it begin? I think delivery by stork would be pretty neat, but the next best thing might look something like this:

Carolyn Dean, MD, ND, who has authored over thirty books on natural health, describes her idea of an ideal, "peaceful pregnancy."[18] She knows that for most of us, "a completely balanced and harmonious life" may not be within our grasp,[19] but let's set that aside for a moment.

"Ideally, both partners would abstain from cigarettes, alcohol, coffee, over-the-counter drugs, and prescription medications for the six months prior to conception," says Dr. Dean. "They would eat organic food that was free of genetic engineering, pesticides, herbicides, hormones, and the other chemical adulterants common in factory-farmed and processed foods. For both partners, stress would be at a minimum, as it would be regulated by prayer and meditation, deep breathing, daily exercise, and a loving graceful attitude toward life and other people."[20] Then, in the ideal pregnancy, these healthy activities would all continue, says Dean. The new mom would pay special attention to her diet, exercise, get regular massages, meditate, and she and her partner would create a safe and secure home environment for their baby that is free of harmful substances like cigarette smoke and toxic cleaning products.[21]

Sounds pleasant, doesn't it? A healthy mom, a healthy baby, and an effortless birth. Yes, this would be ideal. But what if this was also *possible*? What if mothers were able to get as close to the perfect pregnancy as possible? How would they feel? How would their babies fare? How would both mom and baby's health benefit, now and in the future?

If you consider it, there is really nothing *impossible* here. There are many women who could do exactly as Dr. Dean describes. Many others could at least start doing some of it. And many families would reap resounding benefits if they paid such close attention to every part of their health. We can put our health and our baby's health first, and the benefits of such a lifestyle are not limited to pregnancy. Imagine, as my father would call it, "the epidemic of health" that would occur if all Americans strived to live this way.

If it was possible we would also get all the vitamins, minerals, and other nutrients our bodies required through careful selection, preparation, and ingestion of our food. But we don't. Our diets are lacking, to put it mildly, and to make things worse, much of the food available in the grocery store is not made of the choicest, healthiest ingredients. This makes it even more important that vitamin supplements be part of our pregnancy.

Maternal Nutrition and Fetal Development

The health of a baby starts with what the mother consumes, but it doesn't end there. According to the *Journal of Nutrition,* "Promoting optimal nutrition will not only ensure optimal fetal development, but will also reduce the risk of chronic diseases in adults."[22] Want your baby to be healthy now *and* later? Eat right and take your vitamins. "Nutrition is the major intrauterine environmental factor that alters expression of the fetal genome . . . namely, alterations in fetal nutrition and endocrine status may result in developmental adaptations that permanently change the structure, physiology, and metabolism of the offspring, thereby predisposing individuals to metabolic, endocrine, and cardiovascular diseases in adult life."[23]

What we eat not only impacts the healthy development of our baby in the womb but also our child's likeliness of acquiring certain diseases later in life. This idea of "fetal programming" and the potential of "fetal origins of adult disease"[24] means while we are pregnant we make a profound, lifelong impact on our baby each time we eat a meal and choose to take our vitamins. A limited supply of nutrients can permanently change their physiology and metabolism.[25] And, says *Nutrition* journal, "these 'programmed' changes may be the origins of a number of diseases in later life, including coronary heart disease and the related disorders stroke, diabetes, and hypertension."[26] It's a pretty amazing thought, really. And yet doesn't it make perfect sense?

Perhaps it goes even further—a whole lot further than you might think, says Andrew W. Saul, PhD, author and coauthor of many orthomolecular health books, including *The Vitamin Cure for Infant and Toddler Health Problems.* "Ova (human eggs) are formed during the fetal stage of a female's life. In other words, all of a woman's own eggs are actually formed while she was developing inside her mother, before she herself was born," Dr. Saul says. "This means that what your grandmother ate significantly contributed to your anatomy. Think that one over: what looks to be purely a genetic problem may in fact be largely a nutritional one. I call this "dinner table heredity." Just because a problem comes out of the womb does not mean that that problem is genetic and only genetic. Science has known for decades that many a specific birth defect is a direct result of a specific vitamin deficiency."[27]

In a sense, pregnant women literally nourish their own grandchildren. Add the concept of "dinner table heredity" to environmental factors and eating behaviors learned from our parents, and nutrition may be a bigger piece of the puzzle than simply genetics.

If the airplane is going down, we are instructed to put the oxygen mask on ourselves first so we can be conscious to place the mask on our little ones. To take care of them and save them from disease now and in the future, we must take care of ourselves during pregnancy. We must put our nutrition first.

VITAMIN DOSAGES AND STUDY LIMITATIONS

"It is difficult to get a man to understand something when his salary depends upon his not understanding it."
—UPTON SINCLAIR

If we put only a Band-Aid on a broken leg, we might understand why it doesn't heal properly. It's harder to understand how scientists can give a tiny, ineffectual dose of a vitamin and then declare it useless—or worse yet—say it is harmful. There are numerous research studies of vitamins showing their safety, health benefits, and successful treatment of disease when they are given at vastly higher intakes. This includes the efficacy of vitamin treatment during pregnancy.

A tremendous amount of research has been done that proves the value of getting an abundance of vitamins during pregnancy. Much of this research has been ignored. Consider, for example, that the National Library of Medicine, paid for by our taxes, does not even *index* the *Journal of Orthomolecular Medicine*. Censorship is a very large part of the reason we don't get to hear the real story about vitamins. It is one reason why I feel so compelled to write this book.

The RDA and Alleged Tolerable Upper Intake Levels

"RDA= Ridiculously Deficient Amount."
—STEVEN F. HOTZE, MD

Valuable research studies have been marginalized by government declarations of what are supposedly the "safe" intake levels of vitamins, as specified by the U.S. Department of Agriculture's (USDA) Recommended Dietary Allowance (RDA) tables. For example, by setting a tolerable upper intake level of vitamin C as it currently stands at 2,000 milligrams (mg) per day, any study that would seek to use larger amounts in human trials could be deemed unethical, even if the individuals studied require larger doses of the vitamin for it to be effective for their particular condition. For example, let's imagine a tolerable upper intake of water set at eight glasses a day. If a study done on dehydration limits the water intake of its participants to eight glasses a day, and then recruits only ultramarathon runners and other hardcore athletes, the study could potentially show that water did not relieve dehydration effectively. Obviously, athletes might need much more liquid than that to stay hydrated under these conditions. "You can set up any study to fail," says Dr. Saul. "One way to ensure failure is to make a meaningless test. A meaningless test is assured if you make the choice to use insufficient quantities of the substance to be investigated." For example, he says, "If you give every homeless person you meet on the street twenty cents, you could easily prove that money will not help poverty. If you give RDA levels of vitamins, do not expect therapeutic results." There's more. "To a great extent, the problem is in the nature of the research," says nutrition expert Jack Challem. "Single-nutrient studies are by nature reductionist in that they try to isolate the effects of individual nutrients. This approach may work for pharmaceuticals, but nutrients always work in tandem with other nutrients. No right-minded physician would treat or try to reduce the risk of disease with just one nutrient."[28]

Alleged "tolerable upper intake levels," arbitrarily set by our government, limit studies with such "safety" guidelines. Of course, lining up a bunch of pregnant ladies and pumping them full of higher and higher dosages of vitamins to see what happens is unethical. However, limitations set on the study of vitamins are not restricted to the women in the prenatal category.

Additionally, RDAs and tolerable upper intake levels are supposedly based on what "healthy individuals" need. Stress, pregnancy, illness, and much more affects our health. Believing that somehow a healthy diet is enough for everyone to obtain the vitamins and minerals they need is wishful thinking, and it is false. Supplements are needed to supplement a healthy diet, and if you aren't eating healthy foods you need supplements even more.

I have included the RDA and tolerable upper intake levels for the nutrients discussed in this book when available. This is not because I agree with them; it is simply for your information. While there are times the RDA may be sufficient for a healthy individual, there are far more people that would benefit from an ample intake of essential nutrients, not merely the amounts suggested to prevent deficiency.

"Tolerable upper intakes" are believed by many nutritionists to be too conservative and largely theoretical. In his paper "'Safe Upper Levels' for Nutritional Supplements: One Giant Step Backward," Alan R. Gaby, MD, who also has a degree in biochemistry and is an expert in nutritional medicine, says that these limits are excessive and inappropriately restrictive.[29] Such proposed "safety" limits can do more harm than good if folks are scared away from the effective, often larger, doses of vitamins needed for therapeutic results.

Doing It Wrong

Could you hurt yourself with vitamins? You could certainly try. There is a right way and a wrong way to do anything. When we are pregnant, it is understandable to want to know if something could be harmful to us or for our baby. However, "Any discussion of side effects or of toxic reactions without specifying the doses is meaningless, for at zero levels nothing is toxic and at sufficiently high levels everything is toxic, including oxygen and water," says Abram Hoffer, MD.[30] Fortunately for us, vitamins fall in the oxygen and water category. We require them for life. So does our baby.

Vitamins, even in very high doses, are extraordinarily safe. Just because it is *possible* to hurt yourself with vitamins doesn't mean it is likely or that it is easy to do. Vitamin insufficiency and deficiency is far more common than vitamin injury from overdose. This is also true during pregnancy.

And what is a vitamin "overdose" anyway? When the low RDA and alleged "tolerable upper intake levels" are used as guidelines, one could say that any amount of a vitamin in excess of these numbers is too much.

Nonsense. You are far more likely to hurt yourself by not getting enough nutrients than from getting too much.

Unlike with drugs, there is a very large margin for error and, therefore, for safety with vitamins. Minerals are not vitamins, but their safety record is also very good. No matter how you look at it, both vitamins and minerals are vastly safer than any drug on the market.

IF SOME IS GOOD, MORE IS BETTER

A common criticism of vitamin therapy heard from the medical profession and the media is their perceived notion that those who follow the orthomolecular approach think, "If some is good, more must be better."

Abundance happens to be a good thing. When it comes to doses of vitamins, we have these set ideas of what is "small" and what is "large." Orthomolecular physicians know a small dose of a nutrient tends to be an ineffective dose.[31]

Folks who take lots of vitamins are seen as wasting their money. I flatly disagree. Spending money on safe, effective nutrients is worth it. You can spend money on good health, or you will most assuredly spend money on sickness. Cancer is one. Chronic disease is another. Poor nutrition clearly contributes to both.

The facts aren't pleasant. Cancer rates in children are rising.[32] More people will get cancer this year than last.[33] Men, women, and their children will turn to the top medical doctors and brightest scientific minds. They will check into some of the most advanced medical facilities in the country. And tragically, over half a million people will die anyway.[34] Each year.

The fight against cancer and chronic disease starts at home, not in hospitals. Eating lots of fruits and vegetables can protect us against many cancers[35] and chronic diseases.[36] Studies show that a higher intake of fruits and vegetables could cut your risk of cancer approximately in *half*.[37] Incorporating a variety of lots of fruits and vegetables into your diet is, and always will be, a good idea. Don't let anybody tell you otherwise.

Our government recommends making half your plate fruits and vegetables; it's a wonderful goal but it is hard to do. Taking supplemental vitamins can help fill nutritional gaps and provide a measure of what Roger J. Williams, discoverer of pantothenic acid (B_5), would call "nutritional insurance." Prevention of illness is a far better plan than having to treat illness. In my opinion, this is especially true when we are pregnant.

People are told that a balanced diet will give them all the vitamins and minerals they need. They are told they don't need supplements. In fact, they are warned that they are harmful. Is there bias? Well, consider that the presence of major articles concluding that supplements were not safe was 4 percent in journals with the fewest pharmaceutical advertisements and 67 percent in those with the most.[38]

People aren't eating right.[39] Many struggle with illness. Folks are constantly dealing with health issues, and pregnancy is no exception. Fortunately, we have a drug-free alternative for better health right at our fingertips: better nutrition.

When it comes to nutrients, go ahead and get plenty. Some is good, and oftentimes, yes, more is even better.

DRUGS VERSUS VITAMINS

"Let the opponents of vitamin therapy cite the double-blind placebo controlled studies upon which they have based their toxicity allegations. They can't, because there aren't any."
—ABRAM HOFFER, MD, PhD

Over 100,000 people die each year due to pharmaceutical drugs.[40] These are deaths due to medications that are correctly prescribed and taken *as directed*. We are not talking about injury due to doctor's errors, which is another category entirely. "Over 1.5 million Americans are injured every year by drug errors in hospitals, doctors' offices, and nursing homes. If in a hospital, a patient can expect at least one medication error every single day."[41]

Vitamins, on the other hand, have an extraordinary safety record. Vitamins are literally a million times safer than pharmaceuticals. If it seems "easier" to just do as the doctor directs, rely on their judgment of safety, and proceed to take medication during pregnancy, you run the risk of adverse effects far greater than any associated with vitamins or minerals.

BIG BUSINESS SUPPLEMENTS?

You may have heard the supplement industry being accused of being "big business." "My fellow health journalists have an annoying habit, when a negative study on vitamins is published, to point out that vitamin, herbal, and related supplements are a $20 billion a year industry—as if to say all this money is based on deceiving consumers," says nutrition reporter Jack Challem.[42]

Here is some perspective on the situation. If vitamins are "big business", then the pharmaceutical industry is truly gargantuan. "The drug Lipitor, made by Pfizer, generates more than $12 billion in revenues each year worldwide," says Challem. "The annual revenues of Merck, just one of the drug companies, are $23 billion worldwide. The entire pharmaceutical industry, in just the United States, has revenues of more than $200 billion." Such facts are conspicuously absent from the magazine pages and media broadcasts that bash nutritional supplements and celebrate drugs. Let's remember where the money is really going, and who really stands to profit.

An Extraordinary Record of Vitamin Safety

Are you concerned about taking pills during pregnancy? Good. That's just plain smart. You should always pay attention to what goes into your body during pregnancy. So first, we will start with the obvious: nobody dies from taking vitamins. The articles below demonstrate just how remarkably safe vitamins are.

No Deaths from Vitamins—None at All in 27 Years

COMMENTARY BY ANDREW W. SAUL, PhD AND JAGAN N. VAMAN, MD

(Orthomolecular Medicine News Service (OMNS), June 14, 2011) Over a twenty-seven year period, vitamin supplements have been alleged to have caused the deaths of a total of eleven people in the United States. A new analysis of U.S. poison control center annual report data indicates that there have, in fact, been no deaths whatsoever from vitamins . . . none at all, in the 27 years that such reports have been available.

The American Association of Poison Control Centers (AAPCC) attributes annual deaths to vitamins as:

2009: zero	2008: zero	2007: zero	2006: one
2005: zero	2004: two	2003: two	2002: one
2001: zero	2000: zero	1999: zero	1998: zero

1997: zero	1996: zero	1995: zero	1994: zero
1993: one	1992: zero	1991: two	1990: one
1985: zero	1984: zero	1983: zero	

Even if these figures are taken as correct, and even if they include intentional and accidental misuse, the number of alleged vitamin fatalities is strikingly low, averaging less than one death per year for over two and a half decades. In 19 of those 27 years, AAPCC reports that there was not one single death due to vitamins.[43]

Still, the *Orthomolecular Medicine News Service* Editorial Board was curious: Did eleven people really die from vitamins? And if so, how?

Vitamins Not *THE* Cause of Death

In determining cause of death, AAPCC uses a four-point scale called Relative Contribution to Fatality (RCF). A rating of 1 means "Undoubtedly Responsible"; 2 means "Probably Responsible"; 3 means "Contributory"; and 4 means "Probably Not Responsible." In examining poison control data for the year 2006, listing one vitamin death, it was seen that the vitamin's Relative Contribution to Fatality (RCF) was a 4. Since a score of "4" means "Probably Not Responsible," it quite negates the claim that a person died from a vitamin in 2006.

Vitamins Not *A* Cause of Death

In the other seven years reporting one or more of the remaining ten alleged vitamin fatalities, studying the AAPCC reports reveals an absence of any RCF rating for vitamins in any of those years. If there is no Relative Contribution to Fatality at all, then the substance did not contribute to death at all.

Furthermore, in each of those remaining seven years, there is no substantiation provided to demonstrate that any vitamin was a cause of death.

If there is insufficient information about the cause of death to make a clear-cut declaration of cause, then subsequent assertions that vitamins cause deaths are not evidence-based. Although vitamin supplements have often been blamed for causing fatalities, there is no evidence to back up this allegation.

"If vitamin supplements are allegedly so 'dangerous,'
then where are the bodies?"[44]
—Andrew W. Saul, PhD

No Deaths from Vitamins. None. Supplement Safety Once Again Confirmed by America's Largest Database

BY ANDREW W. SAUL, EDITOR

(Orthomolecular Medicine News Service (OMNS), Jan 3, 2014) The 30th annual report from the American Association of Poison Control Centers [AAPCC] shows *zero deaths from multiple vitamins.* And, there were *no deaths whatsoever from vitamin A, niacin, vitamin B_6, vitamin C, vitamin D, or vitamin E.*[45]

It was claimed that one person died from vitamin supplements in the year 2012, according to AAPCC's interpretation of information collected by the U.S. National Poison Data System. That single alleged "death" was supposedly due to "Other B Vitamins." Since the AAPCC report specifically indicates no deaths from niacin (B_3) or pyridoxine (B_6), that leaves folic acid, thiamine (B_1), riboflavin (B_2), biotin, pantothenic acid, and cobalamin (B_{12}) as the remaining B vitamins that could be implicated. However, the safety record of these vitamins is extraordinarily good; no fatalities have ever been confirmed for any of them.

Even if it were to be allowed that the lone alleged fatality claim was correct, one single death in a year associated with nationwide vitamin supplementation is an astonishingly small number. Well over half of the U.S. population takes daily nutritional supplements. If each of those people took only one single tablet daily, that makes 165,000,000 individual doses per day, for a total of over 60 billion doses annually. Since many persons take far more than just one single vitamin tablet, actual consumption is considerably higher, and the safety of vitamin supplements is all the more remarkable.

Abram Hoffer, MD, PhD, repeatedly said: "No one dies from vitamins." He was right when he said it and he is still right today. The *Orthomolecular Medicine News Service* invites submission of specific scientific evidence conclusively demonstrating death caused by a vitamin.

There isn't any. Case closed.

If we want what is safest for our bodies and our babies, it starts with questioning the use of pharmaceutical drugs during pregnancy and looking into natural, safe, and effective alternatives. We have options. We have choice. We don't have to rely on drugs, but we must (and do) rely on nutrients.

An orthomolecular pregnancy means getting optimal doses of nutrients, not merely avoiding nutrient deficiencies. This book will discuss the benefits of optimal, individualized levels of vitamins during pregnancy, vitamin efficacy, and vitamin safety, even in large doses. It's time to take the fear out of taking vitamins.

TAKING YOUR VITAMINS

"The number one side effect of vitamins is failure to take enough of them. Vitamins are extraordinarily safe substances."
—Andrew W. Saul, PhD

Let's answer a few of the common questions I hear about vitamins and pregnancy: how much should we take, how much did I take, do we just urinate out all those nutrients, and is it possible to get enough vitamins through our food.

Can't We Just Get Plenty of Vitamins through Our Food?

Pregnant or not, the idea that we can obtain all the nutrients we need through our diet is substantially untrue. It's a nice legend.

Any trip to your local grocery store will remind you: we have incredible access to a dizzying variety of things we can put in our mouth. Much is edible, but not everything should be.

There's an entire aisle in our grocery stores dedicated to nutritionally void cookies and snacks. Another is reserved for chips and soda. I imagine someone with some design sense knew the two belonged together, just like pasta happens to be on the other side of the aisle from tomato sauce. The bulk "food" aisle is loaded with items we might consider anything but food: plastic bins full of wafer cookies, the everything-dipped-in-chocolate section, and the irresistible mounds of candy that have lured many, child and adult alike, into "just tasting" and committing petty larceny.

Navigating around our directory of pregnancy no-no's, we may avoid every possibly toxic ingestible and every potentially dangerous activity, and still justify why, at the moment, a handful of gummy snacks is okay. We have the overwhelming burden of free will. We have the awesome and weighty responsibility (pun intended, ladies) of bringing new life into the world. We have more motivation than ever to baby our baby and our bodies with the finest foods. Much of the time we are our own audience: we are mere witnesses, watching our bodies contort and change and bulge while marveling that this little person is real, is *living* in there, and living off us.

Some of us will manage spectacular diets during pregnancy. We will eat just the right things. We will turn up our noses at anything that doesn't promote well-being. We will consciously choose to ingest the very best, and eat better now than we have ever before in our lives. After all, it's worth it.

However, more of us will probably do just the opposite. After polishing off two dishes of chocolate mousse today, I can assure you of this with some confidence: it is extremely hard to eat perfectly in pregnancy. Our doctors would probably agree, and I doubt they would give us much grief over the occasional slip up, at least the ones we admit to. (You may just want to keep the one about eating spoonfuls of pure buttercream icing for breakfast to yourself.)

We must consider the possibility that our food choices are not providing our bodies and our babies with the best nutrition, even if we maintain some measure of diligence. There is a reason our doctors want us to take prenatal vitamins before, during, and after pregnancy.

But How Much Should *I* Take?

This is an important and common question. The often unpopular answer is, "It depends." The idea that each of us has unique nutritional needs is called biochemical individuality. If your need is greater, then you may need more vitamins. If your need is not greater, then less may be best. You take the amount of the nutrient that gets the result you seek. You may not be comfortable testing your vitamin requirements while you are pregnant. This is understandable. Discuss your intent to take more vitamins with your doctor, and keep on reading. I'm pretty comfortable with taking larger amounts of vitamins than the average gal, and even I shared my dosage information with my doctor.

How Much Do You Take?

I'm asked this question quite often. For my very first prenatal appointment with my ob-gyn, I was told to write down a list of every over-the-counter drug, prescription medication, or supplement I was taking. I wasn't taking any medicines, but I was taking many supplemental vitamins and minerals. I typed up a reference sheet and this is what I handed to my doctor to look over:

MY DAILY VITAMINS, MINERALS, AND OTHER SUPPLEMENTS	
A (preformed)	5,000 international units (IU)
A (beta carotene)	25,000 IU
B_1, B_2, B_6	100 mg
B_3 inositol nicotinate (flush free)	1,000 mg
B_3 nicotinic acid	250–500 mg
B_{12} and pantothenic acid	50–100 micrograms (mcg)
Biotin	50–250 mcg
Vitamin C	6,000–10,000 mg
Calcium	800 mg
Chromium	400 mcg
D_3 (cholecalciferol)	800–1,200 IU
E	400 IU
Folic acid	800–1,200 mcg
Iron (ferrous fumarate)	18–27 mg
Magnesium (citrate 600, oxide 400)	600–1,000 mg
Omega-3	340 mg
Selenium	50–100 mcg
Zinc	15–30 mg

He took a moment to look over my list and then said, "Wait, are you taking enough folic acid?"

I indicated that I was, and pointed to the line on the sheet. After he confirmed how much folic acid I was taking, he simply said it looked good and put it in my file.

I was stunned. I was pretty certain he'd have a thought or two about how *much* of each vitamin and mineral I was taking, amounts far exceeding the contents of the free prenatal sample he gave me in my new mommy welcome bag, let alone what is indicated in the RDA. But he didn't. To my relief, I found a doctor that was willing to work with me. I took my vitamins with that added confidence.

Other nutrients I did not think to include on my list at the time included choline (as found in lecithin), manganese (4 mg per day), and iodine. I also took probiotics daily. I mention these here for you now just in case you are curious about any additional nutrients I made a point to obtain while I was pregnant.

I often adjust the list to better suit my needs and concerns. For example, I cut down my intake of iron every other day or so by literally cutting the tablet in half, as vitamin C was helping me better absorb the iron I was getting, and the larger daily dose of iron (27 mg) caused constipation. I take more vitamin D now (6,000 IU per day), mainly because I am pregnant in the dead of winter in western New York, with little sunshine available. I eat a plant-based diet, so I occasionally take a 5,000 microgram (mcg) B_{12} tablet, especially if I'm not eating much fish, meat, or other animal products in a given week. Taking 250–500 mg of regular niacin (B_3) is plenty, and I generally skip the 1,000 mg daily dose of flush-free niacin unless stress or anxiety warrants its use. There are also times when I take more vitamin C, especially if I feel "something coming on" or if I am under a great deal of stress. I am constantly adjusting my vitamin and mineral intake to my current needs. I also add nutrients to my list when there is a benefit to be gained. For example, recently, I added CoQ_{10} (coenzyme Q_{10}).

There isn't a prenatal vitamin on the market that is going to provide individualized amounts of nutrients. So, instead of relying on a cookie-cutter style prenatal vitamin, I buy vitamins on an individual basis except when it comes to convenient combinations like B complex. I don't spend a fortune, either. I shop at about three locations, mostly online, and find the best prices for the best quality. For me, superior vitamins are ones that are natural, have no artificial colors, flavors, and fillers, and do not require that you take a serving size of two or three tablets to get the potency indicated on the label. (That gets pretty pricey.) I don't concern myself with brand names. There are lots of quality inexpensive supplements for sale. Sometimes buying a different form is less expensive. For example, buying powdered vitamin C or granulated lecithin saves money, but capsules are worth the extra cash for the sake of convenience. I check for potency per tablet, I check additional ingredients and make sure the tablets are not loaded with junk, I check the expiration date, and I check the price. To keep things as simple as possible, I pre-fill about two weeks' worth of pill cases with the tablets I take in the morning and in the afternoon to avoid having to break out a dozen bottles every time I want to take my vitamins. My husband does the same. It's also more convenient when we travel.

My list of vitamins and minerals is not intended to be a complete or prescriptive list. After all, I'm not a doctor. This doesn't mean you should head off to the store and start taking what I'm taking. This may be obvious, but it bears mention: You should always do your own research, always talk to your healthcare provider, learn your own body and your own nutritional needs, and do what is best for your situation—always. As I have said before, I am continually adjusting my vitamin and mineral intake based on my current needs. Diet, stress—life is ever changing. Be confident to change your supplementation routine along with it.

What my list is meant to do is illustrate a system that, in combination with a good diet and exercise, has worked for me through two healthy, uneventful pregnancies. It is meant to show you that there are ob-gyn doctors who support the use of larger doses of prenatal vitamins. It is a guide for consideration, so you can start a conversation about obtaining your own best intake level of vitamins. It's simply food for thought. Nutrients, actually. The rest of this book will give the details of why I do what I do.

Should I Buy Organic Vitamins?

Sure. If you can afford it, do it. The same is true with eating organic fruits and vegetables. However, organic or not, what is important is that you take them. If it comes to taking nonorganic vitamins or nothing at all, *it is better to take the vitamins.*

Did All My Hard Work Go Straight into the Toilet?

Some folks believe taking vitamins just makes for "expensive urine." That is one way to look at it. Here's another: If you are urinating out excess vitamins, it means you have enough to waste. If your pee starts glowing like a neon highlighter, don't distress. Nutrients in your urine may indicate that you are well-nourished and have some to spare.[46] It also means nutrients have been through your kidneys. What has been in the kidneys has been in your blood. What has been in the blood, your body has absorbed. What has been absorbed is available for you and your baby. Vitamin deficiency is a problem. Abundance, however, is not.[47]

Excreting excess doesn't mean you are done for the day. Like a good meal, vitamin sufficiency doesn't last forever. Your body will be "hungry" for these nutrients again. In the same way your baby needs nourishment many times each and every day, you should be taking your vitamins in several intervals throughout each day, too.

CHAPTER 3

Vitamin C and Pregnancy

"Facts do not cease to exist because they are ignored."
—ALDOUS HUXLEY

Vitamin C is so important during pregnancy. It can't be ignored, and yet it often is. Even worse—vitamin C is made out to be dangerous, which it isn't. Perhaps we are shy about vitamin C because we have heard too many rumors—too many that happen to be false. It's about time C gets the positive press it deserves, and that's exactly what we are going to do here. No more "Loch Ness Monster" science.

VITAMIN C SAFETY

"As the most important antioxidant fuel in the body, there should be no reason to fear the administration of vitamin C during pregnancy."
—THOMAS E. LEVY, MD, JD

Vitamin C is safe. This must be known, first and foremost. When we are pregnant we should be fully conscious of what can help or harm our developing baby. We should know the facts, and then proceed. This is why it is so important to know that vitamin C is not only safe during pregnancy, it is beneficial and essential.

"As the most important antioxidant fuel in the body, there should be no reason to fear the administration of vitamin C during pregnancy," explains Thomas E. Levy, MD, a board certified cardiologist considered to be one of the leading vitamin C experts in the world. "In fact, the metabolic needs of a pregnancy make an increased intake of vitamin C during pregnancy a recommended practice. The mother stays healthier, the pregnancy proceeds more smoothly, and the baby is healthier at birth."

According to two-time Nobel prize-winning chemist Linus Pauling, "Ascorbic acid is not a dangerous substance. It is described in the medical literature as 'virtually nontoxic.'"[1] Vitamin C, even in large doses, is safer than any medicine on the market.[2] It is safer than over-the-counter medications; it's safer than prescription drugs; and nobody is dying from taking too much vitamin C.[3] *The Journal of the American Medical Association* states: "Harmful effects have been mistakenly attributed to vitamin C, including hypoglycemia, rebound scurvy, infertility, mutagenesis, and destruction of vitamin B_{12}. Health professionals should recognize that vitamin C does not produce these effects."[4]

Vitamin C is safe during pregnancy; it is safe during lactation. It is safe for both baby and mom. According to the National Academy of Sciences, "There is no evidence suggesting that vitamin C is carcinogenic or teratogenic or that it causes adverse reproductive effects."[5] And, "No evidence of maternal toxicity of excess vitamin C intakes was found."[6] We are not just talking about a few hundred milligrams here. No issues were found taking over twenty times the U.S. Recommended Dietary Allowance (RDA), 2,000 milligrams (mg) a day, and more.[7] There is safety in larger doses as well. Experience has demonstrated time and time again that routine doses of even 10,000 mg only help and do not harm pregnant women or their babies.[8] Vitamin C does not cause infertility, birth defects, or miscarriage. Vitamin C is not going to harm you or your developing baby, even in large doses. Andrew W. Saul, PhD, coauthor of *Vitamin C: The Real Story*, says, "What vitamin C *does* do is deliver healthier babies."[9]

Pregnancy and Vitamin C: What We Have Known for Years

Vitamin C helps produce healthy, happy babies and support healthy, happy moms. This is not new information. "It has been known for more than thirty years that pregnant women need more vitamin C than other women," says Linus Pauling. "Part of the reason for this extra need is that the developing fetus needs a good supply of this vitamin, and there is a mechanism in the placenta for pumping vitamin C from the blood of the mother into that of the fetus. . . . In normal pregnancy women with the usual low intake of vitamin C have been reported to show a steady decrease in blood plasma concentration" as the pregnancy progresses to full term.[10] Well over half a century ago, Frederick R. Klenner, MD, observed the value of extra vitamin C during pregnancy.

Frederick R. Klenner, MD, and the Vitamin C Babies

Let's get right to it. Dr. Frederick R. Klenner, graduate of Duke University School of Medicine and pioneer of high-dose vitamin C therapy, gave over 300 pregnant women 4 grams (4,000 mg) of vitamin C a day during their first trimester, 6 grams (6,000 mg) during their second, and 10 to 15 grams (10,000 to15,000 mg) during their third.[11] The results? Healthy babies and healthy moms. Baby after baby was delivered without issue. There were no postpartum hemorrhages. Not one. "This is exceptionally significant. For centuries, postpartum hemorrhage was a leading cause of death in childbirth," Dr. Saul says. "Hemorrhage does very often occur in scorbutic (vitamin C deficient) patients" and "Klenner-sized doses of vitamin C prevent hemorrhage and save women's lives. One way it may do this is by strengthening the body's large and small blood vessels. Believe it or not, the press tried to make that out to be a problem, claiming that vitamin C's 'thickening' of artery walls would reduce blood flow. It does not."[12]

Furthermore, there was no cardiac distress. There were no toxic manifestations. The duration of labor was greatly reduced, and labor was less painful. The babies were "robust."[13] The nursing personnel noted that the happiest and healthiest babies were those in Klenner's care and referred to them as the "Vitamin C Babies."[14] Dr. Klenner was also the first doctor to deliver the first set of surviving quadruplets in the southeastern United States, also Vitamin C Babies. Thomas E. Levy, MD, says, "Dr. Frederick Klenner routinely gave many pregnant women about 10,000 mg of vitamin C daily during their pregnancies, and the nurses literally marveled at how healthy his patients and their babies always turned out." Failure to give enough vitamin C during pregnancy is the problem. Dr. Levy explains, "Not supplementing vitamin C during a pregnancy would be expected to increase the chances of complications in the mother and the chances of birth defects and lesser problems in the babies."

Dr. Klenner insisted that not giving vitamin C in large doses during pregnancy bordered on malpractice. As the baby takes vitamin C from the mother, the mother can come up short. Pregnancy takes a lot out of us, and Dr. Klenner would agree: "The simple stress of pregnancy demands vitamin C" and this amount will "vary by individual."[15] However, most women will be told to follow the Recommended Dietary Allowance for pregnant women: 80–85mg a day of vitamin C.[16] There are some obstetricians who will recommend more, but not much more. Prenatal vitamins contain relatively small amounts of C. When our government's "tolerable upper intake level" for vitamin C is set as low as 2,000 mg per day,[17] it is no wonder women worry about taking too much. It's time to stop worrying. Orthomolecular (nutritional) physicians have been strongly critical of so-called tolerable upper limits. Physicians such as Alan R. Gaby, MD, say that such standards have not been science based.[18]

"WAIT, I READ THAT VITAMIN C CAN CAUSE ABORTIONS."

No. It. Does. NOT.

For those of you who did an Internet search about "vitamin C" and "pregnancy" and found a link to a website claiming that vitamin C causes abortions, it simply isn't true. Vitamin C will not terminate a pregnancy. Do a direct search for "vitamin C" and "abortions" and your screen will be plastered with women claiming that 6–30 grams/day (6,000 to 30,000 mg/day) of vitamin C will cause a miscarriage. To make things worse, if you go searching for information to refute the claim, you'll have a hard time finding any.

Perhaps women fear they have few options to turn to with an unwanted pregnancy. Perhaps they look for "home remedies" out of desperation. If this is the case, vitamin C is not going to get them what they are after.

Miscarriages do occur, and more frequently than a hopeful, expectant mother would ever want to contemplate. About one in five pregnancies ends in miscarriage or spontaneous abortion, and this only includes pregnancies that a woman actually knows about—it is estimated up to half of fertilized eggs are aborted before a woman is aware she is pregnant.[19] If you desire to have a child, these statistics are humbling to say the least. Vitamin C, however, is not to blame.

Upon doing some more searching about ascorbic acid induced abortion, I found an article written by two medical students who took an interest in the topic. Their findings? "Any attempt to find a credible source, validated claim, or independent consensus proved futile."[20] Instead, they found research *supporting* the use of vitamins in pregnancy. (Their article is worth a read-through, and its web address can be found in the References section for this chapter.)

It bears repeating: *There is absolutely no evidence that vitamin C causes pregnancy loss.* It's just the opposite: Dr. Frederick R. Klenner worked with women in his practice who had previously experienced as many as five miscarriages. Now, under his care and through the use of supplemental vitamin C, these women were finally carrying a baby to full term—two and three times over. He stated they were all "uneventful" pregnancies, a comforting term, indeed, when previous pregnancy "events" were the devastating loses of children. Abram Hoffer, MD, who since 1953 used daily megadoses of vitamin C with more than a thousand of his patients, in amounts ranging from 3,000 to 30,000 mg, stated that he observed no miscarriages in his vitamin C taking mommys-to-be.[21]

I can also speak from personal experience on the safety of vitamin C. At my first prenatal visit, I handed my ob-gyn a long list indicating all of the vitamins and minerals I was currently taking. "Vitamin C: 6,000–10,000 mg/day" was at the very top of that sheet of paper. He looked it over, and it went into my file for any of the other three ob-gyns in the group to review. Had my doctor been concerned that taking this amount of vitamin C would terminate my pregnancy, I imagine he would have told me so. Instead, he would comment about my good health at my prenatal checkups, saying that I was making his job easy. He was happy that I was healthy.

And let's not forget about the entire animal kingdom. If vitamin C is toxic to pregnancy, earth's creatures would be unable to bear offspring and therefore would all be dead by now. Adjusted for body weight, the RDA would have us believe that we need 10 to 100 times *less* vitamin C than almost any other animal on earth.[22] Based on the research of Irwin Stone and Dr. Pauling, Dr. Saul explains, "Pound for pound, most animals actually manufacture from two to ten thousand milligrams of vitamin C daily, inside their bodies. If such generous quantities of vitamin C were harmful, evolution would have had millions of years to select against it."[23]

A vitamin C caused miscarriage? It's just not true.

VITAMIN C AND HUMAN PREGNANCY VERSUS GUINEA PIGS, MONKEYS, AND GOATS

A fifteen-pound monkey takes in about 600 mg of vitamin C a day from its food.[24] That's about 40 mg of vitamin C per pound of monkey. If an average woman weighs about 160 pounds[25] (and more when pregnant), that's the weight of over ten monkeys. Ten monkeys would get 6,000 mg of vitamin C in their diet each day. I imagine ten pregnant monkeys would likely consume even more.

But the U.S. RDA for vitamin C for an adult woman is only 85 mg per day during pregnancy and 120 mg per day during lactation.

Let's talk guinea pigs. The U.S. Department of Agriculture has stated that "the Guinea pig's vitamin C requirement is 10–15 mg per day under normal conditions and 15–25 mg per day if pregnant, lactating, or growing."[26] An adult guinea pig weighs about one kilogram (2.2 pounds). Guinea pigs therefore need between 10 and 25 mg of vitamin C per kilogram. That means the USDA's standards, if fairly applied to us, would set our vitamin C requirement somewhere between 820 mg and 2,000 mg vitamin C per day.

Practically all animals manufacture their own vitamin C. Just how much they make may surprise you. For example, "A 110 pound goat *makes* over 9,000 milligrams of vitamin C per day," says Dr. Saul. "That would be around 15,000 mg/day for a 180 lb human if we could synthesize it. We can't, but rats can. An average 3/4 lb rat synthesizes 20 to 70 mg/day, or 5,000 to 17,000 mg/day per human body weight.[27] So any animal you can think of consumes, or internally manufactures, vastly more vitamin C than official authority says we need."

VITAMIN C AND THE PREVENTION OF BIRTH DEFECTS

All parents do it. We check for ten little fingers and ten little toes. All of us want to have healthy, happy babies. It is comforting to know that vitamin C can play an important role in the prevention of birth defects.

Exposure to Toxins and Heavy Metals

It is virtually impossible to live a life free of toxins. Our inevitable exposure to environmental pollutants emphasizes the need for an abundance of vitamin C for mothers and children.

Animal studies have shown the protective quality of large doses of vitamin C during pregnancy.[28] Large doses of vitamin C were found to be nontoxic and were protective of early embryos against genotoxic agents, or substances that harm DNA.[29] Hyla Cass, MD, says "Research shows that vitamin C can help reduce harmful effects of aluminum, lead, copper, and radiation."[30]

Pesticide exposure in utero has been linked to developmental delays and autism in children.[31] "Pesticides are diverse in chemical structure, but they are usually susceptible to neutralization by vitamin C," says Thomas E. Levy, MD. "Vitamin C also tends to readily repair the damage done by many pesticides."[32] A developing fetus is especially sensitive to mercury in mom's diet.[33] Pregnant women are advised to eat no more than a couple of small servings (6 ounces each) of low mercury fish a week.[34] Fatty fish is good for us, but fatty fish are known to concentrate toxins in their tissues.[35] "Low-mercury" fish is not "no-mercury" fish, and if we want to benefit from the healthy nutrients present in seafood that are essential to our baby's development and help protect from the developmental damage caused by exposure to heavy metals, it is valuable to know about the protective effect of vitamin C.[36] Dr. Levy states "both acute and chronic exposures to mercury can be effectively treated with vitamin C, and typically most of the damage from such poisoning can be prevented and/or promptly repaired."[37] Of course, our goal is to never get to that point. Pregnant women should avoid mercury as much as possible: we should limit our intake of seafood, and we should also take vitamin C. Practically speaking, whenever I ate fish during pregnancy, I would take extra vitamin C, too.

Lead poisoning in pregnant women may lead to abnormal growth and development of the fetus, and children continually exposed to lead suffer with learning disabilities and behavioral problems.[38] In one study of over 19,500 individuals, higher serum vitamin C levels were associated with significantly lower levels of lead in the blood.[39] Particularly for women who are pregnant or nursing, in another study researchers showed vitamin C may play a role in reducing the content of lead in the placenta and in mother's milk.[40] In this particular study of lead-burdened mothers, combination therapy of vitamin C and calcium phosphate reduced the lead content of mother's milk by 15 percent and decreased lead in the placenta by a whopping 90 percent.[41] Another study found that higher serum levels of the antioxidants vitamin C and E in the mother meant lower levels of lead and may offer protection from lead toxicity in the fetus.[42] "It would seem that 1,000 mg of vitamin C supplementation daily is really the very minimal dose at which some favorable response in lowering blood lead levels can be expected." Dr. Levy says.[43] Considering the remarkable safety of vitamin C, it seems that pregnant women would do well to get at least that much each day. I was comfortable taking far more.

KIDS AND HEAVY METALS (THE TOXINS, NOT THE ROCK BANDS)

According to Thomas E. Levy, MD, "high-dose vitamin C can quickly neutralize a vast array of toxins."[44] This is good news for everybody, especially for our growing and developing children.

"The ability of vitamin C to protect animals from heavy metal poisoning is well established," says the *Orthomolecular Medicine News Service.* "Recent controlled trials with yeast, fish, mice, rats, chickens, clams, guinea pigs, and turkeys all came to the same conclusion: Vitamin C protects growing animals from heavy metals poisoning.[45] Benefits with an animal model do not always translate to equal benefits for humans. In this case, however, the benefit has been proven for a wide range of animals. The odds that vitamin C will protect human children are high."[46]

"There is a virtual epidemic of behavior problems, learning disabilities, ADHD [attention deficit hyperactivity disorder] and autism, and the number of children receiving special education services continues to rise steeply," OMNS continues. "Although not all causes are yet identified, growing evidence suggests that heavy metal pollution is a significant factor, and vitamin C is part of the solution. . . . Few mothers or children can avoid both contaminated air and food, helping to explain why behavior problems are striking rich and poor alike." Part of the solution is nutrition: "[a]dditional vitamin intake, through the use of nutrient supplementation, can help speed up the removal process" of heavy metals.[47]

Antioxidants, Alcohol, and Cigarette Smoke

A teratogen is any substance that can interfere with the development of a fetus and lead to birth defects or developmental malformations. Common examples of teratogens are cigarette smoke or alcohol, both of which can cause severe problems for mom and baby. Moms who smoke during pregnancy have half the levels of ascorbic acid as opposed to nonsmoking mothers.[48] Two things can be learned here. First, we know we shouldn't smoke or drink during pregnancy. Smoking and drinking can have devastating effects for both you and your baby. And second, if exposure to toxins can decrease our levels of such important antioxidants like vitamin C, this means when it comes to C, we need to be sure our bodies have access to plenty. Animal studies show "a variety of antioxidants" such as vitamins C and E, carotenoids, and folic acid "are effective in decreasing the damaging effects of heightened oxidative stress induced by teratogens."[49] In a world where it is impossible *not* to be exposed to harmful substances, it is comforting to know that vitamin C is protective of a developing baby.

VITAMIN C AND ACIDITY

If you are worried about acidity, don't be. Vitamin C is no more acidic than an orange. The next article from the *Orthomolecular Medicine News Service* addresses the acidity of vitamin C and available forms of the vitamin, and may help you pick which kind of vitamin C would be right for you.

Vitamin C and Acidity: What Form Is Best?

(Orthomolecular Medicine News Service (OMNS), December 8, 2009) Vitamin C is commonly taken in large quantities to improve health and prevent asthma, allergies, viral infection, and heart disease.[50] It is non-toxic and non-immunogenic, and does not irritate the stomach as drugs like aspirin can. Yet vitamin C (L-ascorbic acid) is acidic. So, a common question is, what are the effects from taking large quantities?

Ascorbic acid is a weak acid (pKa= 4.2),[51] only slightly stronger than vinegar. When dissolved in water, vitamin C is sour but less so than citric acid found in lemons and limes. Can large quantities of a weak acid such as ascorbate cause problems in the body? The answer is, sometimes, in some situations. However, with some simple precautions they can be avoided.

Acid in the Mouth

First of all, any acid can etch the surfaces of your teeth. This is the reason the dentist cleans your teeth and warns about plaque, for acid generated by bacteria in the mouth can etch your teeth to cause cavities. Cola soft drinks contain phosphoric acid, actually used by dentists to etch teeth before tooth sealants are applied. Like soft drinks, ascorbic acid will not cause etching of teeth if only briefly present. Often, vitamin C tablets are coated with a tableting ingredient such as magnesium stearate which prevents the ascorbate from dissolving immediately. Swallowing a vitamin C tablet without chewing it prevents its acid from harming tooth enamel.

Chewable Vitamin C Tablets

Chewables are popular because they taste sweet and so are good for encouraging children to take their vitamin C.[52] However, some chewable vitamin C tablets can contain sugar and ascorbic acid which, when chewed, is likely to stick in the crevices of your teeth. So, after chewing a vitamin C tablet, a good bit of advice is to rinse with water or brush your teeth. But the best way is to specifically select non-acidic vitamin C chewables, readily available in stores. Read the label to verify that the chewable is made entirely with non-acidic vitamin C.

Stomach Acidity

People with sensitive stomachs may report discomfort when large doses of vitamin C are taken at levels to prevent an acute viral infection (1,000–3,000 milligrams or more every 20 minutes).[53] In this case the ascorbic acid in the stomach can build up enough acidity to cause heartburn or a similar reaction. On the other hand, many people report no problems with acidity even when taking 20,000 mg in an hour. The acid normally present in the stomach, hydrochloric acid (HCl), is very strong: dozens of times more acidic than vitamin C. When one has swallowed a huge amount of ascorbate, the digestive tract is sucking it up into the bloodstream as fast as it can, but it may still take a while to do so. Some people report that they seem to sense ascorbic acid tablets "sitting" at the bottom of the stomach as they take time to dissolve. It is fairly easy to fix the problem by using buffered ascorbate, or taking ascorbic acid with food or liquids in a meal or snack. When the amount of vitamin C ingested is more than the gut can absorb, the ascorbate attracts water into the intestines creating a laxative effect. This saturation intake is called bowel tolerance. One should reduce the amount (by 20–50 percent) when this occurs.[54]

Acid Balance in the Body

Does taking large quantities of an acid, even a weak acid like ascorbate, tip the body's acid balance (pH) causing health problems? No, because the body actively and constantly controls the pH of the bloodstream. The kidneys regulate the acid in the body over a long time period, hours to days, by selectively excreting either acid or basic components in urine.

Over a shorter time period, minutes to hours, if the blood is too acid, the autonomic nervous system increases the rate of breathing, thereby removing more carbon dioxide from the blood, reducing its acidity. Some foods can indirectly cause acidity. For example, when more protein is eaten than necessary for maintenance and growth, it is metabolized into acid, which must be removed by the kidneys, generally as uric acid. In this case, calcium and/or magnesium are excreted along with the acid in the urine which can deplete our supplies of calcium and magnesium.[55] However, because ascorbic acid is a weak acid, we can tolerate a lot before it will much affect the body's acidity. Although there have been allegations about vitamin C supposedly causing kidney stones, there is no evidence for this, and its acidity and diuretic tendency actually tends to reduce kidney stones in most people who are prone to them.[56] Ascorbic acid dissolves calcium phosphate stones and dissolves struvite stones. Additionally, while vitamin C does increase oxalate excretion, vitamin C simultaneously inhibits the union of calcium and oxalate.[57]

Forms of Vitamin C

Ascorbate comes in many forms, each with a particular advantage. Ascorbic acid is the least expensive and can be purchased as tablets, timed-release tablets, or powder. The larger tablets (1,000–1,500 mg) are convenient and relatively inexpensive. Timed-release tablets contain a long-chain carbohydrate which delays the stomach in dissolving the ascorbate, which is then released over a period of hours. This may have an advantage for maintaining a high level in the bloodstream. Ascorbic acid powder or crystals can be purchased in bulk relatively inexpensively. Pure powder is more quickly dissolved than tablets and therefore can be absorbed somewhat faster by the body. Linus Pauling favored taking pure ascorbic acid, as it is entirely free of tableting excipients.

Buffered Ascorbate A fraction of a teaspoon of sodium bicarbonate (baking soda) has long been used as a safe and effective antacid which immediately lowers stomach acidity. When sodium bicarbonate is added to ascorbic acid, the bicarbonate fizzes (emitting carbon dioxide) which then releases the sodium to neutralize the acidity of the ascorbate.

Calcium ascorbate can be purchased as a powder and readily dissolves in water or juice. In this buffered form ascorbate is completely safe for the mouth and sensitive stomach and can be applied directly to the gums to help heal infections.[58] It is a little more expensive than the equivalent ascorbic acid and bicarbonate but more convenient. Calcium ascorbate has the advantage of being non-acidic. It has a slightly metallic taste and is astringent but not sour like ascorbic acid. 1,000 mg of calcium ascorbate contains about 110 mg of calcium.

Other forms of buffered ascorbate include sodium ascorbate and magnesium ascorbate.[59] Most adults need 800–1,200 mg of calcium and 400–600 mg of magnesium daily.[60] The label on the bottle of all these buffered ascorbates details how much "elemental" mineral is contained in a teaspoonful. They cost a little more than ascorbic acid.

Buffered forms of ascorbate are often better tolerated at higher doses than ascorbic acid, but they appear not to be as effective for preventing the acute symptoms of a cold. This may be because after they are absorbed they require absorbing an electron from the body to become effective as native ascorbate.[61] Some types of vitamin C are proprietary formulas that claim benefits over standard vitamin C.[62]

Liposomal Vitamin C   Recently a revolutionary form of ascorbate has become available. This form of vitamin C is packaged inside nano-scale phospholipid spheres ("liposomes"), much like a cell membrane protects its contents. The lipid spheres protect the vitamin C from degradation by the environment and are absorbed more quickly into the bloodstream. Liposomes are also known to facilitate intracellular uptake of their contents, which can cause an added clinical impact when delivering something such as vitamin C. This form is supposed to be 5–10 fold more absorbable than straight ascorbic acid. It is more expensive than ascorbic acid tablets or powder.

Ascorbyl Palmitate   Ascorbyl palmitate is composed of an ascorbate molecule bound to a palmitic acid molecule. It is amphipathic, meaning that it can dissolve in either water or fat, like the fatty acids in cell membranes. It is widely used as an antioxidant in processed foods, and used in topical creams where it is thought to be more stable than vitamin C. However, when ingested, the ascorbate component of ascorbyl palmitate is thought to be decomposed into the ascorbate and palmitic acid molecules so its special amphipathic quality is lost. It is also more expensive than ascorbic acid.

Natural Ascorbate Natural forms of ascorbate derived from plants are available. Acerola, the "Barbados cherry," contains a large amount of vitamin C, depending on its ripeness, and was traditionally used to fight off colds. Tablets of vitamin C purified from acerola or rose hips are available but are generally low-dose and considerably more expensive than ascorbic acid. Although some people strongly advocate this type, Pauling and many others have stated that such naturally-derived vitamin C is no better than pure commercial ascorbate.[63] Bioflavonoids are antioxidants found in citrus fruits or rose hips and are thought to improve uptake and utilization of vitamin C. Generally, supplement tablets that contain bioflavonoids do not have enough to make much difference. For consumers on a budget, the best policy may be to buy vitamin C inexpensively whether or not it also contains bioflavonoids.[64] Citrus fruits, peppers, and a number of other fruits and vegetables contain large quantities of bioflavinoids. This is one more reason to eat right as well as supplement.

SUPPORTING YOUR HEALTH—AND YOUR BABY—WITH VITAMIN C

"My mom is literally a part of me. You can't say that about
many people except relatives, and organ donors. "
—CARRIE LATET

I followed Dr. Klenner's protocol during my first and second pregnancy. I took increasingly larger doses of vitamin C as my pregnancy progressed. I believe it made a huge difference. It also made a difference in the delivery room. (The same is true for my mother, when she was carrying and delivering me.)

Vitamin C and Two Pregnancies

Our first baby was facing up rather than down. The doctor physically reached in and turned her over five times, but the adjustment didn't last.

She stubbornly went back to her previous position, which certainly did not make it any easier to push her out. The doctor warned me her face may be all bruised due to her positioning, with her nose being jammed into my pelvic bone.

There it was. The voice of Larry, our local gym's spinning instructor. "Work. Push. *Push.*" I hadn't been to a spinning class in many weeks, but there he was, nevertheless, in my head. I decided to use it. Work. Push. *Push.*

After three hours of pushing, her heartbeat was still steady, and she was showing no signs of stress. Throughout the whole process, the nurses reassured me several times that she was "relaxed and happy as if nothing was going on." She was born without a mark on her. My husband observed that while other babies screamed in a very full nursery, our child was calm and comfortable. That sounds so much like Dr. Klenner's Vitamin C Babies, that I just thought I'd mention it. All of my daughter's tests came back with flying colors. She was one healthy kid.

My son was another good example of good health. In fact, the hospital pediatrician walked into our room the day after our son was born and told us that he was in such great shape we could head home early, as long as my ob-gyn approved. Keenly aware of the stress that childbirth had on my body the first time around, I prepared for birth the second time by being near saturation (just below bowel tolerance) of vitamin C when I went into labor. I continued to take large amounts of C postpartum. I was taking even more than I had with my first child. My labor contractions were less painful than the first time and my recovery time was faster. We even brought liquid vitamin C to give the baby in the hospital to help him through the stress of being born and healing from his circumcision. Is a second pregnancy and delivery easier that the first? It sure was for me.

The Myth of Rebound Scurvy with Vitamin C during Pregnancy

Scurvy is caused by vitamin C deficiency. "Rebound scurvy, or the rebound effect, is when a person takes a lot of vitamin C, usually with great success, and then abruptly stops taking it. At that instance, symptoms come back, sometimes including a few classic vitamin C deficiency signs. Research shows that such an effect does not occur in the vast majority of situations," says Dr. Saul.[65]

But what about in pregnancy? Could the infants of high-dose vitamin C moms get rebound scurvy?

The answer is no. Infantile "rebound scurvy" is a myth, says Alan R. Gaby, MD.[66] While the notion is still widely believed, consuming large quantities of vitamin C during pregnancy *does not* cause infantile scurvy. "Evidence for the existence of rebound scurvy in infants is somewhere between flimsy and nonexistent," says Dr. Gaby.[67]

For decades, babies have been born to millions of mothers who took large doses of vitamin C, he says, and "not a single new case of rebound scurvy has been reported."[68] He urges the medical community to reevaluate their position. "Uncritical acceptance of this concept [of infantile scurvy] is no longer acceptable; it is time for 'authorities' on vitamin C to take a new look at the evidence."[69]

Dr. Frederick R. Klenner and others have confirmed that vitamin C during pregnancy will make labor shorter, easier, and free of complications.[70] Vitamin C infants are born healthy; our job is to keep them that way. Vitamin C taking moms need not worry about infantile scurvy, but we should not give up on a good thing altogether. "If the baby is used to, and benefiting from, abundant vitamin C, it obviously should be provided for him individually after birth," says Dr. Saul.[71]

There are two ways to make this happen. For one, mom should continue to take vitamin C. If she is breastfeeding, the milk will provide C to the baby. However, varying amounts of C will be found in breast milk, especially if mom is stressed out and healing from birth. Therefore, supplementation for both mom and baby is the solution. "Infants do not need a lot of supplemental C, but they do need it frequently each day for maximum success. 'Success' is easy to define: a healthy, happy baby that eats and sleeps well," says Saul.[72] Dr. Klenner gave newborn infants about 50 milligrams daily.[73]

Not only did I take extra vitamin C after my children were born, I also gave them small doses of tasty liquid vitamin C several times a day, starting in the hospital. My parents used yummy crushed, chewable vitamin C and put it right onto our tongues when my brother and I were babies.

For moms giving babies formula, the same rule applies. There is very little vitamin C found in formula. This is especially true after it has been heated and oxidized during bottle feeding."[74] Even if you see vitamin C on the label, your child may not be getting the amount indicated. To ensure your baby is getting the vitamin C he or she needs, supplementing with small doses throughout the day, every day, is important.

Keeping up with a good thing is a good idea. Think of it like getting a bonus check at work. More money is good. So is supplemental vitamin C for your baby after birth: it's an added benefit. Ensuring a newborn has an adequate intake of vitamin C is important, regardless of how much mom took during pregnancy. And it's safe, too, even for premature babies. Consider this double-blind, placebo-controlled study on vitamin C given to preemies: each day infants received 100 mg per kilogram of vitamin C. The study authors concluded, "ascorbic acid administration to the premature infant is safe."[75]

"PREGNANT—C" QUESTIONS

Here are some common questions many women have when it comes to supplementing with Vitamin C:

Q: Is the Vitamin C in My Prenatal Vitamin Enough?

A: The short answer is no. In both prescription and over-the-counter popular prenatal vitamins, the vitamin C content ranges from about 80 mg to 120 mg. Just because one gal is fine with one amount of vitamin C, does not mean another will not benefit from getting more. As with shoes or underwear, women know there is no "one size fits all." The same is true with vitamin C.

Q: How Much Vitamin C Should I Take?

A: This is, of course, for you to decide. Dr. Klenner's moms fared beautifully taking three to five times the "tolerable upper intake level" of 2,000 mg per day of vitamin C, and had remarkable success. According to pediatrician Lendon H. Smith, MD, "Vitamin C is our best defense, and everyone should be on this one even before birth. Three thousand milligrams daily for the pregnant woman is a start."[76] I took 6,000–10,000 mg of vitamin C daily, as did my mother when she was pregnant with me.

Q: How Much Vitamin C Is Too Much?

A: Side effects of too much vitamin C include stomach distress and loose stool, indicating that the body is saturated with the vitamin. This, however, is temporary, and goes away when the dose is reduced a bit. Of course, we don't want to run around all day with "the runs." If you are, you are taking too much. This is not what we are, er, going for.

"Too much" is really best determined by how you feel. We are all different, and the right dose of vitamin C for one pregnant mom may differ from that of another. If you feel healthy, energetic, and vibrant, take note. If you find yourself with stomach upset or loose stools, you may want to adjust your dosage or chosen form of vitamin C accordingly. Be sure to divide your dose: take smaller amounts several times a day. You'll find any stomach discomfort is minimized by taking your vitamin C along with snacks or meals. You can also purchase buffered vitamin C. Refer back to the article about the different forms of vitamin C for more information.

Your body needs C throughout the day, not just in one abundant blast. You wouldn't feed your baby once a day; babies need nourishment every few hours. In the same way, your body will benefit from getting vitamin C multiple times in a day.

It has been observed that when people undergo surgery or get burned or wounded, the concentration of vitamin C in their blood decreases, indicating a need for more vitamin C under such stressful conditions.[77] When an animal is under stress, it can actually manufacture more vitamin C as needed.[78] We, however, are one of the very few creatures on earth that cannot. We must rely on food sources and supplements. Pregnancy is most assuredly a stress on the body, and we can choose to compensate with supplemental C, or complain about what happens when we don't.

Ascorbic Acid Vitamin C: What's the Real Story?

BY ANDREW W. SAUL, EDITOR

(ORTHOMOLECULAR MEDICINE NEWS SERVICE (OMNS), Dec 6, 2013) Heard anything bad lately about ascorbic acid vitamin C? If you haven't, you may have been away visiting Neptune for too long. For nearly four decades, I have seen that, like all other fashions, vitamin-bashing goes "in" and "out" of style. Lately it has (again) been open season on vitamin C, especially if taken as cheap ascorbic acid. Linus Pauling, the world's most qualified advocate of vitamin C, urged people to take pure ascorbic acid powder or crystals.

Without having met Dr. Pauling, they are also what great-grandma used when she home-canned peaches. Vitamin C powder remains cheap and readily available on the internet. One-quarter teaspoon is just over 1,000 mg. If you encounter a powder that is substantially less potent than that, it may contain fillers. Choose accordingly.

I have told my students for a long time, "If they didn't listen to Linus Pauling, don't be too surprised that they don't line up to hear what you have to say." But Pauling's two unshared Nobel prizes (he is the only person in history with that distinction) are no protection from critics who slam ascorbic acid C without first considering some basic biochemistry.

Atomically Correct

Vitamin C is ascorbic acid, $C_6H_8O_6$, and that's pretty much all there is to it. If you really want to impress your friends, ascorbic acid can also be called (5R)-5-[(1S)-1,2-Dihydroxyethyl]-3,4-dihydroxy-2(5H)-furanone. As I liked to tell my university students, now there is something for you to answer when your parents ask what you learned in school today.

Even if this molecule comes from GMOs [genetically modified organisms], which I disapprove of, it is still molecularly OK. You cannot genetically modify carbon, hydrogen, or oxygen atoms.

There are two ways the atoms can arrange themselves to make $C_6H_8O_6$. One is ascorbic acid. The other is erythorbic acid, also known as isoascorbic acid or D-araboascorbic acid. It is a commercial antioxidant, but cannot be utilized by the body as an essential nutrient.

Acidity

That word "acid" gets us going, but in fact ascorbic acid is a weak acid. If you can eat three oranges, if you can drink a carbonated cola, or if you can add vinegar on your fish fry or on your salad, there is little to worry about. In fact, your normal stomach acid is over 50 times stronger than vitamin C. The stomach is designed to handle strong acid, and nutrients are not destroyed by this strong stomach acid. If they were, all mammals would be dead. Have you ever noticed when you throw up you can feel the burn in your throat? That's stomach acid. A little gross, but we need it to live. People who have a lot of problems with hiatal hernias or reflux can actually regurgitate enough acid over a period of months where they damage and scar the throat.

Vitamin C could not do that on a bet. It's impossible. You couldn't start your car if you put vinegar in your automobile's battery. It requires sulfuric acid, which is a very strong acid. The hydrochloric acid in the stomach is only slightly weaker than car-battery acid. Vitamin C is almost as weak as lemonade. That's a huge difference.

Probiotics

If you eat yogurt or take probiotic capsules, they end up in your stomach. There they are subjected to this strong stomach acid, and survive it easily. Acidophilus bacteria, such as are found in yogurt, are literally so named because they are "acid-loving." Many studies show that eating yogurt and taking other probiotic supplements is a good idea and that it works. If a strong acid does not kill them, then neither will a weak acid.

Furthermore, your body secretes a highly alkaline substance right where your small intestine starts, just past the stomach. This neutralizes stomach acid and automatically keeps the rest of your gut from being acidic. If the body can neutralize a strong acid, ascorbic acid is virtually irrelevant.

Buffering

Ascorbic acid can be buffered, and if you have a sensitive stomach, should be. There are a variety of non-acidic forms. I do not sell vitamins or any other health products, and do not make brand recommendations.

Don't be bluffed or blustered about ascorbic acid. It is cheap and it works. Aside from intravenous sodium ascorbate, the vast majority of research showing that vitamin C is effective in prevention and treatment of disease has used plain ascorbic acid. Yes, the cheap stuff.

Remember what Ward Cleaver, TV father on "Leave It to Beaver," said to his young son: "A lot of people go through life trying to prove that the things that are good for them are wrong."

Q: What Form of Vitamin C Should I Take?
A: Take the form that works best for you. The article included earlier in this chapter, "Vitamin C and Acidity: What Form Is Best?" may help you decide. While it is only a weak acid, ascorbic acid may bother your stomach (especially an empty stomach) unless it is taken along with

something else, like calcium, food, or liquid, as a buffer. When my brother and I were children, this is exactly how our parents gave vitamin C to us. They would mix calcium and magnesium powder together with our powdered vitamin C in juice, or make sure we had eaten first before we took our C. Tablets also work well for both vitamin C and calcium and are more convenient. (We took these once we were older and could comfortably swallow them.) Another good option while you are pregnant is to take calcium ascorbate, a non-acidic form of vitamin C that is very unlikely to cause you any stomach distress. As mentioned above in the article on vitamin C and acidity, calcium ascorbate is a little over ten percent calcium, as you might infer from its name. During pregnancy, calcium supplementation is widely recognized as vital for a growing baby, not only after birth but before. Calcium ascorbate is more expensive, but it may very well be worth it.

Q: Can I Get Enough Vitamin C in My Diet?
A: Just 500 little milligrams of vitamin C would mean eating around seven oranges a day. To score 2,000 mg, we are up to about thirty oranges a day. Need some variety? I suppose you could savor some twenty-four cups of strawberries instead. Or munch down nearly twenty-five cups of raw broccoli. A day. Sheesh.

"Sure. I'm pregnant. No problem. I totally have the time to eat all that. Who needs convenient little tablets of C?"

Yeah, right. I'm tired just thinking about it.

Eat broccoli. Eat strawberries. Eat oranges. Eat all your fruits and vegetables. They are packed with lots of important nutrients, not just vitamin C. But supplementation is necessary if you aim to achieve higher doses of C. Fortunately, supplemental vitamin C is easy to come by and inexpensive.

OBJECTIONS TO VITAMIN C

It's time to put vitamin C in perspective. We have often heard of so-called problems caused by too much vitamin C, many of which are simply not true, and rarely do we hear of vitamin C's remarkable safety and effectiveness. This next article[79] delves into and answers many more questions on the topic.

About "Objections" to Vitamin C Therapy

(ORTHOMOLECULAR MEDICINE NEWS SERVICE (OMNS), Oct 12, 2010) In massive doses, vitamin C (ascorbic acid) stops a cold within hours, stops influenza in a day or two, and stops viral pneumonia (pain, fever, cough) in two or three days.[80] It is a highly effective antihistamine, antiviral, and antitoxin. It reduces inflammation and lowers fever. Administered intravenously, ascorbate kills cancer cells without harming healthy tissue. Many people therefore wonder, in the face of statements like these, why the medical professions have not embraced vitamin C therapy with open and grateful arms.

Probably the main roadblock to widespread examination and utilization of this all-too-simple technology is the equally widespread belief that there *must* be unknown dangers to tens of thousands of milligrams of ascorbic acid. Yet, since the time megascorbate therapy was introduced in the late 1940s by Fred R. Klenner, MD,[81] there has been an especially safe, and extremely effective track record to follow.

Still, for some, questions remain. Here is a sample of what readers have asked OMNS about vitamin C:

Is 2,000 mg per day of vitamin C a megadose?

No. Decades ago, Linus Pauling and Irwin Stone showed that most animals make at least that much (or more) per human body weight per day.[82]

Then why has the government set the "Safe Upper Limit" for vitamin C at 2,000 mg a day?

Perhaps the reason is ignorance. According to nationwide data compiled by the American Association of Poison Control Centers, vitamin C (and the use of any other dietary supplement) does not kill anyone.[83]

Does vitamin C damage DNA?

No. If vitamin C harmed DNA, why do most animals make (not eat, but *make)* between 2,000 and 10,000 milligrams of vitamin C per human equivalent body weight per day? Evolution would never so favor anything that harms vital genetic material. White blood cells and male reproductive fluids contain unusually high quantities of ascorbate. Living, reproducing systems love vitamin C.

Does vitamin C cause low blood sugar, B-12 deficiency, birth defects, or infertility?

Vitamin C does not cause birth defects, nor infertility, nor miscarriage. "Harmful effects have been mistakenly attributed to vitamin C, including hypoglycemia, rebound scurvy, infertility, mutagenesis, and destruction of vitamin B-12. Health professionals should recognize that vitamin C does not produce these effects."[84]

Does vitamin C . . .

A randomized, double-blind, placebo-controlled 14 day trial of 3,000 mg per day of vitamin C reported greater frequency of sexual intercourse. The vitamin C group (but not the placebo group) also experienced a quantifiable decrease in depression. This is probably due to the fact that vitamin C "modulates catecholaminergic activity, decreases stress reactivity, approach anxiety and prolactin release, improves vascular function, and increases oxytocin release. These processes are relevant to sexual behavior and mood."[85]

Does vitamin C cause kidney stones?

No. The myth of the vitamin C-caused kidney stone is rivaled in popularity only by the Loch Ness Monster. A factoid-crazy medical media often overlooks the fact that William J. McCormick, MD, demonstrated that vitamin C actually prevents the formation of kidney stones. He did so in 1946, when he published a paper on the subject.[86] His work was confirmed by University of Alabama professor of medicine Emanuel Cheraskin, MD. Dr. Cheraskin showed that vitamin C inhibits the formation of oxalate stones.[87] "Vitamin C in the urine tends to bind calcium and decrease its free form. This means less chance of calcium's separating out as calcium oxalate (stones)."

Other research reports that: "Even though a certain part of oxalate in the urine derives from metabolized ascorbic acid, the intake of high doses of vitamin C does not increase the risk of calcium oxalate kidney stones. . . (I)n the large-scale Harvard Prospective Health Professional Follow-Up Study, those groups in the highest quintile of vitamin C intake (greater than 1,500 mg/day) had a lower risk of kidney stones than the groups in the lowest quintiles."[88]

Dr. Robert F. Cathcart said, "I started using vitamin C in massive doses in patients in 1969. By the time I read that ascorbate should cause kidney stones, I had clinical evidence that it did not cause kidney stones, so I continued prescribing massive doses to patients. Up to 2006, I estimate that I have put 25,000 patients on massive doses of vitamin C and none have developed kidney stones. Two patients who had dropped their doses to 500 mg a day developed calcium oxalate kidney stones. I raised their doses back up to the more massive doses and added magnesium and B-6 to their program and no more kidney stones. I think they developed the kidney stones because they were not taking enough vitamin C."

Why did Linus Pauling die from cancer if he took all that vitamin C?

Linus Pauling, PhD, megadose vitamin C advocate, died in 1994 from prostate cancer. Mayo Clinic cancer researcher Charles G. Moertel, MD, critic of Pauling and vitamin C, also died in 1994, and also from cancer (lymphoma). Dr. Moertel was 66 years old. Dr. Pauling was 93 years old. One needs to make up one's own mind as to whether this does or does not indicate benefit from vitamin C.

A review of the subject indicates that "Vitamin C deficiency is common in patients with advanced cancer . . . Patients with low plasma concentrations of vitamin C have a shorter survival."[89]

Does vitamin C narrow arteries or cause atherosclerosis?

Abram Hoffer, MD, has said: "I have used vitamin C in megadoses with my patients since 1952 and have not seen any cases of heart disease develop even after decades of use. Dr. Robert Cathcart with experience on over 25,000 patients since 1969 has seen no cases of heart disease developing in patients who did not have any when first seen. He added that the thickening of the vessel walls, if true, indicates that the thinning that occurs with age is reversed. . . . The fact is that vitamin C *decreases* plaque formation according to many clinical studies. Some critics ignore the knowledge that thickened arterial walls in the absence of plaque formation indicate that the walls are becoming stronger and therefore less apt to rupture. . . . Gokce, Keaney, Frei, et al gave patients supplemental vitamin C daily for thirty days and measured blood flow through the arteries. Blood flow *increased nearly fifty percent* after the single dose and this was sustained after the monthly treatment."[90]

What about blood pressure?

A randomized, double-blind, placebo-controlled study showed that hypertensive patients taking supplemental vitamin C had lower blood pressure.[91]

So why the flurry of anti-vitamin-C reporting in the mass media? Negative news gets attention. Negative news sells newspapers, and magazines, and pulls in lots of television viewers. Positive *drug* studies do get headlines, of course. Positive vitamin studies do not. Is this a conspiracy? You mean with unscrupulous people all sitting around a shaded table in a darkened back room? Of course not. It is nevertheless an enormous public health problem with enormous consequences.

150 million Americans take supplemental vitamin C every day. This is as much a political issue as a scientific issue. What would happen if everybody took vitamins? Perhaps doctors, hospital administrators and pharmaceutical salespeople would all be lining up for their unemployment checks.

A skeptic might conclude that there is at least some evidence that the politicians are on the wrong side of this. After all, the US RDA for vitamin C for humans is only 10 percent of the government's USDA vitamin C standards for Guinea pigs.[92] But conspiracy against nutritional medicine? Certainly not. Couldn't be.

VITAMIN C: AN ALTERNATIVE TO ANTIBIOTICS

*"In order to cure infections, an agent is needed to
neutralize ongoing oxidative stress, repair oxidized molecules,
and kill the pathogens, or at least render them more
susceptible to eradication by a healthy immune system.
Vitamin C does all of these things."*
—THOMAS E. LEVY, MD, JD

I was raised to college age without ever taking a single dose of any antibiotic. It's not that I didn't occasionally get sick; I did. But my parents elected to use megadoses of C to treat illness instead of medication. My parents were no fools. They wanted healthy kids. They used vitamin C because it *worked*.

I did the same while I was pregnant. My mother did the same when she was pregnant with me.

A frigid February and a record flu season, along with whatever else was going around, didn't skip our house when I was the size of Indiana in my ninth month. Instead of taking the traditionally prescribed meds, I chose to take large quantities of vitamin C along with the rest of my vitamins, drink several pints of carrot juice a day for a week, and rest as much as possible. Over fifty years ago, physicians and pioneers of high-dose vitamin C therapy such as William J. McCormick, MD,[93] and Frederick Robert Klenner, MD,[94] found that very high doses of vitamin C, by itself, can be used both safely and effectively as an antibiotic and antiviral.[95] "Safe" and "effective" are music to a pregnant gal's ears; at least they are to mine. My husband (who also was not feeling well) and our daughter, not yet age two, (who was just fine but was still exposed to us) also took extra vitamin C, drank plenty of veggie juice, and rested. (Our daughter's carrot juice intake was via her sippy cup in much smaller quantities.) Proactive parenting worked; our daughter got by with just a touch of congestion. My husband and I got better, too, without a prescription and without over-the-counter medications.

People often ask me how much vitamin C did I have to take. My answer is "tons." The key to therapeutic use of vitamin C is one has to take enough. What is "enough" depends on the person and how sick he or she is. The sicker you are, the more vitamin C it takes to get better.[96]

Normally, even when I'm not pregnant, I take 4,000–8,000 mg of C a day. I take it throughout the day in divided doses. In the winter, it's closer to 6,000–10,000 mg a day. When I am sick I can hold much more. By "hold" I mean that I can take vastly higher doses of vitamin C before I reach saturation or bowel tolerance, which means exactly what you think it means. "Bowel tolerance doses are the amounts of ascorbic acid tolerated orally that almost, but not quite, cause diarrhea," says Robert F. Cathcart, MD.[97] When I am ill, I may take 8,000–10,000 mg or more *an hour*. You heard that right. This may sound like a lot, because it is. When I have the cold or flu, I start out the morning with about 8,000–10,000 mg of vitamin C all at once. Experienced vitamin C physicians call this a "loading dose." Then, I wait about an hour. If I still feel awful, I take another 8,000 mg or so. Better yet, I take a smaller amount of C every fifteen minutes until I feel my stomach rumble, a sign that I'm getting close to saturation.

TAKE VITAMIN C AT THE FIRST SIGN OF SICKNESS

Illness in our house rarely ends up in a statement like "I have the flu." We like to tackle illness *before* it becomes a clearly identifiable ailment with its associated list of miserable symptoms. This is done by taking high-dose vitamin C at the first sign of sickness: the first cough or sneeze, runny nose, sore throat, or feeling of malaise. When I was growing up, if anyone in our house coughed, you would hear my father's voice echoing from somewhere in the house: "Take C!" (We heard it often enough for it to become annoying.) This apparent "overprotectiveness" of our health earned him many an out-of-sight eye roll. But it did something else, too. It taught me how to monitor and adjust to my own body's need for vitamin C based on how I feel. Believe it or not, even my young children have a sense for when they need more C. The key to managing illness is to get to it early. Take C *before* there is a problem. An illness doesn't have to get to the point where we feel so awful we must finally resolve to go to the doctor and get a script. Ideally, we don't have to even go. Ideally, we get on top of symptoms so fast with high-dose C, sickness doesn't stand a chance.

Sometimes it takes several hours before I start to get a rumbling tummy. The longer it takes me to get to saturation means that my body is using that extra vitamin C. If I were well, I'd have been on the toilet within an hour after taking that much. Sick bodies can hold an extraordinary amount of vitamin C. If you have been told differently, you have been told wrong. Once there is a rumble (or a loose bowel movement), I ease back my dose to about half of what I was taking, to around 4,000 mg an hour. I continue with this maintenance dose unless two things happen. If I start to feel sick again, I take more. If I get loose bowels, I take less. When I learned to fly a plane, I flew over the trees but below the stars. In a similar fashion, my goal is to take enough vitamin C to be free of the symptoms of the illness (sore throat, cough, what have you), but to avoid experiencing diarrhea. It is common to be gassy after taking larger doses of the vitamin. Tooting away, I would *feel* great, and I would be getting *better*, and doing it *without* drugs. If I let my dosage drop, my illness symptoms would intensify, a sure sign that I needed to get back on the wagon and take more vitamin C. It may take several days to be rid of a bout of cold or flu but I do it without drugs. When my doctor prescribes an antibiotic, I carefully place the prescription in my purse . . . and then I take vitamin C instead.

> Determining the right dosage of vitamin C is like taking off from a cloudy, cold airport in February. The weather on the ground is miserable. As you go up and into the clouds, it is bumpy; you may encounter sleet or rain or snow. But a pilot knows if you keep climbing, you'll come out above the clouds. There, the sun is out. The sky is blue. The bad weather is below you. That is saturation of vitamin C.

Why vitamin C? Because antibiotics are trouble. Antibiotic adverse side effects land over 142,000 people in the emergency room each year, and nearly half of these visits are due to antibiotics commonly prescribed and regarded as safe.[98] Side effects of C? A conspicuous *lack* of visits to the emergency room.

Vitamin C helps your body target illness, but unlike an antibiotic, good bacteria stay alive and healthy. Using antibiotics to fight illness is like dropping a bomb on a city. Antibiotics kill beneficial bacteria and harmful bacteria alike, just as a bomb takes out a primary school as easily as a munitions factory. Hyla Cass, MD, explains, "The word *antibiotic* means 'antilife.' When you take antibiotics, they kill all the bacteria in your system, good and bad . . ." and "[t]hey also make future courses of antibiotics less effective and create antibiotic resistant strains of bacteria."[99]

If we send in an antibiotic army to handle our sicknesses, we inflict constant collateral damage on our good bacteria.

Yes, sometimes antibiotics may be necessary. However, antibiotics are wildly overprescribed and overused. Doctors are quick to give prescriptions, and patients often expect them. This leads to antibiotic resistance and stronger bacteria that are harder to kill. Is the solution of more drugs, stronger drugs, and course after course of antibiotics really the answer?

Side effects from antibiotics include yeast infections,[100] something we are already more prone to experience while pregnant.[101] Yeast (*candida albicans*) thrives in unbalanced environments as caused by antibiotic use.[102] Overuse of antibiotics has led to resistant bacteria. The Center for Disease Control now states that antibiotic drugs "have been used so widely and for so long that the infectious organisms the antibiotics are designed to kill have adapted to them, making the drugs less effective. People infected with antimicrobial-resistant organisms are more likely to have longer, more expensive hospital stays, and may be more likely to die as a result of the infection."[103]

Maternal antibiotic use may not be in the best interests of the baby. A baby's intestinal flora is "considered to be of importance for protection against harmful micro-organisms and for the maturation of the intestinal immune system," says the *Journal of Pediatric Gastroenterology and Nutrition*.[104] More bacteria and more variety of species appear to play a factor. Research suggests the benefits of exposure to mom's good microflora to prevent future illness in her baby.[105] A mother's antibiotic use during pregnancy may also promote obesity in her offspring.[106] As with us, antibiotics take a toll on beneficial bacteria found in infants.[107] Blasting mom or baby with antibiotics isn't in the best health interests of anyone.

Pregnancy is about life and balance. Antibiotics are about killing bacteria. The secret is to have an immune system that is strong, so it can fend for you. Vitamin C can help you do just that. Vitamin C supports your immune system so your body can fight infection, and it can take the place of antibiotics.[108] Thomas E. Levy, MD, says, "Optimal vitamin C dosing should drastically reduce the use of many antibiotics and other medicines."[109]

Using vitamin C to resolve illness involves paying close attention to how you feel. You have to monitor and adjust. It is the rule rather than the exception. When it comes to our health, I really don't think there is any other sensible way to do it.

If you must take an antibiotic, fend off opportunistic side infections by eating yogurt and food or supplements containing probiotics. Do this every day, several times a day, both during and after treatment, to help continually replenish good bacteria. If your doctor fails to tell you about taking probiotics during antibiotic use, you should question your doctor's competence. Take your vitamins, eat lots of vegetables (even better if you can juice them and drink fresh and raw), and drink plenty of water. According to Dr. Robert Cathcart, high-dose vitamin C means needing fewer antibiotics. Dr. Cathcart, who successfully treated over 20,000 patients with very large doses of vitamin C, also observed that high-dose vitamin C, taken along with antibiotics, reduced antibiotic side effects such as allergic reactions.[110] In fact, orthomolecular (nutritional) physicians have been reporting this for years.[111]

"Warning: Keep this medicine out of the reach of everybody!
Use vitamin C instead!"
—LINUS PAULING, PhD

VITAMIN C: LACTATION AND BREASTFEEDING

Getting less than 100 mg per day of vitamin C may mean only a miniscule amount is available for a nursing baby.[112] Your doctor may tell you to keep taking your pre-natal vitamin after the baby is born and to do your best to eat a diet rich in fruits and vegetables. But is that enough?

If we have a sick, stressed-out, overworked mom, (and is there a mom who isn't?) her need for antioxidants like vitamin C increases. Breast milk is pretty amazing stuff. And our breasts are really smart—breast milk changes and adapts to your baby's needs. It has been suggested that there is a regulatory mechanism that limits the amount of vitamin C a baby gets from her mother.[113] But in order for baby to have any, mom needs to have enough, and enough means more. Extra C is good for you, and it is also good for baby. For example, higher levels of vitamin C in mom's milk means a relatively lower risk of allergies in their infant.[114]

Yes, It Is Important

From start to finish, vitamin C, in doses much higher than many would imagine, is a safe and beneficial addition to pregnancy. Vitamin C is proven to help heal wounds faster,[115] (that includes episiotomies and Cesarean sections), prevent and treat infection,[116] reduce swelling and inflammation,[117] and reduce pain.[118] In high doses, vitamin C has anti-histamine, antitoxin, antibiotic, and antiviral properties,[119] without the associated dangers of pharmaceutical drugs. It can protect against high blood pressure, help prevent birth defects, help prevent miscarriage, and more. All of these are good news and good benefits for all pregnancies. If it sounds too good to be true, remember this: like true love, true friend-ship, and a week at a honeymoon resort in the Poconos, nothing is too good to be true.

CHAPTER 4

Vitamin E
and Pregnancy

*"Making the decision to have a child—it's momentous.
It is to decide forever to have your heart
go walking outside your body."*
—ELIZABETH STONE

Discovered by H. M. Evans and K. S. Bishop, vitamin E's name "toco-pherol" was taken from the Greek words for "to carry offspring" or "to bring forth childbirth."[1] Its very name indicates the importance and necessity of vitamin E during pregnancy.

VITAMIN E IS "E"SSENTIAL

Vitamin E is necessary for the proper functioning of many organs, nerves, and muscles.[2] It is an antioxidant.[3] It is also an anticoagulant that can reduce blood clotting.[4] And that's just the beginning.

Wilfrid Shute, MD, and Evan Shute, MD, both obstetricians, were the very first to use high-dose vitamin E during pregnancy. As they repeatedly demonstrated in over thirty years of practice, vitamin E is absolutely essential for a healthy pregnancy. That includes making sure the mother stays pregnant in the first place, because vitamin E protects against miscarriage.[5] There is no question about it: failure to get vitamin E causes spontaneous abortion in animals. Drs. Wilfrid and Evan Shute were so impressed with vitamin E's importance and versatility in obstetrics, they found success in cardiology as well, successfully treating over 30,000 patients with vitamin E therapy.

Vitamin E is protective of our pregnancy and our heart. Abram Hoffer,

MD says, "In one study,[6] Dr. M. Stampfer and his fellow researchers found that during an eight year follow-up, women who had taken at least 100 IU [international units] of vitamin E daily for two years had a 46 percent lower risk of having a heart attack. This was based on a population study involving 87,245 women. . . . They found that there was not enough vitamin E in food; Dr. Stampfer was so convinced by the data he is taking the vitamin himself."[7]

THE SAFETY OF VITAMIN E DURING PREGNANCY

"Toxic levels of vitamin E in the body simply do not occur."
—DR. MARET TRABER, LINUS PAULING INSTITUTE

It only takes one poorly done, highly circulated story about the "dangers" of a vitamin to ensure that many women will be scared off vitamin E supplementation during pregnancy. One "study" suggested that intake above 14.9 milligrams (mg) a day of vitamin E—15 mg or 22.4 IU is the current RDA (Recommended Dietary Allowance)—was associated an increased risk of congenital heart defects.[8]

That's garbage.

Vitamin E does not cause birth defects. It prevents them. This "study" would have us believing that just over two little ounces of sunflower seeds, a handful of almonds, or our daily multivitamin is somehow going to be bad news for baby. Well, ladies, it just isn't so. How did they come up with this ridiculous figure? Based on diet questionnaires given to mothers sixteen months after their babies were born, the authors of the study felt they could "conclude" that during the periconceptual period, around two years prior to the time of their collected data, ingesting small amounts of vitamin E was supposedly risky. First of all, a questionnaire given so long after the birth of the child is quite unlikely to accurately represent mom's diet at the time of conception and early pregnancy. Flaws in study design set aside, many prescription prenatal vitamins contain 30 IU of vitamin E. Over-the-counter preparations may contain 100 IU or more. A "study" like this would have us believe that prenatal vitamins containing vitamin E are supposedly dangerous to our unborn babies. Ladies, just the opposite is true. *There is seventy-five years of material on vitamin E that shows these folks are just plain wrong.* "Pregnancy hasn't changed in 50 years or

50,000 years. Vitamin E's chemical structure hasn't changed in 50 years or 50,000 years either. Old studies are not to be marginalized. They are to be minded," says Andrew W. Saul, PhD.

There is *no evidence* that vitamin E, even in doses up to 1,500 IU a day, is harmful to a pregnant woman or her baby. Vitamin E is an antioxidant. Antioxidants prevent cell damage. Antioxidants protect against birth defects. That negative vitamin E study landed in numerous news reports plastered all over the TV and Internet. Did you read the positive press about vitamin E? Wait, what positive press?

The Safety of High-Dose Vitamin E

A study published in *Reproductive Toxicology* found that doses of 400 IU–1,200 IU per day of vitamin E "does not appear to be associated with an increased risk for major malformations when used during the first trimester of pregnancy."[9] The next year, another study in the same journal also concluded that doses of 400–1,200 IU per day of vitamin E during pregnancy "does not appear to be associated with an increased risk for major malformations."[10]

In an animal study that investigated the impact of an excessive intake of vitamin E, pregnant rats were given 22.5–2,252 mg per kilogram (kg) a day. The authors reported, "No obvious teratogenic effects were observed in the newborn young of the vitamin E-supplemented rats."[11] The survival rate of the pups was unaffected. For the sake of discussion, 1 mg of vitamin E is equivalent to 1.49 IU of the natural vitamin E as alpha tocopherol or 2.22 IU of the synthetic form, dl-alpha tocopherol,[12] the kind that was used in this study. A kilogram is 2.2 pounds. A dose of 22.5 to 2,252 mg per kg or 50 IU to 4,954 IU per kg of synthetic vitamin E would be equivalent to a 160 pound pregnant human female getting over 3,600 IU to a whopping 236,000 IU of vitamin E a day. That's a whole lot of vitamin E; we are not going to take anywhere near that amount. An animal study is not a human study. However, this may provide you with some perspective when you think about the much smaller doses of vitamin E that you are taking to protect against miscarriage.

Vitamin E is safe and nontoxic.[13] Your body is designed to efficiently handle vitamin E, even in large doses, making it almost impossible to take a harmful amount.[14] According to a recent review in the *Journal of Lipid Research,* Professor Maret Traber, internationally recognized vitamin E expert from the Linus Pauling Institute at Oregon State University, says "[t]oxic levels of vitamin E in the body simply do not occur."[15] That goes for vitamin E obtained from both food and through supplements. Excess E is not a health concern—deficiency is. "[I]t's not possible for toxic levels of vitamin E to accumulate in the liver or other tissues," says Dr. Traber. "[P]ast studies which have alleged adverse consequences from vitamin E have misinterpreted the data. Taking too much vitamin E is not the real concern," she says. Rather, "a much more important issue is that more than 90 percent of people in the U.S. have inadequate levels of vitamin E in their diet."[16]

DOSAGE AND FORMS OF VITAMIN E

The current recommended dietary intake for vitamin E is 22.4 IU per day during pregnancy, and 28.5 IU during lactation.[17] The so-called tolerable upper intake levels for pregnancy and lactation have been set at 1,200 IU per day for pregnant women ages fourteen to eighteen and 1,500 IU per day for ages nineteen and older.[18] Wheat germ oil, nuts, and leafy greens are excellent dietary sources of dietary vitamin E. However, it was recognized nearly eighty years ago that ensuring a liberal vitamin E supply in the average daily diet is more difficult than obtaining an adequate supply of any other known vitamin.[19] This remains true. Even with a low RDA, it is very difficult to get this amount of vitamin E in our diets, and most of us still are not succeeding.[20] A study in the *Journal of the American Dietetic Association* found that only 2.4 percent of American women managed to get the Estimated Average Requirement (EAR) of vitamin E from food alone.[21]

Can supplements replace bad diet? They had better, says Dr. Saul.[22] Optimal doses of vitamin E in pregnancy may be much higher. Dr. Saul emphasizes: "Taking vitamin E (at least 200 and perhaps 400 IU daily) greatly reduces the chance of miscarriage. This is no myth: by the end of WW II, there were already dozens of medical studies confirming this."[23]

Your prescription prenatal may not even contain a modest 22.4 IU. While over-the-counter varieties tend to contain more vitamin E, few provide more than 30 IU. To get 200 IU of vitamin E through your diet, you'd literally have to eat six *pounds* of peanut butter or drink down *cups* of oil each day. Of course, this is not advisable during pregnancy, or any other time for that matter. Supplements save time and spare your stomach.

Forms of Vitamin E

What is the best form of vitamin E to take? Any vitamin E is better than no vitamin E, but since you asked, ideally you would choose "d-alpha tocopherol with mixed natural tocopherols and tocotrienols." D-alpha tocopherol is the natural form of vitamin E. The mixed tocopherols are alpha, beta, gamma, and delta tocopherol.

WHICH FORM OF VITAMIN E IS BEST?

BETTER THAN NOTHING   dl-alpha tocopherol: The little "l" after the "d" indicates a synthetic form of E

GOOD   d-alpha tocopherol: Natural vitamin E is more useful to the body than the synthetic form

REALLY GOOD   d-alpha tocopherol with mixed tocopherols: Natural vitamin E with d-alpha, d-beta, d-gamma and d-delta tocopherols

THE BEST   d-alpha tocopherol with mixed tocopherols and tocotrienols: Natural vitamin E that also includes d-alpha, d-beta, d-gamma, and d-delta tocotrienols in addition to the mixed tocopherols

Vitamin E as "dl-alpha tocopherol" (note the little "l" after the "d") is a synthetic form of E that is not as beneficial to your body as the natural form, although it is cheaper than natural vitamin E. (Basically, you are only absorbing half the product. Your body can only use the "d" part, not the "l" part.) Check your vitamin bottle label. Is there a "dl" prefix? You may want to upgrade to the natural form. "Molecular structure determines how the body uses vitamin E," says nutrition expert Jack Challem. "Researchers have found that natural vitamin E assimilates far better than synthetic versions."[24] Natural vitamin E may cost more, but your body can use it more, which makes it worth the extra dough.

If you can't afford the more expensive forms of vitamin E supplements, wheat germ contains natural vitamin E and other nutrients as well, including magnesium, B vitamins, and trace minerals. Sprinkle it on yogurt; add it to a smoothie or shake. The only other appreciable sources of vitamin E are nuts and oils. Nuts are high in good fats, good amino acids, and protein; they're also satisfying. Unsalted, raw, and fresh is best. Pregnancy is already making us enormous, but if you are worried about nuts making you fat, don't. They won't. "Fats don't make you fat," says Hyla Cass, MD.[25] Sugar and nutritionally void processed foods do. Quality fats are good for us, especially during pregnancy. You can find traces of vitamin E in avocados, squash, greens, and organic tofu. Fresh, high-quality vegetable oils or olive oil can also provide a measure of vitamin E.

POST-PREGNANCY BENEFITS OF VITAMIN E

Let's keep a good thing going. Vitamin E is beneficial for you and your baby during pregnancy. It certainly remains important after birth.

Lactation

Your body is smart. It knows what to do with vitamin E, and your breasts are no exception. Mammary transfer of vitamin E is quite efficient.[26] For example, colostrum contains more vitamin E than mature milk.[27] Rest assured: your nursing baby gets the vitamin E it needs from breast milk, as long as you get the vitamin E you need from diet and supplements.

Vitamin E and Healing from Episiotomy, Rips, or Tears

Vitamin E can help sore, dry skin heal, and make it feel so much better. After vaginal birth, nurses will likely give you sprays or ointments or creams to help keep the area down there more comfortable while it mends. Spreading natural vitamin E on the wound may work even better. For more about vitamins, including E, and healing after vaginal delivery or C-section, please see the corresponding sections in the Postpartum Problems chapter.

VITAMIN E CONTROVERSY

The following article from *The Journal of Orthomolecular Medicine*, delves into this surprisingly controversial vitamin. While the original article focused on its use in cardiology, much of it is also relevant for us, as it describes vitamin E's noteworthy history, the safety of high-dose vitamin E for infants, children, and adults, and its importance during pregnancy. These sections are excerpted below. The full article is available online at http://orthomolecular.org/library/jom/2003/toc3.shtml.

Excerpts from *Vitamin E: A Cure in Search of Recognition*

BY ANDREW W. SAUL, PhD

Double Standards

Countless comedians have made fun of the incompetent physician who, when called late at night during a life-threatening disease crisis, says, "take two aspirin and call me in the morning." Now it's no longer funny. Recently, one of the largest pharmaceutical conglomerates in the world ran prime-time national television commercials that declared: "Bayer aspirin may actually help stop you from dying if you take it during a heart attack." The company also promotes such use of its product on the Internet.[28] This statement comes forth after a century of widespread aspirin consumption. Cardiovascular disease remains the number one killer of men and women and there are over a million heart attacks annually in the U.S.A. alone.

If you produced a TV ad that said that megadoses of wheat germ oil, or the vitamin E in it, could save your life by preventing a heart attack, not only would people disbelieve you, you'd also be subject to arrest for breaking federal law. Foods and vitamins may not be advertised as treatments for specific diseases. "All statements of nutritional support for dietary supplements must be accompanied by a two-part disclaimer on the product label: that the statement has not been evaluated by FDA and that the product is not intended to 'diagnose, treat, cure or prevent any disease.'"[29] . . .

A Torrid History

1922 was the year the U.S.S.R. was formed and "Little Orphan Annie" began. Trumpeter Al Hirt and future heart transplant pioneer Christiaan Barnard were born. Alexander Graham Bell died. And vitamin E was discovered by H. M. Evans and K. S. Bishop.[30]

In 1936, Evans' team had isolated alpha tocopherol from wheat germ oil and vitamin E was beginning to be widely appreciated, and the consequences of deficiency better known. Health Culture Magazine *for January, 1936 said, "The fertility food factor (is) now called vitamin E.*

Excepting for the abundance of that vitamin in whole grains, there could not have been any perpetuation of the human race. Its absence from the diet makes for irreparable sterility occasioned by a complete degeneration of the germinal cells of the male generative glands. (T)he expectant mother requires vitamin E to insure the carriage of her charge to a complete and natural term. If her diet is deficient in vitamin E . . . the woman is very apt to abort. . . It is more difficult to insure a liberal vitamin E supply in the daily average diet than to insure an adequate supply of any other known vitamin. "[31] [Emphasis added]

. . . Since the word "tocopherol" is taken from the Greek words for "to carry offspring" or "to bring forth childbirth," it is easy enough to see how Evan Shute and other obstetricians were drawn into the work. As early as 1931, Vogt-Moller of Denmark successfully treated habitual abortion in human females with wheat germ oil vitamin E. By 1939 he had treated several hundred women with a success rate of about 80 percent. In 1937, both Young in England and the Shutes in Canada reported success in combating threatened abortion and pregnancy toxemias as well. A. L. Bacharach's 1940 statistical analysis of published clinical results "show quite definitely that vitamin E is of value in recurrent abortions. "[32] [Emphasis added] And also in 1940, the Shutes were curing atherosclerosis with vitamin E. By 1946, thrombosis, phlebitis, and claudication.

Yet when the MDR's (Minimum Daily Requirements) first came out in 1941, there was no mention of vitamin E. It was not until 1959 that vitamin E was recognized by the U.S. Food and Drug Administration as necessary for human existence, and not until 1968 that any government recommendation for vitamin E would be issued. That year, the Food and Nutrition Board of the US National Research Council offered its first Recommended Daily Allowance: 30 IU. It has been as low as 15 IU in 1974. In 2000, it was set at 22 IU (15 mg) for all persons, including pregnant women. This is somewhat odd in view of a 70-year established research history showing how vital vitamin E is during gestation. It is another curious fact that today, when the public has been urged to increase its consumption of unsaturated fats, the official dietary recommendation for vitamin E is substantially lower than it was 35 years ago. "The requirement for vitamin E is related to the amount of polyunsaturated fatty acids (PUFAs) consumed in the diet. The higher the amount of PUFAs, the more vitamin E is required."[33]

One reason the RDA was lowered is that "dieticians were having difficulty devising diets of natural foods which had the recommended amount (30 IU) of vitamin E."[34] There are about 39 IU of vitamin E in an 8-ounce cup of olive oil. A full pound of peanuts yields 34 IU. Professor Max K. Horwitt, PhD, who spent 15 years serving on The Food and Nutrition Board's RDA committees, said in an interview that "The average intake by adults, without supplements, seems to be about 8 milligrams of alpha tocopherol per day, or 8 tocopherol equivalents. This is equivalent to 12 International Units (IU)."[35] So it might be said that, in the end, the accommodation was not to raise the bridge but rather to lower the river.

Vitamin E is the body's chief fat-soluble antioxidant. It is a powerful one indeed, when you consider that 22 IU is presumed adequate to protect each one of the tens of trillions of body cells in a human being. Even though there has been a veritable explosion in antioxidant research since 1968, the RDA for vitamin E has been decreased.

Postal Fraud

"Any claim in the labeling of drugs or of foods offered for special dietary use, by reason of Vitamin E, that there is need for dietary supplementation with Vitamin E, will be considered false." (United States Post Office Department Docket No. 1/187 (March 15, 1961)

On October 26, 1959, the U.S. government charged an organization known as the Cardiac Society with postal fraud for selling 30 IU vitamin E capsules through the mail. Specifically, the charge was "the operation of a scheme or device for obtaining money through the mails by means of false and fraudulent pretenses, representations or promises . . . that Respondent's product 'E-FEROL 30 I.U.' (containing vitamin E) is therapeutically effective and beneficial in the treatment of heart and cardiovascular diseases for any person so afflicted; that Respondent's said product will prevent heart disease; that "It [vitamin E] is the key both to the prevention and treatment of all those conditions in which a lack of blood supply due to thickened or blocked blood vessels or a lack of oxygen is a part or the whole story of the disease"; that "Vitamin E seems to be a natural anti-thrombin in the human blood stream. . . . It is the only substance preventing the clotting of blood which is not dangerous"; that the book "Your Heart and Vitamin E" tells you "What Vitamin E Is and Does, How It Treats Heart Disease, Its Success in Circulatory Diseases, Your Foods' Deficiency in Vitamin E" . . . That "It (the book) explains medical facts in every-day language concerning the help that is available for sufferers from diseases of the heart and blood vessels such as Coronary Heart Disease, Angina Pectoris, Phlebitis, Buerger's Disease, Diabetes, Strokes, etc."[36]

A four-day hearing in Washington, D.C., generated sufficient testimony to fill "four volumes totaling 856 pages. Seventy-six exhibits were received in evidence . . . for the consideration of the Hearing Examiner. His Initial Decision covers forty-two pages."

It is an oddity of history that, at the height of the Cuban Missile Crisis, the United States of America found both the reason and the resources to prosecute such a case as this. . . .

Dosage and Utility

Vitamin E has many clinically important and seemingly unrelated properties. In their books[37] the Shutes discuss a number of them.

1. Vitamin E strengthens and regulates heartbeat, like digitalis and similar drugs, at a dose adjusted between 800 to 3,000 IU daily.

2. Vitamin E reduces inflammation and scarring when frequently applied topically to burns or to sites of lacerations or surgical incisions. Internally, vitamin E helps to very gradually break down thrombi at a maintained oral dose of between 800 IU and 3,000 IU.

3. Vitamin E has an oxygen-sparing effect on the heart, enabling the heart to do more work on less oxygen. The benefit for recovering heart attack patients is considerable. 1,200 to 2,000 IU daily relieves angina very well. My [A.W. Saul's] father, duly diagnosed with angina, gradually worked up to1,600 IU over a period of a few weeks. He never had an angina symptom again. In this, he had the identical success that thousands of Shute patients had.

Deep Vein Thrombosis (DVT): Anticoagulant Drugs or Vitamin E?

4. "Vitamin E moderately prolongs prothrombin clotting time, decreases platelet adhesion, and has a limited 'blood thinning' effect. This is the reason behind the Shutes' using vitamin E (1,000–2,000 IU/day) for thrombophlebitis and related conditions. The pharmaceutical industry and the medical profession are well aware of vitamin E's anticoagulant property and that 'very high doses of this vitamin may act synergistically with anticoagulant drugs.'[38] However, this also means that vitamin E can, entirely or in part, substitute for such drugs but do so more safely. Perhaps this is best summed up by surgeon Edward William Alton Ochsner, M.D. (1896–1981), who said, 'Vitamin E is a potent inhibitor of thrombin that does not produce a hemorrhagic tendency and therefore is a safe prophylactic against venous thrombosis.'"[39]

5. Vitamin E is a modest vasodilator, promotes collateral circulation, and consequently offers great benefits to diabetes patients.[40] The Shutes used a dose of about 800 IU or more, tailored to the patient. For this, among other reasons, Evan Shute, author of over 100 scientific papers, was literally judged to be a fraud by the United States Post Office Department. The 1961 court decision said, "Vascular degenerations in a diabetic are not effectively treated in the use of vitamin E in any dosage . . . vitamin E has been thoroughly studied and that there is no doubt whatsoever as to its lack of utility."[41]

This statement was premature to say the least. The "thorough study" of vitamin E was not quite completed by 1961. Thirty-eight years later, a crossover study of 36 patients who had Type I diabetes, and retinal blood flows that were significantly lower than non-diabetics, showed that those taking 1,800 IU of vitamin E daily obtained normal retinal blood flow. The patients with the worst initial readings improved the most. "(V)itamin E may potentially provide additional risk reduction for the development of retinopathy or nephropathy in addition to those achievable through intensive insulin therapy alone. Vitamin E is a low-cost, readily available compound associated with few known side effects; thus, its use could have a dramatic socioeconomic impact if found to be efficacious in delaying the onset of diabetic retinopathy and/or nephropathy."[42] Vitamin E also works synergistically with insulin to lower high blood pressure in diabetics.[43]

Quantity and Quality

The most common reason for irreproducibility of successful vitamin E cures is either a failure to use enough of it, or a failure to use the natural form (D-alpha, plus mixed natural tocopherols), or both. For example, in an oft-quoted negative study,[44] researchers who gave 300 milligrams of synthetic vitamin E to patients who had recently had a heart attack saw no beneficial effect. Such failure is to be expected. You can set up any experiment to fail. The Shutes would have used only the natural form, and four times as much.

Natural vitamin E is always the dextro- (right-handed) form. On the other hand, "synthetic vitamin E is a mixture of eight isomers in equal proportions containing only 12.5 percent of d-alpha tocopherol. One mg of dl-alpha tocopherol has the lowest Vitamin E equivalence of any of the common vitamin E preparations."[45]

While personal philosophy is the only possible basis for a decision to conduct a study using only the synthetic form of a vitamin, the use of low dosage is generally explained away by alleging doubts about safety.

Safety

The most elementary of forensic arguments is, where are the bodies? Poison control statistics report no deaths from vitamin E.[46] There is a reason for this. Vitamin E is a safe and remarkably nontoxic substance. Even the 2000 report by the Institute of Medicine of the National Academy of Sciences, which actually recommends against taking supplemental vitamin E, specifically acknowledges that 1,000 mg (1,500 IU) is a "tolerable upper intake level . . . that is likely to pose no risk of adverse health effects for almost all individuals in the general population."[47] The Shutes observed no evidence of harm with doses as high as 8,000 IU/day. In fact, "toxicity symptoms have not been reported even at intakes of 800 IU per kilogram of body weight daily for 5 months" according to the Food and Nutrition Board.[48] This demonstrated safe level would work out to be around 60,000 IU daily for an average adult, some 2,700 times the RDA! . . .

Safety in Children

Children using anti-epileptic medication have reduced plasma levels of vitamin E, a sign of vitamin E deficiency. So doctors at the University of Toronto gave epileptic children 400 IU of vitamin E per day for several months, along with their medication. This combined treatment reduced the frequency of seizures in most of the children by over 60 percent. Half of them "had a 90 to 100 percent reduction in seizures."[49] This extraordinary result is also proof of the safety of 400 IU of vitamin E per day in children (equivalent to at least 800 to 1,200 IU/day for an adult). "There were no adverse side effects," said the researchers. It also provides a clear example of pharmaceutical use creating a vitamin deficiency, and an unassailable justification for supplementation.

Safety in Infants

Overexposure to oxygen has been a major cause of retrolental fibroplasia (retinopathy of prematurity) and subsequent blindness in premature infants. Incubator oxygen retina damage is now prevented by giving preemies 100 mg E per kilogram body weight. That dose is equivalent to an adult dose of about 7,000 IU for an average-weight adult. "There have been no detrimental side effects" from such treatment, said the *New England Journal of Medicine,* Dec. 3, 1981.[50] Nevertheless, the 1989 (sixth) edition of the textbook *Nutrition and Diet Therapy*[51] *advised that "healthy persons stand the chance of developing signs of toxicity with the megadoses that are recommended in these studies." (p. 225) That incorrect statement was dropped in the book's next edition. Instead, the 7th edition (1993) said under "Toxicity Effects" that "Vitamin E is the only one of the fat-soluble vitamins for which no toxic effect in humans is known. Its use as a supplement has not shown harmful effects." (p. 186)*

(Abridged and reprinted with permission from the International Society for Orthomolecular Medicine and the *Journal of Orthomolecular Medicine,* 2003; Vol. 18, Numbers 3 and 4, p. 205–212.)

A bibliography of selected books and papers by Wilfrid and Evan Shute is posted at http://www.doctoryourself.com/biblio_shute.html.

VITAMIN E—SAFE AND NECESSARY

Research has proven that vitamin E is essential for life, and this is inherent in its very name. We can take comfort in its safety and benefits. The evidence has demonstrated time and time again that we should.

CHAPTER 5

Vitamin A and Pregnancy

"Eat real food. Not too much. Mostly plants."
—MICHAEL POLLAN

Vitamin A isn't just a little important during pregnancy, it's a lot important. Vitamin A is vital when it comes to protecting your baby from abnormalities.[1] It is essential for your baby's development and immune function. "Vitamin A, a fat-soluble vitamin stored in the liver, is important for your baby's embryonic growth—including the development of the heart, lungs, kidneys, eyes, and bones, and the circulatory, respiratory, and central nervous systems," says BabyCenter's medical advisory board,[2] and his teeth, too. Andrew W. Saul, PhD, explains, "A baby's tooth enamel is constructed in the womb. Ameloblasts adequately form the enamel in the fetus only if Mom gets enough vitamin A."[3] Vitamin A also helps with baby's resistance to infection and his fat metabolism.[4] In addition to being so important for a developing baby, vitamin A is good for mom. "Vitamin A is particularly essential for women who are about to give birth, because it helps with postpartum tissue repair," says BabyCenter. "It also helps maintain normal vision and fight infections."[5]

Studies that claim vitamin A is harmful get plenty of media attention, but the studies that show its beneficial role, doing just the opposite, are ignored. Did you hear the one about vitamin A causing cancer?[6] Don't worry, it doesn't. In fact, it prevents cancer.[7] Large amounts of vitamin A have also been accused of causing birth defects, and yet vitamin A is essential for normal fetal growth and development. Taking into account the vital nature of vitamin A during pregnancy, conflicting data is confusing and worrisome. Any possible risk can stress out a pregnant mom. It is time to shed some light on the situation.

CONCERNS ABOUT VITAMIN A TOXICITY

You may have heard that very large prenatal doses of vitamin A could cause birth defects. One study from the *New England Journal of Medicine* showed amounts of 10,000 international units (IU) or more of preformed (retinol) vitamin A (yes, form is important, and we'll get to that in a minute) has been associated with birth defects.[8] This study got everyone pretty worried. It was trumpeted, as negative vitamin studies tend to be, but also widely criticized, inciting comments like this one from Martha M. Werler, ScD, Edward J. Lammer, MD, and Allen A. Mitchell, MD: "[w]e do not believe that the results of this study alone provide sufficient evidence of a dose effect for clinicians and the public to be warned of the dangers of any vitamin A dose greater than 10,000 IU."[9] Consider, too, that another study showed that women who consumed more than 10,000 IU a day had only about three-quarters the risk of babies with malformations, as compared with women who consumed 5,000 IU or less.[10] Melvyn R. Werbach, MD, says, "While 10,000 IU of preformed vitamin A is usually the maximum recommended safe intake, there is considerable evidence suggesting that up to 25,000–30,000 IU daily carries only minimal risk, if any."[11] The World Health Organization states, "Recent studies strongly suggest that periconceptional supplements of vitamin A that are close to, but less than 10,000 IU/day, and that are given as a component of a multivitamin, are much more likely to be associated with reduced, rather than increased, risk of malformations."[12]

VITAMIN A DEFICIENCY

We must understand it is much more likely that vitamin A *deficiency* can cause birth defects,[13] not vitamin A intake. A lack of vitamin A is also associated with premature birth and the complications that result from prematurity,[14] night blindness, susceptibility to infection, and impaired growth.[15] It also increases the risk of maternal death.[16] Millions of women worldwide are deficient in vitamin A.[17] That means millions of women and babies could be protected from preventable harm if we could ensure every mom-to-be was getting adequate amounts. Sufficiency of vitamin A should start in the womb and continue after birth for both mother and child. Here's how serious this is: according to the World Health Organization (WHO), vitamin A deficiency is the number one cause of preventable infant blindness worldwide, affecting an estimated quarter to half million children each year. Half of these children, WHO says, will die within a year of losing their eyesight.[18]

It has been said that vitamin A deficiency is rare in the United States. However, says Jack Challem, of *The Nutrition Reporter,* "some evidence suggests that the opposite may be true—that is, that potentially large numbers of Americans may consume levels of vitamin A below the RDA [Recommended Dietary Allowance]."[19] Having access to good food isn't enough. "Despite the fact that vitamin A and beta-carotene rich food is generally available, risk groups for low vitamin A supply exist in the western world," says the *European Journal of Nutrition.*[20] If we aren't getting enough in our food, and we are scared off taking vitamin A supplements, even prenatal vitamins that contain it, we are setting ourselves up for problems. "The American Pediatrics Association cites vitamin A as one of the most critical vitamins during pregnancy and the breastfeeding period, especially in terms of lung function and maturation," the article's authors say. "If the vitamin A supply of the mother is inadequate, her supply to the fetus will also be inadequate, as will later be her milk."[21]

It is extremely unlikely to hurt a developing baby with preformed vitamin A. *The American Journal of Clinical Nutrition* says "[t]he teratogenicity of vitamin A is biologically and physiologically possible," however "its real occurrence in humans seems limited."[22] It's much more likely that you aren't getting *enough* vitamin A. Only about half of Americans are reported to have "adequate" intakes of the vitamin.[23]

How Much Should I Take?

The World Health Organization recommends that women take 10,000 IU of vitamin A each day during pregnancy, regardless of their vitamin A status.[24] The Teratology Society of the United States recommends a more conservative dose, not to exceed 8,000 IU a day of preformed vitamin A.[25] The RDA for pregnancy is 2,500–2,567 IU per day of preformed A (and nearly twice that during lactation) and the so-called tolerable upper level is set at 10,000 IU per day from all sources.[26]

Remember, these suggested amounts refer to preformed vitamin A, or retinol vitamin A. Vitamin A in the form of beta-carotene, even in massive quantities, is completely safe for both mom and baby. We'll talk more about forms of vitamin A next.

FORMS AND SOURCES OF VITAMIN A

First, check what is in your prenatal or multivitamin. Does it say "preformed vitamin A, retinol, or retinoids?" This form of vitamin A is used directly by your body. This is also the kind of vitamin A found in animal products like milk, liver, and eggs, and in fortified cereals and fish oil vitamin A supplements. A three-ounce serving of beef liver, for example, is loaded with about 30,000 IU of preformed vitamin A. I have yet to see a pregnancy warning on a package of liver, but large amounts of preformed vitamin A have been associated with birth defects in the *New England Journal of Medicine* study we talked about before.[27]

So what should we do? Well, first let's put preformed vitamin A from food into perspective. Unless you are a liver lover, you will have a hard time overdoing it on vitamin A from your food alone. A cup of milk has about 500 IU, an egg 260 IU, and fortified cereals have around 500 IU of vitamin A per serving.[28] Unless you are drinking over a gallon of milk every day, an entire box of cereal every day, or over three dozen eggs in your morning omelet, . . . yes, *every* day, you probably aren't going to be getting too much preformed vitamin A from your food. The concern, then, would be getting too much preformed vitamin A from additional supplements, and a simple check of the label will tell you how much you are already taking.

We don't want caution to outweigh the importance of making sure our body and, most important, our growing baby, gets the amount of vitamin A needed. To be on the safe side, which is always preferable during pregnancy, you can cap your intake of preformed vitamin A according to current recommendations and take up to 10,000 IU a day. However, you also have access to another form of vitamin A: beta-carotene, which is completely safe for mom and baby even in high doses.[29]

Hearing the phrase "there is no way this can hurt a baby" may sound shocking, but when it comes to carotene, it happens to be true. Your body is very smart. So is your baby's. It knows when and how to break down beta-carotene into vitamin A, and when not to break it down if you have sufficient A from other sources. There is no risk to your developing baby if you get a lot of beta-carotene in your diet. Pregnancy is a great time to load up on carotene-rich foods. Fruits and vegetables are loaded with carotenoids (a common form is beta-carotene). If your vitamin says "provitamin A carotenoids," it contains this completely safe form of vitamin A. You cannot hurt yourself or a developing baby by eating lots of sweet potatoes, carrots, mangos, squash, broccoli, pumpkin, cantaloupe, and leafy green vegetables. A baked sweet potato has about 22,000 IU of provitamin A. Not a problem. Eat all you want. The worst that will happen if you get too much carotene is you might turn a little orange. It's true—it's called "hypercarotenosis," "carotenemia," or "carotenodermia," and it is completely harmless. While you sport your "fake tan" for a little while, at least you'll know you are getting plenty of carotene in your diet. Vegetable juicing is a great way for mom and baby to get lots of vitamin A. I can pack about nine or ten carrots into a glass of fresh, raw, homemade carrot juice, and I loved to drink it during my pregnancy. Carotene supplements are also available, and many prenatal vitamins will include some or all of their vitamin A in the form of beta-carotene.

There is some concern as to the amount of necessary vitamin A your body will actually convert from beta-carotene. It has been assumed that in healthy people, beta-carotene converts into one-sixth as much vitamin A (retinol),[30] the form your body uses. It turns out our bodies may not be as efficient as previously believed, however. "Recently, researchers have questioned the estimate of the 6-to-1 conversion ratio of beta-carotene to vitamin A. Their newer studies have suggested that the beta-carotene conversion for many people may be as low as 29 to 1. This means that 10,000 IU of beta-carotene would convert to only 344 IU of retinol, instead of the 1,666 IU predicted by the 6 to 1 conversion rate."[31] This just makes it all the more important to eat foods containing vitamin A such as milk and eggs and ample quantities of fruits and vegetables.

CIGARETTES CAUSE CANCER, NOT BETA-CAROTENE

In 2008, authors of a study came to the conclusion that beta-carotene in multivitamin supplements is bad for smokers, stating, "High-dose beta-carotene supplementation appears to increase the risk of lung cancer among current smokers."[32]

Oh, *please.*

Carotene causes cancer? Actually, *smoking* causes cancer. That alleged "high-dose" of beta-carotene was only 20–30 milligrams (mg) a day,[33] the amount you'd find in about six carrots.[34] (Have you seen anybody keel over from eating their vegetables lately? Any carrot casualties?) Antioxidants like beta-carotene prevent, not promote, cancer.[35] Carotene in carrots, and carotene in supplements is extraordinarily safe, and that can confirmed by the American Association of

Poison Control Centers, where you will find that not one individual has ever died from beta-carotene in any form.[36] Ever.

Not only that, but smoking is actually bad for carotene. Smoking destroys the beneficial antioxidant properties of carotene. This makes it likely that smokers need higher doses of antioxidants, like vitamin A, than nonsmokers.[37] Another study showed that cigarette smoking was "significantly related to lower beta-carotene concentrations (even) after supplementation."[38] Now *that* makes sense.

It would appear that smokers need more helpful antioxidants, not less. "A small dose (of beta-carotene) is an ineffective dose," says Dr. Saul. "20–30 mg of carotene a day is too little, too late."[39] Beta-carotene is safe. It is cigarettes that are not.

POST-PREGNANCY VITAMIN A

Achieving adequate levels of A makes a whole lot of sense. There are numerous benefits for both you and your baby both during pregnancy and after you have given birth.

Vitamin A and Lactation

Your nursing baby gets her vitamin A from you. Adequate levels of vitamin A in breast milk is "highly dependent upon maternal diet and nutritional status."[40] If mom doesn't get enough, baby doesn't get enough. "In populations deficient in vitamin A, the amount in breast milk will be suboptimal and insufficient to build or maintain stores of this micronutrient in nursing infants," says the World Health Organization.[41]

The RDA for vitamin A for healthy individuals nearly doubles during lactation.[42] If you find yourself not so healthy and suffering with a postnatal infection, your need for vitamin A may have just gone up. A lack of vitamin A weakens the immune system[43] and, says the journal *Clinical Infectious Diseases,* "[v]itamin A and its metabolites are immune enhancers."[44] Eat plenty of vitamin-rich fruits and veggies and consider the benefits of supplemental vitamin A for both you and your baby.

THE MORAL OF THE VITAMIN A STORY

Read labels. Believe it or not, some prenatal vitamins contain no vitamin A at all. Eat plenty of fruits and veggies. Keep taking your vitamins. There is much to be gained by obtaining optimal levels of vitamin A during pregnancy.

CHAPTER 6

Vitamin D
and Pregnancy

*"Without health there is no happiness.
An attention to health, then, should take
the place of every other object."*
—THOMAS JEFFERSON

Just ten to fifteen minutes of peak sun exposure, without sun block, on an untanned bikini-clad Caucasian will get up to 20,000 international units (IU) of vitamin D_3 coursing through her body.[1] After thirty minutes it will be about 50,000 IU.[2] If this seems like a lot, it may be because you are aware that the Recommended Dietary Allowance (RDA) for vitamin D_3, as of 2014, is still set at only 400 IU for adults and 600 IU for women who are pregnant or lactating.[3] We have to ask ourselves this question: Is all of nature wrong, or is the RDA set way too low?

Bruce Hollis, professor of pediatrics at the Medical University of South Carolina, says, "Recent studies reveal that current dietary recommendations for adults are not sufficient to maintain circulating 25-hydroxyvitamin D (25(OH)D) levels" at or above deficiency levels, "especially in pregnancy and lactation."[4] In other words, getting the RDA of D_3 does just about nothing.[5] Even two to four times the recommended levels, 800–1,600 IU per day, may be insufficient for pregnant gals. For example, pregnant women who were deficient in vitamin D were *still* deficient in D even after receiving 800–1,600 IU of the vitamin throughout their pregnancy.[6] Vitamin D dose matters.

VITAMIN D DEFICIENCY

"Vitamin D deficiency is a major unrecognized health problem."
—MICHAEL F. HOLICK, MD, PhD, Boston University Medical Center

Around half of pregnant American women are deficient in vitamin D[7] even when we take our prenatal vitamins.[8] Some studies say that number is much higher, reaching up to 97 percent in some populations.[9] And we are not alone. "Vitamin D deficiency during pregnancy is a worldwide epidemic; studies have reported a prevalence that ranges from 18 to 84 percent,[10] depending on the country of residence and local clothing customs," says the *American Journal of Obstetrics and Gynecology.*[11]

This is valuable information. Why? Because deficiency in vitamin D can cause a lot of trouble for a pregnant mom and her baby, both now and as baby grows into an adult. And vitamin D sufficiency contributes greatly to the health and well-being of mom and baby.

Currently, studies cite an increase in rickets or soft and weak bones, the classic vitamin D deficiency disease.[12] Michael Holick, MD, explains "In utero and during childhood, vitamin D deficiency can cause growth retardation and skeletal deformities and may increase the risk of hip fracture later in life."[13] And, sadly, this is not all. Jack Challem, of *The Nutrition Reporter,* author and coauthor of many books and papers on health and nutrition, explains that according to a recent analysis published in the *British Medical Journal,* low levels of D have been found to contribute to numerous complications of pregnancy:[14]

> An analysis of thirty-one studies has found that low levels of vitamin D lead to several serious complications of pregnancy. Conversely, women with healthy blood levels of the vitamin have a relatively low risk of those complications. Doreen M. Rabi, MD, and her colleagues at the University of Calgary, Canada, determined that women with low levels of the vitamin were about 50 percent more likely to develop gestational diabetes and about 80 percent more likely to develop preeclampsia. A mother's low vitamin D levels during pregnancy were also associated with an 85 percent greater risk of infants who were small for their gestational age. In addition, mothers-to-be had greater odds of developing bacterial vaginosis and delivering low birth weight infants.[15]

Vitamin D is essential for bone health, to build teeth, to prevent childhood rickets or the softening of bones, which remains a larger public health problem than might be expected[16] and may come as no surprise given the reported levels of vitamin D deficiency worldwide.

"Milder degrees of deficiency are now understood to be one of the causes of a vast array of chronic diseases, including osteoporosis, impaired immune competence, various autoimmune diseases (such as diabetes and multiple sclerosis), several cancers (breast, colon, lung, lymphoma and prostate, among others) high blood pressure, pregnancy complications and cardiovascular disease. All may develop because of, or be exacerbated by, vitamin D deficiency. Asking the body to deal with these disorders without adequate vitamin D is like asking a fighter to enter battle with one hand tied behind his/her back."

—GRASSROOTS HEALTH, A Public Health Organization[17]

BENEFITS OF VITAMIN D

Deficiency of vitamin D is certainly problematic, whereas obtaining optimal levels of vitamin D is certainly positive. "Of great interest is the role it (vitamin D) can play in decreasing the risk of many chronic illnesses, including common cancers, autoimmune diseases, infectious diseases, and cardiovascular disease," says Dr. Holick.[18]

Vitamin D helps your body absorb calcium and phosphorus.[19] Vitamin D reduces inflammation, supports immune function, healthy cell division, and supports the normal, physical development of your baby.[20] Pregnant women who have adequate levels of D have a lower risk of gestational diabetes and preeclampsia, vaginal infections and low birth weight children.[21] Women with sufficient levels of vitamin D, as opposed to those with vitamin D deficiency or insufficiency, are significantly more likely to get pregnant following in vitro fertilization.[22] Research also suggests that adequate levels of vitamin D can be protective against depression during pregnancy.[23] There is a real opportunity here to help women feel better safely and naturally with vitamin D. Antidepressants have been found to be unsafe during pregnancy[24] and no more effective than placebo.[25] Babies who get more vitamin D after birth also benefit from fewer colds and less eczema[26] and a reduced risk of developing asthma as children.[27] Isn't it empowering to know just this one vitamin can help you this much?

HOW MUCH VITAMIN D SHOULD I TAKE?

Generally speaking, if you aren't taking any vitamin D, or getting only the low RDA in your prenatal vitamin, the answer to how much you should take is probably "more." If you inhabit western New York, as I do, and see precious little sunshine much of the year, the answer is probably "more." Vitamin D supplementation is going to be much more necessary if you live in the northern states than in sunny California. But the California girl who slathers on sunblock like you would plaster a wall or decides to wear a giant swim Mumu to cover her blooming belly may want to supplement with vitamin D, too. Will you be pregnant over the winter months? Do you wear hats and protective clothing? Are you overweight? Are you dark skinned? Your answers to these questions (and other similar ones) will be reasons why you'll probably want to buy a bottle of vitamin D. You can always ask your doctor to test your vitamin D level. This is not a routine pregnancy test; you'll have to request it specifically.

According to vitamin D expert and physicist William B. Grant, PhD, 4000 IU per day for pregnant women is probably just about right. "It is extremely important that pregnant and nursing women obtain sufficient vitamin D from solar UVB exposure and/or vitamin D supplements to raise their serum 25-hydroxyvitamin D [25(OH)D] concentration to the range of 40–60 ng/ml (100–150 nmol/l)," says Dr. Grant.[28] "The reasons include the requirement for proper development of the fetus; for the mother, reduced risk of infections such as influenza during pregnancy, reduced risk of vaginal bacteriosis, pre-eclampsia, primary Cesarean section; for the fetus or infant - premature delivery, low birth weight, birth defects, autism, schizophrenia, type 1 diabetes mellitus, rickets. To reach the 40–60 ng/ml takes about 4000 IU/d vitamin D_3."[29] All this protection will cost you less than five cents a day. And sunlight is free.

What Kind of Vitamin D Should I Buy?

If you are going to take an oral supplement, take D_3 rather than D_2. Vitamin D_3 (cholecalciferol) is the form your body naturally makes from skin exposure to sunlight and is regarded as the superior form of vitamin D for many reasons. It is very easy to come by and costs the same as D_2.

What about Vitamin K?

Vitamin D and vitamin K work together. Do you eat fermented foods and plenty of vegetables? Good. Are you avoiding antibiotics? Also good. Between what you eat (K_1 is found in plants like green veggies) and what your friendly gastrointestinal bacteria manufacture (K_2), your levels of the fat-soluble Vitamin K are likely OK during pregnancy, unless a health condition gives your doctor reason to believe otherwise. The intake of vitamin K deemed to be adequate during pregnancy is 75 micrograms (mcg) (for pregnant gals fourteen to eighteen years old) and 90 mcg (for women eighteen years and older).[30] As for safety, "Although allergic reaction is possible, there is no known toxicity associated with high doses (dietary or supplemental) of the phylloquinone (vitamin K_1) or menaquinone (vitamin K_2) forms of vitamin K," says the Linus Pauling Institute.[31] However, "the same is not true for synthetic menadione (vitamin K_3) and its derivatives."[32]

You may not require vitamin K supplementation, but your new baby does. Vitamin K is essential for your newborn. It is needed for normal blood clotting. Most babies are born without sufficient levels of K. This is often remedied via injection, but oral administration works just as well.[33]

Is a Vitamin D Supplement Necessary?

In many cases, yes. Ideally, we would all live in beautiful, cloudless, warm climates and get just enough sun each day, but not too much, so we could naturally make our own vitamin D. The ideal, however, is not the reality. Synthesizing vitamin D from exposure to sun is not always possible or convenient. Sunlight costs nothing, but vitamin D supplements aren't expensive. They are safe and they work. Few food sources of vitamin D are available, and those that contain D do not contain anywhere near the 4,000–6,400 IU found to be of benefit during pregnancy and lactation. For example, in three ounces of salmon, you get about 300–500 IU of vitamin D. "Oddly enough," says Andrew W. Saul, PhD, "fish cannot synthesize vitamin D. They get theirs early in the food chain from planktonic algae, and big fish eat little fish, and we eat them."[34] To limit mercury exposure, we must, however, limit fish. An egg will provide 20–25 IU of vitamin D; a cup of milk, 100 IU. It would be a strange diet indeed that provides plentiful D.

Is There Enough Vitamin D in My Prenatal Vitamin?

Probably not. It is common to find only 400 IU of D per "serving size," and only 200 IU per tablet. I imagine more prenatal vitamins will now contain the recently updated daily recommendation of 600 IU of vitamin D. Based on current research, this amount, too, is inadequate.[35] It would be a shame to give a false sense of confidence to those women that see they are getting "100 percent" of their D when more could be necessary and beneficial.

VITAMIN D SAFETY

Vitamin D is safe and beneficial for mom and baby in amounts ten times that of the current RDA.

More Vitamin D Is Safe during Pregnancy

Current research points to the safety of much larger doses of D during pregnancy. A study of hundreds of pregnant women showed that 4,000 IU of vitamin D a day during pregnancy is safe, and it effectively raises circulating vitamin D for both mom and baby.[36] Professor Bruce Hollis and colleagues have conducted several studies showing the value of increased vitamin D. They write:

> Vitamin D supplementation of 4,000 IU/day for pregnant women was safe and most effective in achieving sufficiency in all women and their neonates regardless of race while the current estimated average requirement was comparatively ineffective at achieving adequate circulating 25(OH)D. . . . These findings suggest that the current vitamin D EAR [estimated average requirements] and RDA for pregnancy women issued in 2010 by the Institute of Medicine should be raised to 4,000 IU vitamin D per day so that all women regardless of race attain optimal nutritional and hormonal vitamin D status throughout pregnancy.[37]
>
> [There is] strong evidence of the positive effects of vitamin D on birth outcomes without any hint of adverse effects. The daily intake of vitamin D to accomplish these results was 4,000 IU.[38]

Healthier babies? Healthier moms? That's exactly what vitamin D is helping to do. As Hollis and his colleagues explain, "4,000 IU/day vitamin D3 during pregnancy will 'normalize' vitamin D metabolism and improve birth outcomes including primary cesarean section and comorbidities of pregnancy with no risk of side effects."[39] In other words, supplementing with 4,000 IU of daily D can significantly decrease the complications of cesarean sections (and reduce the likelihood you'll need one in the first place), reduce premature births, decrease your chances of having high-blood pressure, preeclampsia, and diabetes during pregnancy as well as help protect you from colds, flu, and vaginal infections.[40]

If you want the benefits of vitamin D, your body has to have enough. Sufficient levels of D not only mean the absence of deficiency disease; sufficiency means the presence of health benefits.

As of 2014, the so-called tolerable upper intake for vitamin D is set at only 4,000 IU a day for women who are pregnant and lactating.[41] This is double the upper intake level that was set prior to 2010. However, the recommended dietary allowance for pregnant and lactating women remains at just 600 IU of vitamin D a day. Though this is a slight increase from the previously set 400 IU a day, current research finds both amounts to be insufficient.[42] Clinical evidence proves the benefits and safety of a much higher intake of vitamin D.

More Vitamin D Is Safe during Lactation

The more vitamin D you take, the more that is available for your nursing baby. Of course, tender, delicate baby skin should not be overexposed to sunlight. Baby relies on mother's milk or supplementation to get adequate vitamin D. This is extremely doable, and extremely safe.

The breastfeeding infants of moms who took 4,000 IU of vitamin D each day (about ten times the RDA) "had a substantially improved nutritional vitamin D status due to the transfer of vitamin D into the mothers' milk with no adverse events."[43] This dose was safe for mom. It was safe for a nursing baby. Another clinical trial demonstrated that 4,000 IU a day of vitamin D was "more effective" at raising vitamin D levels than 2,000 IU a day for breastfeeding moms, with no vitamin D-related adverse events for either mother or child.[44] A study of 6,400 IU of supplemental vitamin D a day significantly increased maternal circulating 25(OH)D and supplied sufficient D to their breastfed infants, and was, once again, completely safe for all involved.[45]

The Vitamin D Council recommends babies get 1,000 IU of vitamin D each day. "If you take a supplement of 6,000 IU of vitamin D each day you shouldn't need to give your baby any vitamin D supplement. Your breast milk has enough vitamin D for your baby," they say. "If you aren't taking a supplement or getting a good amount of sun exposure, or if you're taking less than 5,000 IU/day of vitamin D," or you aren't nursing, "you should give your baby a vitamin D supplement." Liquid drops work well. And they recommend that you (and baby) don't miss a day. "Breast milk will clear itself of vitamin D very quickly unless you're regularly getting enough."[46]

Is Vitamin D Dangerous?

The short answer is no. But, like with many vitamins, vitamin D has been the subject of much controversy over the years. In *The Journal of Orthomolecular Medicine*, in an article entitled "Vitamin D: Deficiency, Diversity and Dosage," Dr. Saul writes:

Vitamin D: Deficiency, Diversity and Dosage

DR. ANDREW SAUL, PhD

"As with all vitamins, there is ongoing and ever-protracted debate about vitamin D's safety and effectiveness. In the end, the issue really boils down to dosage. Because vitamin D can be made in the body, given sufficient sunlight, it has been considered more of a hormone than a vitamin. This terminology is likely to prejudice any consideration of megadoses, and that is unfortunate. Government-sponsored "tolerable" or "safe upper limits" (UL) for vitamin D have been established, perhaps based as much on speculation as on available facts. . . ."

. . . Vitamin D has sometimes been regarded as the most potentially dangerous vitamin. In his 2001 article "Vitamin Toxicity," Mark Rosenbloom, MD, writes that, for vitamin D, "Acute toxic dose is not established, and chronic toxic dose is more than 50,000 IU/day in adults. In children, 400 IU/day is potentially toxic. A wide variance in potential toxicity exists." There were no fatalities cited.[47]

The Merck Manual's assessment is somewhat different: "Vitamin D 1000 μg (40,000 IU)/day produces toxicity within 1 to 4 months in infants, and as little as 75 μg (3,000 IU)/day can produce toxicity over years. Toxic effects have occurred in adults receiving 2,500 μg (100,000 IU)/day for several months."[48]

The Merck Manual's lowest "toxicity" figure for "infants" of 3,000 IU is substantially higher than Dr. Rosenbloom's "potentially toxic" figure of 400 IU for presumably older and larger "children." "Potentially toxic" is very different than "toxic." Moreover, "toxic" is very different than "death." The choice to use the word "toxic" may serve to convey a false impression of immediate and mortal danger. There are numerous symptomatic warnings before serious toxic effects occur. Merck says, "The first symptoms are anorexia, nausea, and vomiting, followed by polyuria, polydipsia, weakness, nervousness, and pruritus. (Eventually) renal function is impaired. . . . Metastatic calcifications may occur, particularly in the kidneys. In Great Britain, so-called hypercalcemia in infancy with failure to thrive has occurred with a daily vitamin D intake of 50 to 75 μg (2000 to 3000 IU)."[48] Though the details and duration of intake are not stated, a body-weight comparison suggests that if an infant weighed 10 pounds, that would be the dose equivalent of approximately 32,000 to 48,000 IU per day for an average adult.

A widely-used nutrition textbook[50] that I taught from said that 2,000 IU daily for an adult is toxic (p. 220–221). In this same textbook, on the same page, there was an error that, by the author's own standard, could likely be fatal to the reader's baby. A "Caution" statement on page 221 indicated the daily vitamin D requirement for an infant as 10 MIL-LIGRAMS. This is 1,000 times the correct figure, which is 10 micrograms. 10 milligrams is 400,000 IU; 10 micrograms is 400 IU. That textbook typo is a far greater mistake than any health nut would ever make. By the next edition, the mistake had been corrected. . . .

. . . It is instructive to note that as far back as 1939, some truly enormous doses of vitamin D were in fact found to be far less deadly than one might expect. In several countries, most infants, including preemies, survived 200,000 to as many as 600,000 units of vitamin D given in a single injected or oral dose. These are incredibly high quantities, especially when they are considered in relation to a premature infant's body weight.[51] Pregnant women have likewise been given two huge oral doses of vitamin D (600,000 IU) during the 7th and 8th months. . . .)"[52]

. . . It may readily be conceded that huge but occasional doses are insufficient to produce toxicity because vitamin D is fat-soluble, stored by the body, and it takes many months of very high doses to produce calcification of soft tissues, such as the lung and kidneys. "Overdose," "toxic," and "fatal" are very strong, yet very different terms that are often used interchangeably by critics of vitamin supplementation. Most overdoses are not toxic, and most toxicities are not fatal. . . .

. . . Hypervitaminosis articles are popular with the media, sometimes even making it into the pages of the *Wall Street Journal.* On April 30, 1992, David Stipp reported that between 1990 and 1992, "a series of patients with vitamin D overdoses began turning up at Boston hospitals." One of these patients subsequently died from drug complications, and the case went to court.[53] "Essentially, this was a product liability action against the producer of dairy products, specifically milk which contained excessive amounts of Vitamin D. The plaintiff's decedent purportedly suffered from elevated levels of Vitamin D in her bloodstream which required medication which in turn allegedly compromised her immune system, leading to her death."[54] This is the one and only vitamin D-related death I could find confirmation of anywhere, and even this one was not directly due to the vitamin, but rather to side effects of medication.

A physiology textbook later stated that "At least 19 cases of vitamin D toxicity were reported in the Boston area during 1992. Symptoms included fatigue, weight loss, and potentially severe damage to the kidneys and cardiovascular system. The problems resulted from drinking milk fortified with vitamin D. Due to problems at one dairy, some of the milk sold had over 230,000 units of vitamin D per quart instead of the usual 400 units per quart. The incident highlighted the need for quality control in the production, and care in the consumption, of vitamin supplements."[55]

Such a conclusion is inaccurate. The incident might just as well be taken to be an unintentional proof of vitamin safety, even in ridiculously high overdosage situations. It is certainly noteworthy that 580 times the normal amount of vitamin D produced, at most, one alleged fatality over a two-year period. Furthermore, there was a total of fewer than two dozen toxicity reports, for the entire Boston metropolitan area, after large numbers of people had been ingesting close to a quarter of a million units of vitamin D per liter of milk day after day, month after month, for up to two years. This borders on the extraordinary. Events such as this demonstrate that the margin for error with vitamin D is very large indeed. Though the news reported about the vitamin's toxicity, the real story was the vitamin's safety. The scientific literature confirms the vitamin's value.[56]

(Abridged and reprinted with permission from the International Society for Orthomolecular Medicine and the *Journal of Orthomolecular Medicine,* 2003; Vol. 18, Numbers 3 and 4, p. 194–204.)

The safety of vitamin D, even in high doses, has been well established. Absurdly huge doses of vitamin D taken every day for an extended period of time could potentially be an issue, but it would be singularly difficult to hurt yourself with vitamin D. Hollis and his colleagues explain, "[T]here is no evidence in humans that even a 100,000 IU/d dose of vitamin D for extended periods during pregnancy results in any harmful effects"[57] for mom or her unborn baby. Another study demonstrated that a single dose of 200,000 IU of vitamin D given to treat deficiency during the third trimester caused no signs or symptoms of toxicity.[58]

As with any nutrient, take the minimum amount of the vitamin that gets you the positive results you seek. Let your doctor help. Ask to have your serum levels of vitamin D checked periodically, now and after supplementation. Is the amount you are taking enough? If not, adjust accordingly. But remember, you have to ask for the test. Currently, the Vitamin D Council and the Endocrine Society sets the safe maximum amount of daily D supplementation at 10,000 IU daily for pregnant and lactating women and 2,000 IU daily for babies.[59]

TESTING YOUR VITAMIN D LEVEL

*"People's minds are changed through observation
and not through argument."*
—WILL ROGERS

The American Congress of Obstetricians and Gynecologists states, "At this time there is insufficient evidence to support a recommendation for screening all pregnant women for vitamin D deficiency," even though in the very same report they say "recent evidence suggests that vitamin D deficiency is common during pregnancy" and "infants of mothers with or at high risk of vitamin D deficiency are also at risk of vitamin D deficiency."[60] So much else is tested during pregnancy. Why not test something as important as vitamin D?

During my second pregnancy, when I learned more about optimal dosages of vitamin D, I took about 5,000 IU each day and continued this dose while I was breastfeeding. This did not include the amount I obtained through my diet. Some might think this is rather a lot. I did.

Early one November I had a vitamin D test, or 25(OH)D test, done; it came back at 53 ng/ml. My doctor said my level of D was just a bit on the low side. Others would say that's just about right. A vitamin D level that falls between 50–70 ng/ml is considered "optimal" according to recent clinical research[61] and ranges of 40–60 ng/ml are considered "necessary."[62] During summer months I am often outside and getting plenty of sunshine, but this is just about impossible during cloudy winter months, so I supplement instead.

Personally, I'm aiming to achieve *the best possible* levels of vitamin D, not just the *adequate* amount. So, like many folks who take a vitamin D test, I learned that what we may think is "a lot" may merely turn out to be "adequate." I've since upped my dosage of D from 5,000 IU to 6,000 IU a day when I'm not in the sun. Even more important than numbers, I care about how I feel. Although this is subjective, not objective like a test, how you feel matters. Larger doses of vitamin D in the winter have helped me *feel better,* just like sunshine makes me feel great in the summer. Speaking of which, studies have shown that simply exposing your skin to the sun will achieve vitamin D levels of 60–80 ng/ml. This is healthy, natural, and safe.

Sun Exposure and Skin Cancer

*"The adverse effects of UV irradiance are easy to see and relate to UV; the beneficial effects are difficult to determine as they occur after many years, and may be masked by other factors such as diet, smoking, etc. **However, the health benefits are much stronger.**"* [Emphasis added]
— WILLIAM B. GRANT, PhD, Physicist and Vitamin D Expert

We've been told again and again that we should avoid excess sun and wear sunblock. We have heard that chronic unprotected exposure to ultraviolet (UV) radiation increases the risk of skin cancer.[63] We have slathered on "protective" lotions and creams, and, as a result, our vitamin D levels have decreased.[64]

Interestingly, exposure to sunlight may indeed *prevent* skin cancer.[65] Low levels of vitamin D is a "major risk factor for melanoma."[66]

The answer appears to be quite simple: make a point to get a reasonable amount of sunshine each day, or make up for what you lack with vitamin D supplements. We don't need to burn our skin to a crisp in order to get our daily dose of vitamin D. Some daily sun exposure is a good idea. Excess isn't. Get outside. Skip the sunblock for fifteen to twenty minutes, and when you can't get your daily dose from sunlight, take vitamin D regularly. Supplements are a safe and inexpensive way to provide the vitamin D our body and that little body inside us craves.

If you are curious what your vitamin D test results mean and are wondering how much vitamin D to take (now that you know!), there are result-determinate dosage recommendations available at the Vitamin D Council webpage. I found an article that helped me figure out how much vitamin D I should take at https://www.vitamindcouncil.org/further-topics/i-tested-my-vitamin-d-level-what-do-my-results-mean/.

CHAPTER 7

The B Vitamins and Pregnancy

"Nobody knows anything about the area of dietary supplementation, but the National Institutes of Health knows for sure it's impossible."
— RUTH F. HARRELL, PhD, Medical Tribune, 1981

When it comes to our health, it's hard to get people excited about prevention. Unless, of course, you're pregnant. Sure, there are folks interested in avoiding health issues with good nutrition, but pregnant women (and their expectant partners) are especially keen on keeping their baby healthy and safe. One simply has to browse the multitude of pregnancy books; there is an overwhelming amount of information for new parents who want to ensure the best possible outcome for their child. I'm glad you are also reading this one.

The B vitamins are absolutely essential for a healthy pregnancy. Between what you eat and your prenatal vitamin, it is easy to score plenty of some B vitamins. However, you may not be getting enough of others, and your optimal, individualized dose may be quite different than what your current prenatal vitamin provides.

The B vitamins are remarkably safe. In nearly three decades of reports from American Association of Poison Control Centers (AAPCC), there has been not one confirmed death whatsoever from any B vitamin.[1] It is very unlikely that you can hurt yourself or a developing baby with the Bs, unless you don't get any.

VITAMIN B BASICS

B vitamins work best when they're taken together. This is true for all of them. They need each other, like pregnant mom and baby. To get the complete set of B vitamins, a good B complex may do the trick, as may your prenatal vitamin. Then you can supplement with additional amounts of particular B vitamins as needed.

B vitamins are water soluble, so excess is excreted in urine. This may present a colorful bathroom experience. For example, riboflavin (B_2) may turn your urine electric yellow. Don't worry: that's normal. Of course, it is always a good idea to keep a watchful eye on your byproducts for anything out of the ordinary. But this harmless side effect simply shows that the body is flushing out excess. Having an abundance of essential vitamins is a good thing. It is deficiency that is a problem.

Our body's ability to excrete excess B vitamins in urine provides for a very wide margin of error and for safety. Due to this efficient process, B vitamins like riboflavin are not stored in your body and must be replaced with diet, or diet and supplements combined.

VITAMIN B$_1$—THIAMINE

Thiamine (also known as thiamin) is essential for your baby's brain development. It enables you and your baby to convert carbohydrates into energy. Thiamine is also involved with the proper functioning of the nervous system, muscles, and heart.[2] Inadequate thiamine intake or absorption can cause fatigue, weakness, psychosis, and nerve damage.[3] On the other hand, adequate intake is necessary, safe, and beneficial.

The positive impact of thiamine on childhood learning and development has been known for decades. In the 1940s, Ruth Flinn Harrell investigated nutritional supplementation on learning ability. She found that "a liberal thiamine intake improved a number of mental and physical skills of orphanage children."[4] In the 1950s she researched the "effect of mothers' diets on the intelligence of offspring" in her study "A Study of the Influence of Vitamin Supplementation of the Diets of Pregnant and Lactating Women on the Intelligence of Their Children." She concluded, "supplementation of the pregnant and lactating mothers' diet by vitamins increased the intelligence quotients of their offspring at three and four years of age."[5] In the 1980s Dr. Harrell was still researching this topic. She and her colleagues showed in a study published in *Proceedings of the National Academy of Sciences* that high doses of vitamins improved the intelligence and educational performance of kids who were learning disabled, including those who had Down syndrome.[6]

John B. Irwin, MD, board-certified by the American Board of Obstetrics and Gynecology, has found large doses of thiamine and other nutrients to be safe and beneficial for the treatment and prevention of complications during pregnancy. He found thiamine to be of particular importance. "Large doses of thiamine (100 mg [milligrams] daily) have been essentially 100 percent effective in preventing toxemia of pregnancy in my patients," Dr. Irwin says.[7] He reports that "[i]n the over 1,000 prenatal patients who have been given this protection, there has been no prematurity, no growth retardation, no fetal death, no premature separation of the placenta, and no reason to do cesarean delivers because of fetal heart irregularities."[8] What an incredible impact.

Pregnancy and lactation require an increased intake of thiamine.[9] However, the Recommended Dietary Allowance (RDA) for thiamine is a mere 1.4 mg per day for women who are pregnant or lactating.[10] A tolerable upper intake level has not been established for thiamine. There are "no well established toxic effects from consumption of excess thiamin in food or through long-term, oral supplementation (up to 200 mg/day)," says the Linus Pauling Institute.[11] A dose of 100 mg a day may still seem high when compared to such a low RDA. Paired with these words of caution from the National Institutes of Health—"[n]ot enough is known about the safety of using larger amounts during pregnancy or breast-feeding"[12]—there are women who will assuredly shy away from this highly essential, nontoxic[13] nutrient that could do far more good than it has ever done harm to anyone. Extra thiamine is very safe during pregnancy. Once again, deficiency, not abundance, is an issue. "The cost of a full pregnancy supply of thiamine is less than ten dollars, there are no adverse reactions, and you cannot overdose on it with pills even if you try," says Dr. Irwin.

Dr. Harrell and Dr. Irwin know that nutrients work best together. They found supplementation with a variety of vitamins and minerals to be protective and beneficial during pregnancy. You may wish to get your thiamine as part of a B complex vitamin. Mine contained 50 mg of thiamine per tablet, and I took it twice daily throughout both pregnancies. Will thiamine be in breast milk? You bet. And your child will be all the smarter for it.

Thiamine deficiency, in particular, is commonly seen among alcoholics, as alcohol inhibits the body's ability to absorb this nutrient as well as many others.[14] It is possible that the deficiency of thiamine and other B vitamins can be a cause of fetal alcohol syndrome (FAS).[15] We need thiamin and other B vitamins to metabolize carbohydrates (like alcohol). While there is no safe level of alcohol consumption when we are pregnant, thiamine consumption during pregnancy is very safe. Food sources of thiamine include legumes, vegetables, and seeds.

VITAMIN B$_2$—RIBOFLAVIN

Vitamin B$_2$ is extremely safe. Zero toxic side effects—none—have ever been reported in humans.[16] Alan Gaby, MD, says, "[N]o toxic effects have been reported in animals given an acute oral dose of 10,000 mg/kg [kilogram] of body weight, or after long-term ingestion of 25 mg/kg/day (equivalent to 1,750 mg/day for a 70 kg human)."[17] This study was not specific to pregnancy, but that does not make this essential vitamin any less safe.

Riboflavin is not hard to obtain. Your diet probably provides plenty. It is found in yogurt, milk, eggs, nuts, enriched flour, mushrooms, and green veggies like peas, spinach, and broccoli. The current RDA for B$_2$ is 1.4–1.6 mg a day for pregnant and breastfeeding women respectively.[18] Your prenatal vitamin probably contains at least that much. However, therapeutic doses, like the 400 mg per day that has been used to safely and effectively reduce migraine headache attacks,[19] would be nearly impossible to obtain from food alone.

If you suffer from migraines, perhaps trying a vitamin with an admirable safety record is a better option than resorting to drugs. Extra riboflavin may also be of interest for women with an increased risk for preeclampsia. A study of 154 pregnant women found that "those who were deficient in riboflavin were 4.7 times more likely to develop preeclampsia than those who had adequate riboflavin nutritional status."[20] This may be another good reason to acquire additional B$_2$ during pregnancy.

B₂ OR BOTOX? MANAGING MIGRAINES DURING PREGNANCY

For women that get migraine headaches, like myself, a vitamin solution is far more desirable that a drug solution. Vitamins are certainly safer and likely more effective. For example, let's discuss the latest drug for headaches, Botox (botulinum toxin type A). The U.S. Food and Drug Administration went ahead and approved Botox for migraine "a little more than a month after the company agreed to pay $600 million to settle allegations that it had illegally marketed the drug for unapproved uses like headaches for years," says *The New York Times*.[21] Animal studies have demonstrated the risk of birth defects with use of botulinum toxin,[22] but this risk has not been shown (yet) in humans *because those studies have not been done.* Still, women are using it, and doctors are still administering it. [23] On the Botox website it says, "[I]t is not known if BOTOX® can harm your unborn baby."[24] So far "studies" seem to consist of women who have used Botox during pregnancy and researchers conclude, "Well, it didn't hurt that kid!"

Botox is marketed to folks who spend fifteen or more days each month with a headache, and is advertised to prevent up to nine headache days a month. Well, a placebo, an inert pill that should do absolutely nothing, prevents up to seven. *Seven.* This is stated right on the front page of the Botox website.[25]

Botox might not even work for you. Studies report that Botox does "not differ from placebo-treated subjects in measures of headache frequency and severity."[26]

And it can kill you. On the front page of Botox's advertisement webpage, in popular magazines, and in the repetitive commercials I see while I catch up on primetime TV online, among other cautions it states: "problems swallowing, speaking, or breathing, due to weakening of associated muscles, can be severe and result in loss of life. You are at the highest risk if these problems are pre-existing before injection. Swallowing problems may last for several months."[27]

The cost? Hold onto your wallet. Doctors report that injections cost about $300 a pop, and closer to $600 for a total treatment, but based on the total number of "units" and injections you may receive, industry analysts say Botox treatment would cost closer to $1,000 to $2,000 per treatment session,[28] which will supposedly last a few months. This high cost may not surprise those folks already paying a premium for migraine headache drugs (Botox's targeted clientele), but $6,000 a year is a hefty investment. What does a bottle of riboflavin cost? About five to eight bucks. A three month's supply will set you back about $28, without the risk of dying or fetal deformities. Side effects include electric yellow-orange pee and fewer migraines. No worries. Vitamin B_2 is totally harmless.

Migraines are truly awful. I can understand that anyone suffering for half a month every month with migraines is desperate. There are many alternatives to drugs that are both safe and effective. To read more about what can be done to reduce the severity, duration, and number of migraines while pregnant, look at the section in the Pregnancy Issues chapter.

For women receiving Botox for cervical dystonia, consider looking into the benefits of vitamin D, vitamin E, B_{12}, and magnesium.[29]

VITAMIN B₃—NIACIN

Vitamin B_3 (niacin or niacinamide) is essential during pregnancy. Niacin is also a fantastic, safe, drug-free option for managing stress, anxiety, headaches, and insomnia. The value of niacin is even greater for women who suffer with mood disorders, especially those who must discontinue antidepressant or antianxiety medication during pregnancy because of the increased chance of birth defects.

Niacin and Mood

Abram Hoffer, MD, who published over thirty orthomolecular health books, was a pioneer in the use of niacin for schizophrenia and anticholesterol treatment. In 1952, Dr. Hoffer proved that niacin cured schizophrenia[30] with the first ever double-blind, placebo-controlled studies in the history of psychiatry. He continued to demonstrate its efficacy for over the next fifty years. Hoffer explained, "Vitamin B_3 is made in the body from the amino acid tryptophan. On the average 1 mg of vitamin B_3 is made from 60 mg of tryptophan, about 1.5 percent. Since it is made in the body it does not meet the definition of a vitamin; these are defined as substances that cannot be made. It should have been classified with the amino acids, but long usage of the term vitamin has given it permanent status as a vitamin. . . . [T]he amount converted is not inflexible but varies with patients and conditions. For example, women pregnant in their last three months convert tryptophan to niacin metabolites three times as efficiently as in non-pregnant females."[31]

A Case of Depression, Anxiety, Schizophrenia, and Pregnancy

A patient called by the name Mrs. L.T. (born 1955) is featured in a paper Dr. Abram Hoffer wrote for the *Journal of Orthomolecular Medicine* entitled "Chronic Schizophrenia Patients Treated Ten Years or More."[32] Suffering from schizophrenia with bouts of severe depression and anxiety attacks, Mrs. L.T.'s therapeutic nutritional program before she became pregnant included nicotinamide (niacinamide), 1 gram three times a day; ascorbic acid (vitamin C), 12 grams daily; pyridoxine (B$_6$), 250 mg daily; zinc citrate, 50 mg daily; Ludiomel, 100 mg daily; Prozac, 40 mg daily; and Chlorpromazine, 200 mg daily.

Prior to pregnancy, Mrs. L.T. weaned off her medication and continued with her nutritional program. In her own words, she says:

> I completed a normal pregnancy with the birth of a beautiful baby boy. I maintained my vitamin program throughout the pregnancy, having managed with doctor's guidance to wean off all medications in the year prior to becoming pregnant. I have been medication free ever since, a total of four years, keeping on with the diet, vitamins and lifestyle. . . .
>
> Ever since I'd become well, I had been trying to figure out a way to help other schizophrenics. Surely what had worked for me would work for some of them as well.

At the time, Mrs. L.T. joined the Friends of Schizophrenia Society. When Mrs. L.T. attributed the majority of her recovery to her use of vitamins, the reaction was less than positive. Dr. Hoffer said that in the group, "Other patients were interested but the professional people were not. . . . They were convinced that tranquilizers were all that one could offer and that taking vitamins was a waste of time."[33]

Unfortunately, this response from "professionals" is still common today. It couldn't be the vitamins that helped. That can't be it. (Insert sarcasm.)

This is only one story. Many more women could benefit from vitamin supplementation if their doctors simply presented nutrition as a treatment option, as Dr. Hoffer did.

Antidepressants and Antianxiety Medications during Pregnancy

Do a search for "antidepressant" or "antianxiety and pregnancy" and the Google screen fills with lawyers looking for your business. The happy little bouncing Zoloft bubble with his adorable cowlick (remember him?) will likely be in court for his role in the doubling of the number of babies born with heart defects.[34] Are many babies being affected? Enough to get litigators interested.

Shouldn't we test a drug's safety on a relatively small group of pregnant women first before it can be sold to all pregnant women in the mass market? Wait a minute. That sounds kind of unethical. Apparently, it is more ethical to give millions of pregnant women access to a drug rather than to first study its consequences in smaller, controlled groups of pregnant women.

A Baby Is Hurt. Who Is Responsible?

In 1999, a twenty-two-year-old regular cocaine user gave birth to a stillborn child. "She became the first woman in the United States to be tried and convicted of homicide by child abuse based on her behavior during pregnancy and was given a twelve-year prison sentence," said The American Congress of Obstetricians and Gynecologists in an article called "Maternal Decision Making, Ethics, and the Law."[35] Of course, using illicit drugs while pregnant is a horrible thing to do because they are dangerous to both mother and child.

But then there are pharmaceutical drugs. Are women protected from legal action because they could not have known any better if a prescription medication would harm their child? Are doctors protected? Are drug companies?

Actually, the drug companies are protected. The government has shielded generic drug manufactures[36] and, for that matter, vaccine manufacturers[37] from lawsuits. If you are harmed by a defective generic drug, you cannot sue the drug maker.[38] Considering that about 80 percent of prescriptions are for generics,[39] this provides immense protection for drug companies and no protection for consumers or their children. If your child is injured or killed due to vaccinations, you cannot sue the vaccine manufacturer even if the manufacturer could have chosen to make the vaccine safer.[40] Who is ultimately responsible for harm done to a baby? What an awful question to even have to consider. In the end, only the child and her family are the ones that must cope with the physical, mental, and emotional harm that can so often be caused by pharmaceutical drugs and vaccines.

A developing baby does not know the difference between a legal drug or an illegal one. A drug is still a toximolecular substance, meaning its molecular structure is foreign to the body. Orthomolecular substances are natural to the body. They are the molecules our body and our baby's body are made of. Which do you think is safer?

Instead, these drugs are made accessible to all, and we find out through trial and error whether or not babies will be harmed. History has shown that the medical industry appears content to operate this way. Prescription drugs are given during pregnancy when, at least initially, there is insufficient data to indicate whether this may hurt the fetus. Then, after there is a problem, *there is already a problem*. There is no going back once your baby is born with a defect. It is there. It is real. "Surgery," "suffering," or "death" are words we never want to associate with "baby," and yet families are put in this position time and time again. Many studies link the use of antidepressants called selective serotonin re-uptake inhibitors (SSRIs) during pregnancy with birth defects.[41]

Antidepressants and Birth Defects

Alwan and his colleagues looked at the risk of birth defects associated with SSRI use and published their results in 2007 in the *New England Journal of Medicine*. In the study of 9,622 infants born with birth defects versus 4,092 without, they reported that "[m]aternal SSRI use was associated with anencephaly" (a large part of the brain or skull is missing, which usually results in miscarriage or death after birth), "craniosynostosis," (the sutures between the bony plates of the skull close earlier than normal, causing an unusually shaped head which often requires surgery), "and omphalocele" (the baby is born with internal organs outside of the body, requiring surgery).[42] Their conclusion: "Associations were observed between SSRI use and three types of birth defects, but the absolute risks were small, and these observations require confirmation by other studies"[43] When "confirmation is needed by other studies" it makes me think of the babies that will have been born with a problem before precautions are taken to reduce exposure to potentially harmful drugs.

So the research continues.

That same year, another study by Louik and his colleagues published in *NEJM* comprised of 9,849 infants with defects and 5,860 infants without "showed significant associations between the use of sertraline (the generic name for Zoloft) and omphalocele . . . and septal (heart) defects."[44] It also showed significant associations "between the use of paroxetine (Paxil) and right ventricular outflow tract obstruction defects."[45] In response to Alwan, they conclude, "Our findings do not show that there are *significantly* [my emphasis] increased risks of craniosynostosis, omphalocele, or heart defects associated with SSRI use overall."[46] Instead, their findings "suggest that individual SSRIs may confer increased risks for some specific defects, but it should be recognized that the specific defects implicated are rare and the absolute risks are small."[47] There is that word "small" again.

So *overall,* SSRI use is not associated with birth defects, but *specific* SSRI's may increase the risk of *specific* defects. To make this clearer, Louik's study reports, "[W]e found a doubling of the risk of septal defects associated with sertraline use . . . and a tripling of the risk of right ventricular outflow tract obstruction defects associated with paroxetine use" and "the latter finding is supported" by Alwan even though Louik's study "did not confirm" Alwan's "previously reported associations between overall use of SSRIs and craniosynostosis, omphalocele, or heart defects."[48] Once again, note the word "overall." I guess they just want to breeze by that "doubling" or "tripling" stuff that occurs with *certain* SSRI's.

Maybe "overall" isn't what moms need to hear. Maybe they need to hear about the specific risks associated with the specific drug they take. Would each study propose to cancel the other out because their results were different? One study found one set of problems; the other revealed a different set of problems. Both found problems. Both found an association with the SSRI paroxetine and heart defects. Both studies associate SSRI use with an increased risk of serious birth defects, but instead of words of caution, their conclusions marginalize the danger, saying the actual risk is small.

For example, if 80 out of 10,000 babies are born with heart defects,[49] a "doubling" or "tripling" of risk for specific heart defects may only affect a small number of children. But a risk is only small as long as it is not your baby that suffers. If your child is born with a life-threatening birth defect, his risk is 100 percent—and it's too late. Prevention of birth defects, rather than this wait-and-see approach, is a far safer and kinder road to travel.

There are a humbling number of studies that show the dangers of SSRI use during pregnancy.[50] I've only highlighted two. A large study of over 493,000 babies in the *British Medical Journal* found "an increased prevalence of septal heart defects among children whose mothers were prescribed an SSRI in early pregnancy, particularly sertraline and citalopram (aka Celexa)."[51] In a study of 1.6 million infants, SSRI use late in pregnancy resulted in a twofold increased risk of a child being born with persistent pulmonary hypertension, a birth defect that affects breathing.[52] Numerous studies report birth defects, heart defects, premature births, small birth weight, pregnancy complications, miscarriage, limb malformations, delivery complications, and health issues for newborns whose mothers used antidepressants during pregnancy.[53]

One recent study found that boys with autism were three times more likely to have been exposed to SSRIs in utero than boys without autism, the strongest association occurring with first-trimester exposure.[54] SSRI use during pregnancy may also contribute to the development of attention deficit hyperactivity disorder (ADHD).[55] With antidepressants ranking way up there as the second-most prescribed drug (second only to antibiotics),[56] and research showing antidepressants are no more effective than placebo,[57] I feel it is imperative that women are offered natural, safe alternatives to effectively treat depression during pregnancy. Yes, it is important to treat depression, but there are safer options than drugs, options we have not heard about in our doctor's office.

Our babies are not guinea pigs. Neither are we. Warnings eventually surface, and pregnant women are shuffled away from one drug only to be "tested" out on others. Few other options, besides psychotherapy, are likely to be offered by doctors when a woman is pregnant and depressed. What we hear at the doctor's office is not the whole story. Our goal is the same: happy, healthy moms and babies. The question is: What is the best way to help make that happen?

A Nutritional Alternative to Antianxiety and Antidepressant Medications

Niacin deficiency can cause depression, fatigue, anxiety, and psychosis.[58] Adequate intake of niacin is preventive and curative. All forms of niacin are helpful for managing your anxiety.[59] Niacinamide especially is the form of B_3 "most effective for the treatment of anxiety disorders," say Dr. Abram Hoffer and Jonathan Prousky, ND.[60] Niacinamide has "therapeutic effects similar to benzodiazepines," the drugs most often prescribed to reduce anxiety, but niacinamide does not come with all of the negative side effects.[61]

> *The reason that one nutrient can cure so many different illnesses is because a deficiency of one nutrient can cause many different illnesses. This has led to something of a vitamin public relations problem. When pharmaceuticals are versatile, they are called "broad spectrum" and "wonder drugs." When vitamins are versatile, they are called "faddish" and "cures in search of a disease." Such a double standard needs to be exposed and opposed at every turn.*
> —ABRAM HOFFER, MD, PhD, ANDREW W. SAUL, PhD,
> HAROLD FOSTER, PhD, in *Niacin: The Real Story*

Niacin is also therapeutic for depression.[62] According to Dr. Hoffer, taking 1,000 mg of vitamin B_3 three times a day often cures mild to moderate depression.[63] It must be understood that B_3 is just one of the important nutrients needed for the treatment of anxiety and depression. There are many more. Nutrients need each other; they are all important. Those taking B_3 should also take a B complex vitamin, since the Bs work best together. Furthermore, "[n]utrients such as the B vitamins are most successful when taken regularly, taken in relatively high doses, and taken in conjunction with vitamin C, the essential fatty acids, and the minerals magnesium and selenium," says the Orthomolecular Medicine News Service.[64] For more information about the specific nutrients helpful in the treatment of depression, check out the Postpartum Problems chapter.

Niacin for Migraines, Cholesterol, and Toxin Reduction

The value of niacin during pregnancy is not limited to its therapeutic use in cases of depression, anxiety, or schizophrenia. Other benefits include cholesterol management, help for migraine headaches, and even reduction of toxins in the body.

I was opposed to taking pain relievers during my two pregnancies, but with each child I had a single migraine episode. While nursing, I experienced closer to one migraine a month. Lack of sleep and stress are my triggers, both of which are inherent to being a mother of a toddler and a newborn, with the infant nursing throughout the night. I have learned from experience that a niacin flush reduces the intensity of my migraine pain. I can often stop a migraine with a niacin flush *before* it starts. If the headache has already set in, niacin will not cure my headache but flushing makes the pain more tolerable, which is a welcome compromise. When it is not an option to be comatose on the couch with a migraine, niacin helps me work through the pain. To read much more about nutritional options for managing migraines during pregnancy, including the use of niacin, see the migraine section in the Pregnancy Issues chapter.

Your cholesterol levels will naturally be higher during pregnancy. This is normal. If weeks after birth your cholesterol levels remain high to the point where your doctor is concerned, niacin may be just what you are looking for. The authors of *Niacin: The Real Story* say that niacin lowers low-density lipoprotein (LDL) cholesterol, and "the only substance that significantly elevates HDL is niacin."[65] Niacin also "lowers triglycerides, lowers Lipo A [lipoprotein(a)], lowers the anti-inflammatory factor C-reactive protein and therefore is the best substance known for these important therapeutic effects."[66]

Niacin expert Dr. Todd Penberthy says niacin is a powerful detoxifying agent,[67] another valuable benefit of niacin for conscientious moms.

Niacin Safety

If there is a choice between taking a nutrient or a drug, always choose the nutrient. Niacin is safer than any drug. Nobody has ever died from taking niacin, and no known toxic dose exists for humans.[68] Vitamins, including B$_3$, are remarkably safe. "Although vitamin supplements have often been blamed for causing fatalities, there is no evidence to back up this allegation,"[69] report Andrew W. Saul, PhD, and Jagan N. Vaman, MD. The American Association of Poison Control Centers (AAPCC) attributes eleven deaths to vitamins over the course of twenty-seven years (1983–2009). When the members of the Orthomolecular Medicine News Service looked into these alleged deaths, they found no evidence that a vitamin had ever been the cause. Pharmaceutical medicines, on the other hand, taken as directed, kill over 100,000 people every single year.[70] "Niacin does not require a prescription because it is that safe," says Dr. Saul.[71]

Niacin: The Real Story explains niacin toxicity:

> The toxic dose for dogs is about 5,000 mg per 2.2 pounds (1 kilogram) of body weight. We do not know the toxic dose for humans since niacin has never killed anyone.[72] . . .
>
> . . . Between 1940 and 1950, when the toxicity of niacin and niacinamide were studied, the LD50 (lethal dose 50%) of rats was determined. The LD50 is the amount of a compound that will kill one half of the population of animals used to test toxicity. If 100 mice are given the drug and half die, that dose is the LD50. For niacin the LD50 is very high, about 4.5 grams per kilogram. This is equivalent to 225 grams (nearly half a pound) for a 110 pound female and 360 grams for a 176 pound male, approximately 100 times the normal recommendation. Whether anyone will ever find an LD50 for people is extremely unlikely.[73]

Dr. Hoffer explains that niacin and niacinamide "have no toxic effects and must be considered non-toxic; they have very few minor side effects."[74] Despite the myth you may have heard, niacin does not cause liver damage.[75] "[N]iacin will often increase liver function tests but these increases do not arise from liver pathology,"[76] says Hoffer. Niacin is not habit forming.[77] Niacin can to some extent increase blood sugar, but according to Dr. Hoffer and his extensive clinical experience, "several thousand milligrams daily, long-term, raised blood sugar only slightly if at all."[78] Niacin could possibly cause a drop in blood pressure, but generally speaking, "niacin does not lower blood pressure very much if at all," say the authors of *Niacin: The Real Story*.[79] This is a wonderful opportunity to use common sense. If you plan to take large, therapeutic doses of niacin each day, work with your doctor. Dr. Hoffer says, "[A]s with any substances, they (niacin and niacinamide) must be used with care."[80] In other words, use common sense. From Drugs.com: "There are no reports of adverse effects of niacin or niacinamide on the human fetus."[81] No deaths, no toxicity, no adverse effects. These are words worth repeating. This means not only is niacin almost certainly not going to kill you, it isn't likely to hurt you or your baby either. Taking vitamin B$_3$ along with the other B vitamins, and at least a similar-sized dose of vitamin C, also reduces the likelihood of side effects.

Still, the RDA for niacin was set at a mere 18 mg a day during pregnancy and only 17 mg a day for lactation, with a tolerable upper intake level set at a ridiculously low 35 mg a day.[82] Hoffer, Saul, and Foster say this is "preposterous" and that "[t]here is no clinical or laboratory evidence whatsoever that proves that niacin, or any other vitamin, is dangerous at double the RDA" and that "Orthomolecular (nutritional) physicians consider the current RDA for niacin of only 18 mg or less to be way too low for optimum health."[83]

> Niacin is so safe and so essential that your body and your baby's body
> *makes* it from tryptophan. Therefore, the only question is dose.

The FDA has placed niacin in "category C" and therefore, it states on Drugs.com: "Niacin may be harmful to an unborn baby when the medication is taken at doses to treat high cholesterol or other conditions. Tell your doctor if you are pregnant or plan to become pregnant during treatment."[84] So, wait—is niacin safe? Is it any wonder we are confused? Most drugs are also placed in "category C." Yes, *most*.

Categorizing and profiling vitamins just like drugs because it is convenient for a bureaucrat or profitable for a pharmaceutical lobby is wrong. Vitamins *are not* drugs. They don't belong in the same category. Niacin does not belong on a list that contains Prozac (fluoxetine), Zoloft (sertraline), Ventolin (albuterol), hydrocodone, and Percocet (acetaminophen and oxycodone). Niacin is so safe and so essential, that your body and your baby's body *make* it from tryptophan. Your body does not make a single drug. Therefore, the only question is dose. With drugs, *there is no safe dose;* even the recommended doses are dangerous. Even when used as directed, prescription drugs kill lots of people.[85] Vitamins (that includes niacin) don't.[86] Let's shift our attention of risk to where the risk actually is.

Niacin Use during Pregnancy

In medical research, animal data is not human data. It is true that there is a lack of human studies on supplemental niacin and niacinamide during pregnancy. The data that is available does not support that B_3 is toxic to pregnancy. In fact, it is just the opposite. Still, conflicting reports circulating about the safety of niacin during pregnancy demand that we take a closer look.

According to Melvyn Werbach, MD, 50–100 mg per day of niacin may be useful to prevent premature and low birth weight babies. He notes, "maternal niacin intake early in pregnancy may be directly associated with infant birth weight and size."[87]

The Expert Group on Vitamins and Minerals, United Kingdom,[88] cites a study[89] in the journal *Obstetrics and Gynecology,* where niacin deficient pregnant women were reportedly given up to 2,000 mg of niacin a day without evidence of fetal toxicity. In an animal study, oral administration of niacin to pregnant rats "during the period of organogenesis [the period of internal organ development] at doses up to 200 mg/kg/day was without adverse effects. At 1,000 mg/kg/day maternal body weight gain, placental and fetal weights were slightly depressed. No effect on survival, on litter size nor morphological changes upon 'in utero' development were observed."[90] A kilogram is 2.2 pounds. For the purpose of comparison, 200 mg per kg of niacin a day would be like a 160 pound woman taking over 14,500 mg a day. Pound for pound, these researchers reported no adverse effects with this high dose given to rats. The 1,000 mg per kg a day shown to have an effect on the weight gain of both mother rat and her fetus would be a truly enormous dose of over 70,000 mg a day of niacin for a 160 pound human female. Of course, taking such dosages during pregnancy would be unwarranted and foolish, but it may give us some perspective as to the safety of niacin during pregnancy.

Now, let's talk niacinamide. Niacinamide does not cause birth defects, and may do just the opposite. Research professor at University of Central Florida, Todd Penberthy, PhD, explains, "There have been lots of animal toxicity studies for nicotinamide (niacinamide), but not nicotinic acid (niacin). Basically there is no teratogenicity concern and in fact nicotinamide can prevent urethane induced teratogenicity and even cleft palate formation in genetic models of CF[91] to some degree." This, of course, is good news.

When it comes to flush-inducing doses of niacin, Dr. Penberthy explains, "It is PGE2 (prostaglandin E2) that initiates labor contractions and the niacin flush is caused to dramatic increases in PGD2 (prostaglandin D2) and PGE2." However, he says "There is no evidence of which I am aware that indicates that the niacin flush can actually lead to induction of labor." But "[I]f it (niacin) is inducing premature labor, you would think someone would have made the connection by now."[92] While I can only speak for myself, I took niacin and flushed through two pregnancies, and both of my children were born abundantly happy and healthy, each weighing over eight pounds. My daughter was born a week after her anticipated birthday. My son was born exactly on his due date.

Niacin Side Effects

Dr. Hoffer emphasized that it is important to understand that when you take niacin, you will have a flushing sensation. This is a tingling or itchy, warming sensation, accompanied by redness on the skin, which may have the appearance of a splotchy rash. These side effects are harmless and temporary.[93] "With continued use the flush gradually recedes and eventually may be only a tingling sensation in the forehead. If the person stops taking the vitamin for a day or more the sequence of flushing will be re-experienced. Some people never do flush and a few only begin to flush after several years of taking the vitamin," Hoffer says.[94] Niacinamide is unlikely to cause a flush. For those women uncomfortable with flushing, niacinamide may be a good alternative.

When you have taken too much niacin or niacinamide, first you will experience nausea. Since many pregnant gals will already be suffering with morning sickness, determining a maximum therapeutic and tolerable dose of B$_3$ (especially niacinamide) based on nausea alone may be difficult. This is why the flush associated with regular niacin may come in handy. Are you flushing? Then you've taken enough. The goal is to achieve a slight flush, not one that has you crawling out of your skin. With a little practice, you will be able to determine the dose that is best for you.

Vomiting may result if you experience nausea and continue to take niacin without reducing your dose.[95] You are taking too much, and it is time to cut back on your B$_3$ intake. Taking in excess of 5,000 mg a day of niacin makes me nauseous, so I don't do that. I learned this years ago, before I became pregnant, when I was trying to find the right dose for managing a migraine headache. The migraine headache prevented a full on flush, my usual indicator, but the side effect of nausea told me I had taken too much. You can think of this as a "built in safety valve."[96]

Therapeutic Dosages of Niacin

Dr. Hoffer split niacin dosages into two categories, with "Category 2" of specific interest to women who are pregnant or lactating. He wrote:

> *Category 1.* These are people who are well or nearly well, and have no obvious disease. They are interested in maintaining their good health or in improving it. They may be under increased stress. The optimum dose range varies between 0.5 to 3 grams daily. The same doses apply to nicotinamide (niacinamide).

> *Category 2.* Everyone under physiological stress, such as pregnancy and lactation, suffering from acute illness such as the common cold or flu, or other diseases that do not threaten death. All the psychiatric syndromes are included in this group including the schizophrenias and the senile states. It also includes the very large group of people with high blood cholesterol levels or low HDL when it is desired to restore these blood values to normal. The dose range is 1 gram to 10 grams daily. For nicotinamide the range is 1 1/2 g to 6 g.[97]

Dr. Hoffer's daily dose recommendations may feel like a wide range and seem like quite a lot, but this is because the amount of B$_3$ will differ greatly based on an individual's need. Usually, Dr. Hoffer's therapeutic dose range of B$_3$ was 1,000 mg three times daily.[98] Note the word "therapeutic." If you do not suffer from a mood disorder, then you may not need anywhere near that amount.

"THE TV TOLD ME I'D BETTER NOT TAKE NIACIN"

The media has a way of only getting half the story when it comes to supplements. With niacin, they appear to have none of it. If after the latest media vitamin scare you, too, felt unsure about the safety of niacin, read the article "Laropiprant Is the Bad One; Niacin Is/Was/Will Always Be the Good One" by W. Todd Penberthy, PhD.[99] You will find that the non-FDA-approved drug Laropiprant, not niacin, causes problems for folks. "[N]one of the headlines mentioned Laropiprant, which is quite clearly the real culprit that caused the side effects reported," says Dr. Penberthy.[100] The media just flat out got it wrong.

If you need some reassurance about niacin safety right now, here's some: niacin is an essential nutrient and is far safer than any drug on the market. "Niacin has been used for over 60 years in tens of thousands of patients with tremendously favorable therapeutic benefit,"[101] says Penberthy.[102] "Most important, after 60 years of use the safety profile for niacin (especially immediate release niacin) remains far safer than the safest drug."[103] His article concludes, "Nutrients such as niacin you need. Media misinformation you don't."[104]

How Much Niacin Should I Take?

It depends. Not everyone will need large amounts of niacin. If you have no treatment reason to take niacin, megadosing is not the answer. The amount in your prenatal vitamin and B complex may be enough. Evaluate your need. Are you suffering from depression? Anxiety? High cholesterol? Having trouble quieting your mind so you can fall asleep? If so, your need for niacin may be greater. Certainly, a few hundred milligrams a day can benefit everyone. Those seeking to address a health issue may benefit from more.

As the medical industry would have you always weigh the risks and benefits of medication, so you should with vitamins. I believe the benefits of niacin supplementation during pregnancy far outweigh any (unlikely) risk. Vitamins have a spectacular safety record in comparison to any antidepressant or antianxiety medication.

Work with your doctor. Take time to look into this for yourself. And start small: try taking just 25 mg of niacin after each meal. Gradually increase your dose over subsequent days until you achieve a flush. Dr. Saul explains, "As a general rule, the more you hold, the more you need. If you flush early, you don't need much niacin. If flushing doesn't happen until a high level, then your body is obviously using the higher amount of the vitamin."[105] If you are taking niacin for mood or headache, do you feel better? Your answer determines your next step.

If you cannot tolerate the flush, try taking niacinamide instead. Once again, start small and see how you feel. As research biochemist Richard Passwater, PhD, would recommend, take the smallest dose of a nutrient that gets you the positive health result you seek.[106]

For the management of stress, anxiety, and resulting migraines, or to help me relax so I can get back to sleep, I take enough niacin to get the job done. My personal daily (divided) dose of niacin hovers around 250–500 mg, an amount I took during both of my pregnancies and during lactation. On stressful days I may take closer to 1,000 mg of flush (regular) niacin in divided doses. The flush is my indicator that I have had a sufficient amount for the time being. I happen to prefer regular niacin because I like knowing when I've taken enough, and I happen to like the flushing feeling. It makes me feel warm and relaxed. I may take 150 mg of flush niacin in the morning (approximately a third of a 500 mg tablet, which I just break off with my teeth), another 150 mg at lunch, and another 150 mg at bedtime. If I wake up in the middle of the night and have trouble sleeping, I take another 150 mg of niacin each time on an "as needed" basis. When I feel anxious, overstressed, have difficulty sleeping, or if my moods become erratic, I know I need extra niacin. Other days, what is available in my multiple vitamin and B complex is enough. If I have eaten or taken vitamin C, I can "hold" more niacin; in other words, it takes a larger dose to achieve a flush. If I haven't taken extra niacin in a while or I take it on an empty stomach, I may flush within minutes. I may choose to take niacinamide if I am going to be in public and would prefer not to explain why I am colored red. I take up to 1,000 mg a day of niacinamide and avoid flushing altogether on an as-needed basis. Dr. Hoffer explains, "As is always the case with nutrients, each individual must determine their own optimum level."[107] Be sure to also take a B complex vitamin each day in addition to the extra niacin you are taking. Food sources of B_3 include tuna, crimini mushrooms, turkey, chicken, legumes, and vegetables.

TYPES OF NIACIN

There are basically three types of niacin. When you buy a bottle, no matter what the description is on the label, flip it over and read the supplement information on the back. This will give you a better idea of what exactly is in the bottle. To learn more than you will in this brief summary, you may want to read *Niacin: The Real Story.*

1. **Niacin (nicotinic acid)** This is regular, plain old niacin. In this form, niacin causes a flushing reaction, that feeling of being warm, red, and tingly all over. To sidestep this side effect, take your niacin with food and with vitamin C, or take a different form of the vitamin (below). This type of niacin generally does not cause nausea, even in doses of several thousand milligrams a day, and is the best form for managing cholesterol. It is also effective for reducing anxiety and improving mood.[108] ("Nicotinic acid" has nothing to do with nicotine, by the way.)

2. **Niacinamide (nicotinamide)** This form of B_3 usually does not cause a flush. It is also not effective for the reduction of cholesterol. Its benefits include its antianxiety effects and its ability to treat arthritis. In doses of several thousand milligrams a day, it is more likely to cause nausea than other forms of B_3.[109]

3. **Inositol Hexaniacinate (inositol hexanicotinate)** This form of B_3 is not likely to cause flushing or nausea. It is still possible to flush but it may be delayed. This form is effective for mood disorders. It may be referred to as "sustained-release," "no-flush," "flush-free," or "timed-release" niacin; however, certain preparations of nicotinic acid can, too. This matters because nicotinic acid in a "timed-release" formula may cause upset stomach, whereas inositol hexaniacinate usually will not. Manual, regular doses of nicotinic acid (not timed-release) may cause less stomach distress.[110]

Niacin during Lactation

Lactating mothers want their milk to be safe and beneficial for their babies. Drugs are notoriously unsafe. We certainly don't want these in our breast milk. Vitamins, however, have a remarkable safety record. If niacin was beneficial to you during pregnancy, there is much reason to believe it will also be of benefit during lactation.

Taking small doses of regular niacin and being mindful of the dose it takes to produce a flush will help determine the amount that is best for you. If you suffer from mood disorders such as the baby blues or postpartum depression, B vitamins like niacin are going to come in handy. You can read more about therapeutic nutritional options for postpartum depression in the Postpartum Problems chapter.

VITAMIN B$_5$—PANTOTHENIC ACID

By definition, most of us get plenty of pantothenic acid. Discovered back in 1933 by Roger J. Williams, PhD, the name of the vitamin itself is derived from the word "pantothen," meaning "from everywhere." Pantothenic acid is present in all cells in all forms of life. This, of course, makes it easy to obtain, and it means that it is extremely rare for anyone to be deficient.

"Little is known regarding the amount of dietary pantothenic acid required to promote optimal health or prevent chronic disease," says the Linus Pauling Institute, but "[a] varied diet should provide enough pantothenic acid for most people."[111]

According to the very conservative National Institutes of Health, an adequate intake of pantothenic acid is 6 mg a day while you are pregnant, and 7 mg a day while breastfeeding.[112] A tolerable upper intake level has not been set and pantothenic acid is not known to be toxic in humans.[113] Good sources of B$_5$ include broccoli, avocados, eggs, chicken, milk, lentils, sunflower seeds, cheese, and sweet potatoes.

VITAMIN B$_6$—PYRIDOXINE

Want to puke less? Helpful for morning (all day) sickness including both nausea and/or vomiting),[114] B$_6$ (pyridoxine) is probably in your prenatal multivitamin. For example, prescription products like Prenate Essential, Prenate Elite, NataFort, and Nestabs have between 10–50 mg per tablet. Over-the-counter prenatal supplements also contain extra B$_6$ in varied amounts.

Are you getting enough? Well, how do you feel? If you are suffering over the sink every a.m., and many of the hours in-between, taking closer to 75 mg a day might be in order if you have severe morning sickness.[115]

You'll have a tough time obtaining extra B$_6$ through food. A cup's worth of chickpeas will get you about 1 mg of B$_6$, as will three ounces of yellowfin tuna. Even if you like fish, the four to nine *pounds* per day you'd have to indulge in to get that extra B_6 you may benefit from is not a healthy or reasonable way to go.

Less morning sickness is certainly desirable, but B_6 is also very necessary during pregnancy for other reasons. In infancy and during pregnancy, vitamin B_6 is involved in brain development and immune function.[116] There's more. "Vitamin B_6 plays a vital role in the function of approximately 100 enzymes that catalyze essential chemical reactions in the human body," says the Linus Pauling Institute.[117] In animal models, severe deficiency of B_6 caused "omphalocele, exencephaly, cleft palate, micrognathia, digital defects, and splenic hypoplasia,"[118] which are a lot of fancy terms for really awful deformities. Right there is good reason to take your prenatal vitamin.

While severe deficiency is uncommon in humans, insufficiency is not.[119] The current RDA for B_6 is 2.0 mg a day for pregnant women,[120] an amount that seems laughably low, especially given that getting over twice that amount each day may still not be enough.[121] It might make you feel like you are doing something wrong if you take more that the RDA. But you aren't doing anything wrong. You are fine. You are right. B_6 is a beneficial and essential nutrient. Safe, therapeutic doses will be twenty to fifty times or more the highly conservative RDA.

Vitamin B_6 Safety

High doses of B_6, one to six *thousand* milligrams a day every day for months or even years, may cause neurological symptoms such as temporary nervousness, tingling, and numbness. However, these side effects are temporary and go away once supplementation stops. B_6 is water soluble and is not stored in the body for long. It is also important to note that in these cases, B_6 was given by itself, without the other complementary and important B vitamins. Taking up to 200 mg of B_6 a day, along with the other B vitamins, means it is extremely unlikely you will experience any side effects.[122]

"A sensory neuropathy has been reported in some individuals taking large doses of vitamin B_6. Most people who suffered this adverse effect were taking 2,000 mg/day or more of pyridoxine, although some were taking only 500 mg/day. There is a single case report of a neuropathy occurring in a person taking 200 mg/day of pyridoxine, but the reliability of that case report is unclear," says Alan Gaby, MD. "[P]yridoxine neurotoxicity has been known to the medical profession for 20 years, and because vitamin B_6 is being taken by millions of people, it is reasonable to assume that neurotoxicity at doses below 200 mg per day would have been reported by now, if it does occur at those doses. The fact that no such reports have appeared strongly suggests that vitamin B_6 does not damage the nervous system when taken at doses below 200 mg per day."[123] Therefore, setting a tolerable upper intake level at only 100 mg/day[124] is unwarranted.

We are unlikely to experience side effects taking 200 mg a day of B_6 and it certainly won't kill us. According to chemist Linus Pauling, "Vitamin B_6, pyridoxine, has no known fatal dose."[125] To improve health without the risk of toxicity, he recommends 50–100 mg or more a day, noting that 5,000 patients receiving 200 mg B_6 daily had no observed side effects.[126]

How do these amounts line up with current recommendations for women who are pregnant? For morning sickness, the American College of Obstetrics and Gynecology recommends women take up to 100 mg a day in divided doses.[127] It may also be comforting to know that a recent study of 192 pregnant women who were given 50 to 500 mg of B_6 each day during their first trimester for the treatment of nausea and vomiting showed no increased risk of birth defects in their babies.[128] For women asking themselves if the 100 mg a day they are taking for nausea and vomiting will harm their baby, the answer is no.

A retrospective study in the *Journal of Orthomolecular Medicine* reported that John Ellis, MD, and Jean Pamplin, authors of the book *Vitamin B_6 Therapy,* "observed that high dose pyridoxine can alleviate pregnancy-induced oedema [swelling] as well as carpal tunnel syndrome precipitated by pregnancy and it was standard for him to prescribe 200–300 mg per day."[129]

Additionally, pregnancy appears to increase the need for B_6. Women with preeclampsia show even lower levels of B_6 than healthy pregnant gals, which suggests they may require more of the vitamin.[130] Folks with Crohn's disease or other malabsorption conditions tend to have lower levels of B_6 and may also have trouble getting enough.[131]

It boils down to this: if you are puking your guts out, 40–100 mg a day of B_6 is highly advisable, and up to 200 mg a day is very unlikely to cause you (or your baby) any problems. B_6 has been shown to significantly help morning sickness.[132] The Linus Pauling Institute says, "Vitamin B_6 itself is considered safe during pregnancy."[133]

"B₆? I HEARD IT WILL DECREASE MY MILK FLOW" OR "I WANT TO STOP MY MILK FLOW NOW. WILL B₆ HELP?"

Speaking from personal experience, this was not the case for me. Before, during, and after pregnancy, and all while breastfeeding, I took 100 mg of B_6 a day. I always produced enough breast milk to feed my baby (and several additional babies). It certainly didn't slow down my flow one iota.

The word on the street is that B_6 can help relieve engorgement in doses of 200 mg a day for several days. But "relieving" engorgement is not "stopping" milk production, so if that's your intent, you may be disappointed. However, engorgement is uncomfortable and if a little more of a safe nutrient can ease that ache, it may be worth giving it a try.

VITAMIN B₉—FOLIC ACID AND FOLATE

Are you pregnant? Are you thinking about becoming pregnant? Are you *not* thinking about becoming pregnant? Whatever your baby plans are, it is strongly recommended that a folic acid supplement be part of your daily routine. "Your body needs folic acid to make normal red blood cells and prevent a type of anemia. Folic acid is also essential for the production, repair, and functioning of DNA, our genetic map and a basic building block of cells. So getting enough folic acid is particularly important for the rapid cell growth of the placenta and your developing baby," says Baby-Center's medical advisory board.[134]

The March of Dimes urges that all women of childbearing age take a multivitamin that includes 400 mcg of folic acid: "Folic acid helps prevent NTDs (neural tube defects) only if taken before pregnancy and during the first few weeks of pregnancy, often before a woman may even know she's pregnant. Because nearly half of all pregnancies in the United States are unplanned, it's important that all women take folic acid every day."[135] This, they say, could "help reduce the number of pregnancies affected by NTDs by up to 70 percent."[136]

Folic acid isn't just important before and during the early stages of pregnancy. It is important all nine months. In addition to an increased risk for NTDs, *The American Journal of Clinical Nutrition (AJCN)* says that "[d]uring pregnancy, low concentrations of dietary and circulating folate are associated with increased risks of preterm delivery, infant low birth weight, and fetal growth retardation."[137] On the plus side, there is evidence that folic acid, as part of a multivitamin, may reduce the risk of cleft lip and cleft palate;[138] however, much higher doses (6,000 mcg of folic acid) may be needed to confer this benefit.[139] A multivitamin with folic acid may also reduce the risk of heart defects.[140] In addition, the *American Journal for Obstetrics and Gynecology* says "[s]upplementation of multivitamins containing folic acid in the second trimester is associated with reduced risk of preeclampsia."[141]

The RDA for folic acid during pregnancy is 600 mcg.[142] Your doctor may recommend more. Your prenatal vitamin may contain 800–1000 mcg. It may sound like a lot, but it isn't. A microgram (mcg) is only one thousandth of a milligram (mg), and a milligram is a thousandth of a gram (g). Still, it would be extremely difficult to obtain the amount of folate you need during pregnancy from food alone. Even if you do, it is still important that you take a folic acid supplement.[144] If there is one thing doctors now agree about when it comes to nutrition and pregnancy, "take folic acid" seems to be it. Yet many women remain deficient. Even when the intake of folic acid from supplements is included, 19 percent of fourteen to eighteen-year-old female adolescents and 17 percent of nineteen to thirty-year-old women do not meet average requirements.[144] Scary thought.

Obtaining folate from fresh, raw veggies, such as leafy greens, is best. We need the greens regardless; it's just nice that they happen to contain folate, too. Our government recognizes the importance of this essential nutrient and the risks of folate deficiency. Since we don't eat enough folate-containing vegetables, the government fortified pastas, cereal, and other grains with folic acid to ensure we get more, knowing full well we eat more grains than greens.[145]

If you supplement with folic acid in its bioactive form of metafolate or metafolin, you may be one step ahead.[146] However this form is far more expensive; taking enough of the cheap stuff and eating greens works, too. Pregnant women would do to well to get folic acid and folate in any form. Period.

Safety of Folic Acid

The benefits of folic acid supplementation during pregnancy are immense. The risks are next to none. Folic acid is nontoxic.[147] It is water soluble and excess is excreted in urine. Fears about folic acid seem to center around the possibility of its potential to hide the need for B_{12}. "Large amounts of folic acid can mask the damaging effects of vitamin B_{12} deficiency" or intensify it "by correcting the megaloblastic anemia caused by vitamin B_{12} deficiency without correcting the neurological damage that also occurs," says the National Institutes of Health.[148] B_{12} deficiency (pernicious anemia) can result in nerve damage, and of course this is to be avoided.[149] But how much folic acid would you have to take to hide pernicious anemia? The *Journal of Obstetrics and Gynaecology Canada* states, "Folic acid 5 mg (5,000 mcg) supplementation will not mask vitamin B_{12} deficiency (pernicious anemia), and investigations (examination or laboratory) are not required prior to initiating supplementation."[150] It is curious then why our tolerable upper intake level is set at only 1,000 mcg per day.[151]

The need for one essential nutrient, B_{12}, does not cancel out the need for another, folic acid. They are both important. Both must be obtained during pregnancy. Having pernicious anemia does not mean you should stop taking folic acid. It means you should start taking B_{12}, too.

As for concerns about folic acid and zinc function, folic acid does not appear to inhibit maternal uptake or function of zinc.[152] AJCN says, "Large, well-conducted clinical trials have found no adverse effects of folic acid on pregnancy through zinc antagonism or any other mechanism, although they have shown a clear benefit in reducing the risk of NTDs."[153]

Folic acid does NOT cause cancer

The media may try to scare you off taking folic acid supplements by quoting garbage science that suggests folic acid causes cancer. "If you look at the research suggesting a human cancer connection,[154] it does not say that folate in food causes cancer. The research only points to folic acid, as specifically as found in supplements,"[155] Dr. Saul says. "No, folic acid does not cause cancer."

Here's why: "There is virtually no difference whatsoever between the two forms of this nutrient," says Saul. "Folate and folic acid are different only in whether the carboxylic acid groups have dissociated or not. Folic acid's molecular formula is C19, **H19**, N7, O6. Folate is C19, **H18**, N7, O6. The difference? Folate has one less hydrogen cation (H+). A hydrogen cation is a proton. A single proton. I have never seen evidence that protons cause cancer."[156]

"Decades ago," says Saul, "one teacher gave me wise advice that spans all disciplines: 'Look at your answer. Does your answer make sense?' So when research suggests that the vitamin folic acid somehow causes lung or colon cancer, it is time to hit the books. It may even occasionally be necessary to hit them right out of the way, and use common sense instead."[157]

Sometimes very important "details" are left out of what you hear in the media. For example, "[a]s for lung cancer, the research accusing folic acid also happens to show that 94 percent of the study subjects who developed lung cancer were either current or former smokers," says the Orthomolecular Medicine News Service.[158]

Oh.

In other words, smoking causes cancer, not folic acid.

Well, everybody makes mistakes. Even Fox News.[159] While they were content to jump on the "vitamins cause cancer" bandwagon, Fox News now reports just the opposite. Referring to a recent study on folic acid published in *The Lancet* that included thirteen trials and nearly 50,000 people,[160] the article states, "there was no increased risk of individual cancers—including colon, prostate, lung or breast cancer—attributed to folic acid."[161] This was true even when the nutrient was given in very high doses. The article continues to say, "Most trials used daily doses of folic acid between 0.5 and 5 milligrams (500–5,000 mcg). In the one study that used a much larger dose, 40 mg (40,000 mcg) daily, there was still no difference in cancer diagnoses."[162]

No, folic acid does not cause cancer.

The U.S. Food and Drug Administration (FDA) and Folic Acid

If a vitamin is safe, effective, and necessary for the healthy development of a baby, as clearly is the case for folic acid, why did we have to wait so long for the FDA to get around to confirming it? Now, it would be hard to imagine anyone would argue against the importance of folic acid during pregnancy. But there was a time when folic acid was still under review by the FDA, and was rejected for the prevention of neural tube defects. This excerpt from Dr. William Kaufman's article (below) shows the safety and efficacy of folic acid during pregnancy and, unfortunately, the slow response of the FDA's approval of the vitamin for the prevention of birth defects:

What Took the FDA So Long to Come Out in Favor of Folic Acid?

BY WILLIAM KAUFMAN, MD, PhD

Folic acid (or folate) is frequently referred to in the news media, so I will make some comments about it. . . .

Folic acid is an inexpensive chemical with a vitamin-like action. One can buy at retail 250 tablets containing 800 micrograms of good quality folic acid for about $6.00. These tablets contain four times the folic acid in today's RDA (recommended daily allowance). One tablet costs a little over two cents.

Who is most susceptible to general folic acid deficiencies? Pregnant woman, fetuses, premature infants, and elderly people. Women with a systemic folic acid deficiency can develop, in addition to other health problems, pre-cancerous changes in the uterine cervix. In addition. some women (users of oral contraceptive agents or smokers) who do not have a systemic folic acid deficiency can develop areas of localized folic acid deficiency in the uterine cervix. Areas of localized folic acid deficiency on the uterine cervix also may become pre-cancerous. Pre-cancer in both types of women, can become cancer. However, the administration of adequate amounts of inexpensive folic acid can effect a cure of the pre-cancerous areas. Then, perhaps the woman may be able to change her diet to include foods rich in folates and sustain such a cure. But it is often hard for a woman to make a sustained improvement in diet. Poor women simply cannot afford the improved diet. In both such types of women, it would seem wise to use inexpensive, adequate pill-a-day folic acid maintenance therapy in addition to as good a diet as they can afford and get themselves to eat.

A folate deficiency in a pregnant woman may cause a special kind of anemia, a premature separation of the placenta, spontaneous abortion, bleeding, an abnormal fetus including those with a neural tube defect, anacephaly, spina bifida, and low-weight babies. Not only do these sad events cause misery to the mother, father, and family but they simultaneously cause a large drain on medical resources as well as an enormous economic drain on Medicaid and on other sources for financing medical care. It would appear that these complications of pregnancy can be largely prevented by good nutrition and appropriate folic acid supplementation for the entire duration of the pregnancy from conception onward. And, this leads me to comment on the FDA's (initial) rejection(s) of an application for approval of the use of folic acid therapy for the prevention of neural tube defects as being premature.

The FDA is charged with making sure that the drugs they approve for prescription use are both safe and effective for specific therapeutic use.

The FDA has recently publicized a change in policy. It now plans to speed up the new drug approval process. This will enable giant pharmaceutical companies to sell expensive drugs with many side effects much earlier than is now possible, which will result in less careful scrutiny of the safety and efficacy of such new drugs.

Nutritional substances such as vitamins and minerals are not drugs. Folic acid is a vitamin. However, there is a section of the FDA regulations that states that any substance can be considered to be a drug if a claim is made that it can improve function or structure in an individual or prevent illness. Because of this, folic acid was legally characterized as a drug, the sponsor had to subject folic acid to the regulations governing the application of a new drug application.

The FDA (had previously) rejected a new drug application for the use of folic acid intended to prevent neural tube defects in the fetus of a pregnant woman who had such a tragic event in a previous pregnancy. (For years) they had considered this New Drug Application to be premature. This is a way of saying that the FDA considers the data submitted in the folic acid New Drug Application was inadequate and that the sponsor must spend time, possibly years, gathering more data. [*Editor's note: This is precisely what indeed happened with folic acid. See note below.*] In the meantime, women who have had the misfortune to have had a fetus with a neural tube disorder in a previous pregnancy could not, for a long time, legally be prescribed folic acid with the view of possibly reducing her risk of having another neural tube defect fetus in future pregnancies.

About the Safety of Folic Acid

Folic acid has been used for over forty years as a vitamin and has been found safe in the treatment of men, non-pregnant women, and in pregnant women who have had folic acid deficiencies. Folic acid has been used to remove pre-malignant lesions on the uterine cervix and thus prevent cancer.

Even a very high daily oral dose (10 milligrams, which is 10,000 mcg) that is 50 times the present RDA (Recommended Daily Allowance) taken by 27 non-pregnant women for four months was safe and there were no adverse side effects. The much lower oral doses commonly used in treatment of folic acid deficiencies are also safe and effective.

There are no folic acid adverse side effects excepting the following:

1. Folic acid in huge doses administered to epileptic persons may block the anti-epileptic action of their drugs and cause them to have an increase in epileptic attacks (this is unlikely to occur with lower doses of folic acid);

2. it may rarely decrease zinc absorption of zinc but this does not lower blood zinc levels because of decreased urinary excretion of zinc; and

3. the patient may have concurrent deficiency in both vitamin B_{12} and folic acid, a condition that requires concomitant treatment with both vitamin B_{12} and folic acid. Therefore, folic acid alone cannot be effective.

Thus, folic acid is safer than most of the drugs, if not all the drugs, the FDA has approved for prescription use.

About the Probable Effectiveness of Folic Acid in the Prevention of Neural Tube Defects in the Fetus

While the FDA may (have been) bureaucratically and legally right in rejecting the application for the use of folic acid for the prevention of neural tube defects as being premature, from a humane and practical point of view it is wrong.

Neural tube defects are terrible complications of pregnancy. A mother who has had this calamity happen to her infant in a previous pregnancy is at considerable risk of having it happen again in subsequent pregnancies.

Many published reports in the medical literature indicate that giving such a woman folic acid in sufficient amounts can greatly lower the risk of recurrences of such extremely damaged fetuses. Some other medical reports disagree. A meta-analysis of all these published papers would probably show that there is enough favorable evidence to show that folic acid can reduce the risk of having a fetus damaged by neural tube defects. In view of all the circumstances, the FDA should give this application provisional approval to since folic acid is an exceedingly safe vitamin.

I am now suggesting how such provisional approval could get the FDA the additional data they want and currently not deprive women at risk of having neural tube defects infants of possible freedom from the recurrence of this calamity through the use of folic acid.

This provisional approval should be subject to the following conditions:

a. that the non-epileptic woman who has had a previous fetus with neural tube defects start the agreed upon dose of folic acid before conception and continue it throughout her entire pregnancy;

b. that she will agree not to indulge in alcohol before conception and throughout her entire pregnancy and if she does, she will inform her physician how much and how often she partakes of alcohol (alcohol will negate folic acid action);

c. the obstetrician or nurse midwife who delivers the infant will make a full report about the pattern of folic acid oral usage, whether or not alcohol has been indulged in during the pregnancy and the amounts and frequency of intake, and the condition of the infant on birth to the FDA.

The data on controls (women who have had neural tube defect babies in a prior pregnancy and who have become pregnant again but who did not take folic acid during the current pregnancy) should be collected under the direction of the Surgeon General of the U.S. Public Health Service, who could make it mandatory that all hospitals which supply obstetric care in the United States compile data report the condition of every baby at birth born to a mother who had not been treated with folic acid during her pregnancy but has had a previous pregnancy ending with a neural tube defect infant. This data would give some reliable measure of how great the risk is of having subsequent neural tube defect babies when folic acid treatment was not given during the pregnancy. This information combined with the prospective information reported to the FDA on the incidence of neural tube defect babies occurring in women treated with folic acid, in turn, would make it possible to assess accurately how effective folic acid is in lowering the risk of occurrence of such tragedies.

Editor's Note: FDA did ultimately approve folic acid as preventive for neural tube defects such as spina bifida. It took them almost ten years to do so. In each of those years, at least 1,200 babies were born with neural tube defects. That makes some 12,000 birth defects that FDA failed to prevent because of unwarranted caution over a substance that is vastly safer than any drug that they have ever approved.

Dr. Kaufman is a pioneer of orthomolecular medicine. This article has been abridged and reprinted with the kind permission of Charlotte Kaufman.[163]

VITAMIN B_{12}—COBALAMIN

Vitamin B_{12} can't kill you, unless you don't get any. B_{12} is required for neurological function, DNA synthesis, and the proper formation of red blood cells.[164] Like veggies? Good. But B_{12} is found primarily in animal based products like eggs, cheese, meat, fish, and milk. If you are a strict vegetarian or vegan, it is especially important that you seek out fortified foods and supplemental B_{12} and even more so when you are pregnant and nursing.

Oral B_{12} is not easy to absorb. Moreover, some women may have pernicious (harmful and destructive) anemia or the inability to absorb B_{12} through what they eat. "People who have pernicious anemia can't absorb enough vitamin B_{12} from food. This is because they lack intrinsic factor, a protein made in the stomach. A lack of this protein leads to vitamin B_{12} deficiency," says the National Institutes of Health.[165] In the old days, this condition could literally kill you. Nowadays, B_{12} can be administered directly via shots, oral tablets, and with nasal sprays. For cases of pernicious anemia, about 1 percent of oral vitamin B_{12} can still be absorbed.[166] However, your doctor may also administer intramuscular B_{12} shots to bypass your gut's faulty absorption system.

You may be nervous about the seemingly large amount of B_{12} you are eating or taking relative to the RDA. The RDA for B_{12} is set at 2.6–2.8 mcg a day for women who are pregnant or lactating.[167] Don't be. Because of its low toxicity, no tolerable upper intake level has been set by the United States Food and Nutrition Board.[168] Just three little ounces of clams have about 84 mcg of B_{12}. The American Pregnancy Association supports eating two 6-oz servings of clams each week.[169] This would provide, on average, about 24 mcg of B_{12} daily, over nine times the RDA during pregnancy.

Vitamin B_{12} supplements are safe, and inexpensive, too.[170] Like the rest of the B vitamins it is water soluble, so excess is excreted in urine. There is really no reason to avoid getting adequate amounts. The benefits are many, and the risks are next to none. Researchers have reported that "[n]o adverse effects have been associated with excess vitamin B_{12} intake from food and supplements in healthy individuals."[171] In healthy folks, oral administration can be as effective as an intramuscular shot.[172] Sublingual tablets (the kind that dissolve under your tongue) can do the trick. Look specifically for methylcobalamin. B vitamins work best together, so along with that extra B_{12}, see to it that you are getting the other Bs. A B complex supplement can provide just what you are looking for.

Prevention is always the best medicine, and when it comes to B_{12}, it would seem that is the only way to operate. Here's why: the body can store B_{12} for some time, making deficiency difficult to spot. Symptoms of a problem may not be apparent for years. A B_{12}-deficient mom may not realize it, and without testing, her doctor might not realize it either. Babies receive B_{12} through the placenta and through breast milk. If mom is deficient in B_{12}, less is available for baby. Low reserves of the vitamin can lead to deficiency within months of birth.[173] Severe and permanent neurological damage can result. Why risk it? Taking this safe and essential vitamin can provide peace of mind, and protect the mind of your baby, too.

BIOTIN

Biotin is made by bacteria in our large intestine. This, among others, is a very good reason to keep our gut flora as healthy and balanced as possible, with a good diet consisting of plenty of vegetables and probiotics or fermented foods and avoiding antibiotics.

Biotin deficiency is rare. However, pregnancy is a special case. It is estimated that at least one third of pregnant women are marginally deficient in biotin.[174] If you develop brittle nails, hair loss, or skin rashes, investigate your biotin intake. According to the Linus Pauling Institute and the research of Donald Mock, MD,[175] biotin is broken down more rapidly during pregnancy and a "substantial number of women develop marginal or subclinical biotin deficiency."[176] This matters because subclinical biotin deficiency has been shown to cause birth defects in some animals.[177] Ensuring that a safe, water soluble nutrient like biotin[178] is in your prenatal is a must. There is no evidence that biotin has ever hurt anybody, including pregnant women.[179] In pregnancy especially, it appears that biotin deficiency, not biotin abundance, is the concern. Obtaining at least 30–35 mcg of biotin a day during pregnancy and lactation is a good idea.[180] Your prenatal may contain biotin; check and see. I found quite a few that contain 300 mcg or more, and some contain less or have none at all. Over-the-counter biotin supplements commonly contain 1,000–5,000 mcg. Food sources include yeast, eggs, salmon, and avocados.

Biotin Safety during Pregnancy

You may be warned off against taking supplemental biotin during pregnancy. This warning appears to stem from the potential for excess biotin to cause miscarriage in rats. Let's take a closer look at the numbers. In rats, a 50 and 100 mg per kg dose of biotin given via injection was reported to cause miscarriage.[181] That would be equivalent to a 160 pound woman getting over 3.5 to 7 *million* micrograms of biotin injected into her body. We aren't aiming to swallow anywhere near that amount. Based on this information, women should not be deterred from biotin dietary supplements. Of note, another study done on excessive biotin intake and mice showed "no differences" in the rates of miscarriages between the study group and the control group, and excess biotin "did not disturb normal reproductive functions and embryonic development."[182] Oral doses, in the amounts present in our biotin supplements, should not make us worry.

CHOLINE

Choline is an essential nutrient, but not, strictly speaking, a vitamin. However, it is usually grouped along with the B vitamins. The B vitamins are very important for helping your brain function normally. In animal studies, choline has been found to improve brain function.[183] Pregnant rats given choline showed improved memory in their babies, and this remained true even when the young 'uns were elderly.[184] What is good for babies is likely helpful for moms, too. For those women that feel a bit fuzzy-brained and forgetful during pregnancy, this may be just the nutrient they are looking for.

Moms may benefit from choline in other ways, too. It may be more difficult to sleep during pregnancy. Choline may help you stay asleep. Another benefit is feeling better. "Acetylcholine is the end neurotransmitter of your parasympathetic nerve system. This means that, among other things, it facilitates good digestion, deeper breathing, and slower heart rate. You may perceive its effect as 'relaxation,'" says Dr. Saul.[185] Your body knows how to make its own acetylcholine from choline. The trick is to get enough choline so your body can do this.

When we are pregnant and lactating, choline becomes even more important. "The demand for choline is especially high during pregnancy and lactation because of transport of choline from mother to fetus," says Steven H. Zeisel, MD.[186] This transfer of choline depletes the mother's plasma choline.[187] "Thus," he says, "despite enhanced capacity to synthesize choline during pregnancy, the demand for this nutrient exceeds the supply and stores can be depleted. Because human milk is rich in choline, lactation further increases maternal demand, resulting in extended depletion of tissue stores."[188]

Research suggests that choline is important for our growing baby. Dietary intakes of choline are associated with a reduced risk of neural tube defects (NTDs).[189] "Shaw et al.[190] found that women in the lowest quartile for dietary choline intake had four times the risk of giving birth to a child with a neural tube defect, compared with women in the highest quartile of intake," says Dr. Zeisel.[191] As with folic acid, more choline meant a reduced risk of NTDs. Choline deficiency could contribute to heart defects, as shown in an animal study[192] suggesting that choline intake may help prevent problems of the heart. Additionally, in a mouse model of Down syndrome, babies of mothers fed excess choline during pregnancy and lactation "dramatically improved attentional function" of the adult offspring.[193] Their "heightened reactivity to committing an error" was also normalized, in other words, they were more emotionally relaxed.[194] Decrease the risk of birth defects, improve baby's attention, and help him or her feel better? All seem like really good reasons to seek out ways to incorporate choline into our prenatal diet.

Choline is in many foods. For example, wheat germ, eggs, soy, meat, quinoa, broccoli, nuts, milk, seeds, lentils, seafood, and cauliflower are all food sources of choline. Another place choline can be found is in lecithin, as phosphatidyl choline. Lecithin makes up about 30 percent of the dry weight of your brain . . . and your baby's brain, too. It's a combination of several valuable substances. A tablespoon (7.5 grams) of lecithin granules contains about 2,200 mg of essential fatty acids (such as linoleic acid), 1,700 mg of phosphatidyl choline, and 1,000 mg of phosphatidyl inositol.[195] Lecithin is an emulsifier that helps our body absorb fat-soluble vitamins like vitamin E. It also helps keep cholesterol from becoming a problem, helps prevent arteriosclerosis, aids in the absorption of vitamin A and thiamine (B_1), and is protective against cardiovascular disease.[196] You can find soy lecithin granules or capsules. Lecithin is cheaper in the granular form, but capsules have the added advantage of being convenient and taste-free. I don't mind the flavor of lecithin (it's kind of nutty) but I don't like the texture and it sticks to my teeth. During pregnancy I opted to take lecithin in capsule form, and take granules when they could be added to food that would make it easier to get it down, like a smoothie. Lecithin supplements are generally derived from soy. If you want another option, sunflower lecithin is available.

You may have heard that lecithin could be helpful in preventing ligament pain during late pregnancy, and that lecithin helps breastfeeding mothers steer clear of clogged ducts. I found extra lecithin helped me in both areas.

Lecithin is nontoxic. It has no known harmful effects.[197] But pregnant women may be discouraged from taking lecithin and told that there isn't enough scientific evidence to support its use. I, however, was very satisfied with the science and safety of added choline in my diet, including choline obtained from lecithin, and my doctor was also supportive.

THE B VITAMINS:
IMPORTANT FOR A HEALTHY PREGNANCY AND BABY

All of the B vitamins are important during pregnancy and can make a critical difference in the health and development of your baby. You can be more relaxed, avoid depression during pregnancy and postpartum, eliminate or manage migraines, and lessen the nausea many women experience. Your baby will have a much better chance for healthy development without birth defects, and even for better health and cognitive function later in life. There's just no question about it.

CHAPTER 8

Minerals and More

"In an ancient Chinese system, doctors were only paid when the patients were healthy. When they were sick, the doctors had to work without pay to make them healthy again. Imagine what our health care system would look like if that system were in effect today."
—WILLIAM B. GRANT, PhD

No, minerals are not vitamins. However, the goal of this book is to help demystify nutrient supplementation during pregnancy. Since, your prenatal vitamin includes minerals, it seems only logical that this book should, too.

The amount you need of any particular mineral varies greatly from really tiny to "Wow, that seems like quite a lot." Regardless of the quantities needed, they are all important. Like vitamins, minerals should be taken together because they need each other. Your prenatal vitamin likely contains a combination of essential minerals. So do fruits and veggies. Eating lots of fruits and vegetables does a really nice job of providing a variety of nutrients, especially when it comes to micro or trace minerals, the minerals of which you only need a small amount. But food is only as good as the soil it is grown in. One of the best ways to ensure you are getting trace minerals in your diet is to eat organically grown foods, like from your own garden. Better soil means better vitamin, mineral, micronutrient, and enzyme content, and don't let anyone try to tell you differently.

Eating right is a great place to start, but supplements are still a good idea in addition to that healthy diet. For example, macro minerals, like magnesium, are more easily obtained through simple supplementation. The following alphabetical list provides information about the importance of minerals and other nutrients during pregnancy.

MINERAL MEASUREMENTS IN PERSPECTIVE

Amounts of minerals in supplements vary greatly. This is simply because we require more of some and less of others. Selenium, iodine, and chromium, for example, are trace or microminerals. We only need a little bit. Trace minerals are usually measured in micrograms (mcg). A microgram is a thousandth of a milligram (mg).

Then there are macrominerals, like magnesium and calcium. Macrominerals will often be measured in milligrams. We require relatively large amounts of macrominerals, but the "relatively large" is in comparison to the micrograms we need of microminerals. A milligram is a thousandth of a gram (g). A gram is about a quarter teaspoon. Therefore, a milligram is about a *thousandth* of a quarter teaspoon, and a microgram is about a *millionth* of a quarter teaspoon, a very tiny amount indeed.

BORON

Boron is a trace mineral and you only need a little bit. Along with calcium, magnesium, and vitamin D, boron is essential for bone strength and bone growth.[1] Fruit and vegetables are the main sources of boron in your diet[2] and likely provide an adequate amount of boron during pregnancy, as long as you actually eat them. About 3 mg a day should do the trick.[3] It is considered safe for pregnant or breastfeeding women aged nineteen to fifty years old to take 20 mg a day and fourteen- to eighteen-year-olds to take up to 17 mg a day.[4]

CALCIUM

Calcium is well regarded and strongly recommended during pregnancy, and for good reason. Your baby has a whole skeleton to grow. She requires calcium to build strong bones and teeth, grow her muscles, nerves, and a healthy heart, and to develop normal heart rhythm.[5]

Your growing baby needs calcium, and she is going to get it from somewhere. Pregnant women are encouraged to get 1,000–1,300 mg/day of calcium.[6] If mom doesn't get enough calcium, the baby actually "robs" the mineral from her bones.[7] Feed the demand. Have you checked to see how much your prenatal contains—maybe 120–600 mg? Chronically consuming suboptimal amounts of calcium (less than 500 mg a day) may mean that you will have increased bone loss during pregnancy.[8] The good news is calcium is easy to come by and we absorb calcium better while we are pregnant, especially during the second and third trimester.[9] Calcium (1,200–1,500 mg a day) may also help prevent pregnancy-induced high blood pressure,[10] and 1,000 mg/day may also help with leg cramps during pregnancy.[11] Getting two to three times this amount (2,500–3,000 mg a day) is regarded as safe in women who are pregnant or lactating.[12]

Focusing on calcium alone without considering intake of magnesium would be a mistake. *It is equally important to get enough magnesium.* Carolyn Dean, MD, says, for example, that "calcium appears to help leg cramps, at least initially, because excess calcium forces magnesium to be released from storage sites."[13] "But," she says, "[I]f someone is magnesium-deficient, the excess calcium can begin to cause more problems."[14] Calcium is readily attained through food, but acquiring adequate magnesium proves much more difficult. Pregnant women should be sure to get enough of both. (You can read more about magnesium requirements and pregnancy later in this chapter.)

Consuming yogurt and other forms of dairy can be a simple way to get the additional recommended amount of calcium in your diet. If you are lactose intolerant, you may still be able to eat yogurt and aged cheeses. Are you craving pickles? Your desire for foods prepared with vinegar could be your body's way of telling you it's time to evaluate your calcium intake. For example, hundreds of women taking 1,200 mg a day of calcium significantly reduced their cravings for sweets and salt during PMS.[15] The same kind of thinking may apply to pregnancy, and suggests that women should assess their calcium intake if confronted with cravings.

If you aren't getting enough calcium through food, supplementation may be necessary. Two forms of calcium are readily available: calcium carbonate and calcium citrate. Calcium carbonate should be taken with food while calcium citrate, the preferred form, is well absorbed in general, and without a meal. Calcium will not work properly without magnesium so they are equally important.[16] As is vitamin D. Vitamin D helps you absorb calcium. Divide your doses and take calcium every day along with both magnesium and vitamin D.

CHROMIUM

Chromium is a trace mineral that helps with glucose metabolism by working with insulin.[17] This may be of particular importance for women who are diabetic or develop gestational diabetes during pregnancy. Women with gestational diabetes who supplemented daily with 4 mcg (that's micrograms) of chromium picolinate for every 2.2 pounds of body weight (this would mean a 165 pound woman would take 300 mcg a day), "had decreased fasting blood glucose and insulin levels compared with those who took a placebo."[18] While not referring to its use specifically in pregnancy, in *Orthomolecular Medicine for Everyone,* Dr. Abram Hoffer, MD, supports taking 200 mcg a day of chromium.[19] I took 400 mcg a day of chromium during pregnancy and my doctor did not object. To help treat depression, Malcolm N. McLeod, MD, recommends taking anywhere from 400–1,000 mcg of chromium picolinate daily, or about 4 mcg per pound of body weight.[20]

Chromium can help even out the highs and lows of blood sugar. When our blood sugar crashes, we often head for unhealthy quick fixes like sugar and simple carbohydrates. Chromium can help curb carbohydrate cravings,[21] reduce overeating, and reverse the feelings of depression.[22]

You are supposed to gain weight during pregnancy. This is normal and necessary. Your calorie needs go up, but good calories from nutritious food are best, of course. Chromium does not have magical powers to keep you from eating crap. You still need to eat right. You still have to keep access to good food available so that when you are hungry you do eat, and there is something you want to eat that's actually good for you and readily available with minimal prep.

The adequate intake of chromium during pregnancy has been set at 29 to 30 mcg daily and 44 to 45 mcg for lactating women.[23] But nearly 90 percent of us are eating chromium deficient diets.[24] Chromium is depleted throughout pregnancy and is secreted in our milk when lactating, and most foods contain very little.[25] For example, an apple provides 1 mcg of chromium and a cup of mashed potatoes has only 3 mcg.[26] One of the better food sources is broccoli: a half a cup provides 11 mcg.[27] Brewer's or "nutritional" yeast is a good food source of chromium and can help increase energy and improve mood. Chromium picolinate is also available in supplement form.

Dietary chromium is safe. According to the National Academies of Sciences, "No adverse effects have been convincingly associated with excess intake of chromium from food or supplements."[28]

"It is far safer to take chromium than not to take it," says Dr. McLeod. His extensive, in-depth review of the medical and scientific literature has convinced him that chromium picolinate is safe "both immediately as a single dose and after taking it for an extended period, if not taken in amounts that exceed 1,000 mcg per day."[29]

COPPER

Getting a little copper is important (1 mg per day during pregnancy),[30] but this is a mineral you won't need to supplement. Copper deficiency is rare and excess copper consumption is more likely.[31] Since most folks have copper pipes running through their homes, you could use a countertop water filter pitcher that removes some copper for you. "Elevated copper levels are correlated to various mental and neurological illnesses including schizophrenia, depression, autism, tardive dyskinesia, and memory loss," says Carl C. Pfeiffer, MD.[32] This is of special importance for women who are pregnant. Here's why: "Excess copper is associated with pregnancy," says Dr. Hoffer, and "this may be a factor in postpartum psychosis, toxemia of pregnancy, and depression that sometimes follows the use of birth control pills."[33] Fortunately, elevated copper can be addressed with nutrient therapy. "In combination with ascorbic acid (vitamin C), zinc is used to reduce high serum copper levels," says Hoffer. For treatment of excess copper, taking vitamin C, a combination of zinc and manganese (in a 20:1 ratio), and eating a high fiber diet is recommended.[34]

IODINE

Iodine sufficiency is extremely important during pregnancy and lactation.[35] How much your baby gets depends on you. You need iodine to make thyroid hormones, which in turn regulate your metabolism, and are crucial to your child's brain development and nervous system. The scary side of very serious iodine deficiency during pregnancy is it can permanently harm our developing baby, causing mental retardation, stunted growth, and atypical sexual development.[36] In less severe cases, it could present itself as lower-than-average intelligence (IQ).[37] This deficiency may not be obvious. We want to try to protect the health of our growing baby and help him reach his fullest potential. Seeking out iodine in food and supplements while we are pregnant can help do that.

You don't need a lot of iodine but you most assuredly need a little. Iodine *sufficiency* is our goal during pregnancy. Iodine has a negative safety connotation with mothers and children because tincture of iodine, which is used topically as an antiseptic, is poisonous if ingested. However, the amount of iodine essential for good health is very small and very necessary.

Japanese women may consume quite a bit of iodine compared to their American counterparts. "In Japan, the average Japanese woman is eating 13.8 mg of iodine per day while the average American woman consumes 100 times less iodine per day (approximately 0.138 mg per day)," says Jorge D. Flechas, MD.[38] However, Alan Gaby, MD, author of *Nutritional Medicine*, says this is a "significant overestimate." Studies that specifically investigated iodine intake in the Japanese population show an average intake of 330–550 micrograms a day, not 13.8 milligrams.[39] The U.S. government's "safe upper limit" for iodine is set at 1,100 micrograms (1.1 milligrams) per day.[40]

We don't all have to jump the next plane to Tokyo in an attempt to get adequate iodine, but we can make a conscious effort to obtain the small recommended amount of iodine through our pregnancy diet and supplements. Japanese women aside, it is far more common for women to not get enough iodine. "Iodine deficiency is epidemic in developing countries and parts of Europe," says Lyn Patrick, ND. They aren't alone. Dr. Patrick says, "Recent evidence shows iodine deficiency is also strikingly common among adult women in the United States."[41]

According to the American Academy of Pediatrics, about one-third of American women are deficient in iodine during pregnancy, and only about 15 percent of pregnant and lactating women take supplements with adequate levels of iodine.[42]

Insufficient iodine may not present us with obvious symptoms like a goiter. While pregnant women may not show overt symptoms of iodine deficiency, intake may still be insufficient.[43] Let's not wait and see. According to the National Institutes of Health, "During pregnancy and early infancy, iodine deficiency can cause irreversible effects."[44] You can easily avoid this possibility.

"Iodine is very crucial in the first three years of life from the development of the fetus inside the womb until two years after birth," says Dr. Flechas. "In the development of a child's IQ, I feel that it would be very advantageous for the mother to supplement her diet during pregnancy and, if she is nursing the child, for the first two years after pregnancy."[45] Food sources of iodine include iodized salt, eggs, fortified grains, seafood, and dairy products.[46]

During pregnancy, I was a fan of sushi rolls with cooked seafood wrapped with seaweed, which can be a good source of iodine;[47] I ate yogurt every day and periodically ate fish, and we use iodized salt in our cooking. Supplementation of iodine is still recommended *in addition* to the iodine you obtain from food. Currently, the American Thyroid Association advises that women take an additional 150 micrograms of iodine each day during pregnancy and lactation,[48] for a total of 250 mcg a day from diet and supplements combined.[49] The RDA recommends 220 mcg a day during pregnancy, and 290 mcg a day while lactating.[50] Check to see if your prenatal vitamin contains iodine. Only about half of them do, and the dosage level varies greatly from brand to brand.[51]

IODINE SKIN APPLICATION

No iodine in your prenatal? Smearing a small amount of tincture of iodine right onto the skin may be an effective alternative. (I do this every month or so.) "[S]kin application of iodine is an effective if not efficient and practical way for supplementation of iodine with an expected bioavailability of 6 to 12 percent of the total iodine applied to the skin," says Guy E. Abraham, MD.[52]

IRON

Whether you are building a building or building a baby, you need enough good building materials. Growing a baby requires much more blood than when you're not pregnant, and that means you need iron. Iron is needed to make hemoglobin, and you need hemoglobin to transport oxygen throughout your body. Iron helps keep your immune system strong, and low levels of iron may increase the risk of pregnancy complications such as low birth weight and premature birth.[53] The daily recommendation for iron during pregnancy is 27 mg; this number drops to 9–10 mg a day during lactation.[54] Your doctor will likely test you for iron-deficiency anemia at your routine pregnancy checkups. Your doctor recommended iron dose may vary based on your needs.

Form matters when it comes to iron. Ferrous sulfate will likely make you feel sick to your stomach, something a pregnant woman surely does not need. "Many doctors still prescribe this cookie-tossing form of iron, in too large an amount, and without enough supplemental 'C' for absorption," says Andrew W. Saul, PhD. "And constipation is almost guaranteed with ferrous sulfate. Use ferrous fumarate, ferrous gluconate, or especially carbonyl iron instead." If your prenatal vitamin makes you feel sick or throw up, investigate the form of iron it contains and see how much you are getting. If it contains nausea-causing ferrous sulfate, switch to a different form of iron. If you are getting more than 27 mg of iron a day and suffering side effects, talk to your doctor. You may need more, or less may be sufficient. You could ask to have your iron levels tested again when taking a lower dose. At the same time, consider taking more vitamin C to help you better absorb the iron you are getting. Iron is important, and the last thing we want to do is stop taking our vitamins and minerals while we are pregnant because we can't stomach them. It is worth finding a supplement and dosage that works best for you.

Personally speaking, I found taking less iron (in the form of ferrous fumarate, about 18–20 mg per day), dividing my dose, taking it with extra vitamin C (6,000–10,000 mg a day), and taking it with food worked best for me during pregnancy. I gained the necessary benefits of supplemental iron without experiencing iron-deficiency anemia, unpleasant gastrointestinal side effects like constipation, or iron-induced nausea.

Calcium, zinc, and vitamin E may affect iron absorption, so you may want to take your iron at a different time of day than those supplements. Food sources of iron include red meat (stick with the grass-fed organic variety if you can), turkey, lentils, beans, spinach, and fortified, preferably organic, cereals.

IRON OVERDOSE AND CHILDREN: PRECAUTION IS ONE THING, PANIC IS ANOTHER

Many mothers may worry about their kids ingesting too many iron supplements. While we should always protect our kids from potential injury, the preeminent poison in our household is not found in the form of iron tablets.

Unlike drugs, excess intake of vitamins is very unlikely to cause the death of your little one. Although iron, a mineral, is not as safe as vitamins, it accounts for fewer deaths than laundry or dishwashing detergent.[55] This doesn't mean we should leave iron tablets strewn about our kitchen. A fatal dose of iron is typically more than 250 mg per kilogram (kg), or 2,500 mg (or more) for a twenty-two pound child.[56] However, doses as low as 60 mg per kg or (the equivalent 600 mg for that same twenty-two pound child) have been reported to cause death.[57] If a twenty-two pound child chows down half a bottle (thirty tablets) of Flintstones children's multivitamins with iron, he will be exposed to 450 mg of iron (15 mg per tablet). He may be uncomfortable, but it's probably not going to kill him. Usually, a danger of iron overdose arises when children ingest adult iron supplements, namely prenatal vitamins, which may contain a whole lot of iron and rightfully deserve additional careful storage. "Until iron supplements were put in child-proof bottles, on average there were one or two fatalities per year attributed to iron poisoning from gross overdosing on supplemental iron," says Dr. Saul. Still, "[m]inerals have an excellent safety record," he says, "but not quite as good as vitamins."

Child resistant bottles work, but only if adults close them up properly. Unit-dose packaging of iron has been regarded as an effective way to reduce the risk of iron overdose in children under the age of six.[58] However, in 2003, the U.S. District Court decided that the Food and Drug Administration did not have the authority to regulate a unit-dose packaging requirement for iron tablets.[59] Did this needlessly expose children to potentially harmful iron tablets?

The facts may surprise you. The Centers for Disease Control and Prevention (CDC) reports that in 2009, 824 children died from poisonings.[60] This is a terrible statistic, but iron was not to blame. According to the American Association of Poison Control Centers (AAPCC), not a single child died due to dietary iron supplement overdose in 2009.[61]

In fact, according to the AAPCC, there have been no deaths whatsoever from children's multivitamin supplements in the ten-year span from 2000 to 2010, even those that contain iron.[62] Over the past ten years, three deaths have been attributed to adult multivitamin supplements containing iron, a number that would include both children and adults.[63] There was one death due to iron in both 2009 and 2010, but the AAPCC specifically notes these fatalities were not due to iron from nutritional supplements.[64]

The toxic pills in our homes are not vitamin or mineral supplements; they are drugs. According to the CDC, among children in the United States, "Between 2000 and 2009 there was an 80 percent increase in the poisoning death rate, largely due to prescription drug overdoses."[65] (And no, it's not your prescription prenatal vitamins we are talking about here.)

The moral of the story: don't make it easy for your child to get a hold of high-potency iron tablets. Keep iron supplements tightly capped and out of reach.

However, *it is even more important that you keep your prescription drugs tightly capped and out of reach of children.*

Our family goes one step further. We avoid taking prescription drugs in the first place. We don't keep them in the house at all.

MAGNESIUM

Numerous studies have found that magnesium supplementation reduces the risk of complications of pregnancy and also improves the health of the baby.[66] Magnesium is commonly used for the treatment of toxemia, and especially eclampsia-associated seizures,[67] and prenatal exposure to magnesium may significantly reduce the risk of cerebral palsy and mental retardation.[68] Additionally, it is a muscle relaxant that effectively treats leg cramps during pregnancy[69] and it also regulates insulin and blood sugar levels and may be helpful for combating gestational diabetes.[70]

Dr. Carolyn Dean, MD, ND, author of *The Magnesium Miracle* says, "Clinical trials have demonstrated that mothers supplementing with magnesium oxide have larger, healthier babies and lower rates of pre-eclampsia, premature labor, sudden infant death, and birth defects, including cerebral palsy."[71] And while she recommends you always check with your healthcare provider before adding any supplement to your diet, she reminds us that "magnesium has a long history of safety for both mother and child."[72] It may come as no surprise then that many researchers suggest pregnant women make magnesium supplementation part of their healthy pregnancy protocol to prevent complications during pregnancy, delivery, and postpartum.[73]

Magnesium in Our Prenatal . . . or Not

The current recommended dietary intake of magnesium for women who are pregnant is between 350–400 mg a day, and 310–360 mg/day while breastfeeding.[74] Looking over some of the most commonly prescribed prenatal supplements, I found they only contained 30–45 mg of magnesium, if they contained any at all. Over-the-counter prenatal vitamins didn't look much better: they only contained 125–200 mg of magnesium. Not only is this too little, it's the wrong form. Often the poorly absorbed "magnesium oxide" is listed on these labels.

"Right," you say, "but it's a supplement, which means it is supposed to *supplement*—not replace a good diet already rich in a variety of healthy foods." All right. Let's see where we can make up for what our prenatal isn't providing.

Magnesium in Our Meals . . . or Not

About 50 percent of magnesium in food and water is absorbed.[75] Foods that contain magnesium include wheat bran, nuts, spinach, soybeans, oatmeal, beans, and potatoes. However, we would need to get six to seven servings of these foods *each day* to make up for the magnesium that our prenatals are lacking. Would it be possible? Maybe. Would it be easy? Maybe not. It would certainly be hard to *continually* provide your pregnant body with this necessary nutrient, every single day, even if you paid very close attention to your diet. It may come as no surprise then that the average pregnant gal is not getting their recommended dietary allowance of magnesium.[76] That accounts for about half of us.[77]

Is this a big deal? It sure could be. Low magnesium status during pregnancy could mean elevated blood pressure, reduction in weight of the fetus, and placental and renal lesions.[78] It could also mean premature labor, preeclampsia, and could "potentiate the development of gestational diabetes."[79]

Does It Really Matter What Form of Magnesium I Take?

There are many forms of the mineral available. There are pills, powders, oils, and salts. However, just because the number of milligrams of magnesium on the label seems impressive doesn't mean your body is soaking up the benefits, unless the mineral is actually being absorbed. For example, "Only about 4 percent of magnesium oxide is absorbed and utilized in the body," says Dr. Dean. She explains that the best forms of magnesium are magnesium taurate, magnesium glycinate, magnesium citrate, magnesium malate, magnesium orotate, and magnesium oil, but "weight for weight dollar for dollar, magnesium citrate may be the best buy for general use" as it is inexpensive and easily absorbed.[80] Magnesium citrate is pretty easy to come by in tablet or powder form. It is absorbed by your body about twice as well as sulfate or carbonate.[81] Take it in the morning or in between meals to enhance absorption.[82] Epsom salt, also known as magnesium sulfate, is inexpensive, easy to come by, and easy to use. Adding a cup or two to a weekly bath can provide magnesium transdermally, meaning it will be absorbed through the skin.

How Much Magnesium Should I Take?

It depends on your needs. Let's start with the basics. It is recommended that pregnant women get between 350–400 mg of magnesium a day.[83] Magnesium obtained through diet alone is probably not enough. "Many researchers and clinicians recommend that pregnant women have a red blood cell magnesium test or EXATest and take 300–600 mg of supplemental magnesium," says Dr. Dean.[84] If we only absorb about half of the magnesium available in food, and somewhere between 4 and 50 percent from supplements,[85] and our prenatal vitamins only have a fraction of the magnesium we need, seeking additional sources of the mineral may be necessary. Are you suffering from constipation? Migraines? Leg cramps? Symptoms of preeclampsia? Anxiety? Twitches? Oversensitivity to noises? Insomnia? That's a mighty long list, but there's a mighty long line of people with these symptoms. This may be your pregnant body's way of saying you need more magnesium. "There is no way of knowing how many factors correlate with anyone's magnesium deficiency," says Dean, but "everyone could benefit from extra supplementation."[86] For most of us, the only side effect of too much magnesium is loose stools, which is the way our bodies excrete excess, but it is also a sign you should take less.[87] Somewhere in the middle is where we want to be, and that is "symptom free." As with most nutrients, your need will vary dependent on one factor: you. If you want to know your magnesium status, you could request to have it tested. Research supports this idea.[88] You don't have to wait until there is a problem. You can manage your magnesium now.

MANGANESE

Manganese is a trace mineral essential for the development of a healthy baby.[89] Deficiency, although rare,[90] "is associated with growth impairment, diabetic-like carbohydrate changes, and increased susceptibility to convulsions. About one third of epileptic children have low blood manganese," says Abram Hoffer, MD.[91] Low levels of manganese have also been associated with schizophrenia.[92]

Manganese is an essential nutrient; getting a small amount of manganese from a varied, healthy diet is important.[93] "The body contains 10–20 mg of manganese," says Dr. Hoffer. "A healthy person excretes 4 mg per day, and the average diet contains 2–9 mg per day."[94] The current intake of manganese considered adequate during pregnancy is 2 mg a day and increases slightly to 2.6 mg a day while lactating.[95] If you are eating the right foods, you are likely obtaining sufficient manganese. Nuts, seeds, whole grains, beans, and tea are all dietary sources of manganese.[96] Manganese-deficient soils, processing, and cooking decrease the amount actually present in what you eat. Additionally, only a very small portion of the manganese obtained in your diet is actually absorbed.[97]

Manganese Safety

Obtaining too little manganese is unhealthy. So is obtaining way too much. Exposure to excessive environmental manganese, such as in industrial settings or contaminated groundwater, can be toxic. For example, air that welders and smelters breathe contaminated with manganese dust can cause neurotoxicity.[98] Children are more susceptible than adults to the negative effects of excessive manganese.[99]

According to the Linus Pauling Institute, "Manganese toxicity resulting from foods alone has not been reported in humans, even though certain vegetarian diets could provide up to 20 mg/day of manganese. . . . There is presently no evidence that the consumption of a manganese-rich plant-based diet results in manganese toxicity."[100]

SELENIUM

You only need a little selenium, but you need that little a lot. Selenium is a trace mineral. It reduces inflammation and stimulates your immune system to fight infection; it is also important for reproduction, DNA production, and proper thyroid gland function.[101]

Selenium can help protect against exposure to toxic heavy metals. According to University of Victoria professor Harold Foster, PhD, "Pregnant women need special protection because their fetus may be poisoned in the womb, so interfering with its development."[102] Therefore, "[i]n addition to vitamin C, nutrient minerals are also protective against heavy metal toxins," he says. "For example, selenium is antagonistic to (and so protective against) arsenic, mercury, and cadmium."[103]

In women with thyroid peroxidase antibodies, taking 200 mcg a day of selenium may reduce postpartum thyroid inflammation (postpartum thyroiditis).[104]

The current RDA is 60–70 mcg (that's micrograms) a day for pregnant and lactating women (the amount in one Brazil nut) and 400 mcg a day has been set as the tolerable upper intake level, which, believe it or not, is just about right.[105]

ZINC

Zinc is a trace mineral important for all aspects of a baby's growth and development.[106] It plays an important role in brain function, reproduction, and helps defend against infection, and may help protect against premature birth.[107] Zinc is also vital for the prevention of birth defects.[108]

If your prenatal doesn't contain any zinc, consider that pregnant women should be getting 11–12 mg a day.[109] "Because zinc is so crucial for a healthy pregnancy—and a healthy baby—it may be just as important for pregnant women to take zinc as it is for her to take iron and a daily multivitamin," says Ian E. Brighthope, MD.[110] Food sources of zinc include beef, crab, baked beans, fortified cereal, dark-meat poultry, and, lest we forget, oysters. Cooked oysters are regarded as safe to eat during pregnancy and they are packed with zinc and iron.

The conservative tolerable upper intake level for zinc has been set at 34 mg a day for ages fourteen to eighteen, and 40 mg a day for adults nineteen or older.[111] The American Pregnancy Association places oysters in the "low mercury" category and says pregnant women can "enjoy two 6-oz servings per week."[112] Just three ounces of cooked oysters provides 74 mg of zinc.[113] Consuming two six-ounce servings of oysters a week, regarded as safe by the American Pregnancy Association, would provide 296 mg of zinc a week, or the equivalent of about 42 mg a day. If you are eating oysters, you probably won't need that zinc supplement. I make sure to take my zinc with food. On an empty stomach, it can make me feel queasy, something we experience enough during pregnancy.

OTHER IMPORTANT NUTRIENTS

They aren't minerals; they aren't vitamins; but the following nutrients are important, too.

COENZYME Q_{10}

Coenzyme Q_{10} (CoQ_{10}) is both an antioxidant and a micronutrient.[114] It is fat soluble and found in virtually all living cells.[115] Even though CoQ_{10} is generally regarded as safe,[116] due to a lack of studies in pregnant and lactating women, the recommendation I see most commonly given to us is, "Don't take it."

I challenge that.

Our bodies literally make CoQ_{10}. CoQ_{10} is necessary for the basic functioning of our cells.[117] It is found in small amounts in many foods, but particularly in meat, fish, and nuts.

CoQ_{10} may be helpful during pregnancy. Low levels of coenzyme Q_{10} are associated with preeclampsia,[118] and in doses of 200 mg a day, coenzyme Q_{10} may reduce the risk of preeclampsia in women at risk for the disorder.[119]

CoQ_{10} (100 mg a day) may also be helpful for migraine headache sufferers,[120] and while this isn't specific to pregnancy, CoQ_{10} may be worth looking into if you are looking for medicine-free migraine therapy. For more nutrition based migraine help, you may want to read the section on migraine in the Pregnancy Issues chapter.

If you are at risk for preeclampsia, or you suffer with debilitating headaches, taking a nutrient that your own body finds essential enough to produce sounds a lot better than resorting to drugs. There's certainly no harm in looking into it. A helpful hint: it is better to take CoQ_{10} in the morning, as taking it late at night may cause insomnia.[121]

OMEGA-3 FATTY ACIDS

Omega-3 fatty acids are essential to your baby's development.[122] They are also essential for you, especially if you want to feel better now and after baby is born. Low omega-3 intake increases your risk for postpartum depression[123] and supplementation can help prevent depression.[124] In fact, women who eat plenty of omega-3-rich food during their third trimester can cut their risk of postpartum depression *in half.*[125] That's pretty impressive.

Your baby requires omega-3s for the development of her nervous system; breast milk production further depletes mom's omega-3 supply.[126] Both of these demands result in diminishing omega-3s in subsequent pregnancies.[127] Because the typical American diet is "greatly lacking" in omega-3s,[128] pregnant women would be well advised to optimize their omegas.

> A study of pregnant North American women showed that the average dietary intake of DHA was only about 80 mg a day; 90 percent of the women consumed less than 300 mg of DHA daily.

Eating fatty fish, like salmon, is one way to get a dose of essential fatty acids. However, potential mercury exposure means our doctors tell us to limit our intake to two low-mercury fish servings a week, and rightly so. Perhaps even more caution is warranted while we are pregnant. Seek out "wild caught" fish or organic options to reduce your exposure to heavy metals. Take vitamin C every time you eat seafood. (Please see the section on Exposure to Toxins and Heavy Metals in the Vitamin C chapter). You can look into non-fish dietary sources of omega-3s such as the occasional serving of cold-milled flaxseed or take fish oil or krill oil supplements for a safe, virtually mercury-free dose of omega 3s.[129] As with any supplement, the quality of the product depends on the quality of the producer. If you are concerned about purity, you can always contact the supplement manufacturer and ask.

Look for a tablet that contains both docosahexaenoic acid (DHA) and eicosapentaenoic acid (EPA). Both EPA and DHA are important for you and your baby. The American Pregnancy Association says, "Although EPA and DHA naturally occur together and work together in the body, studies show that each fatty acid has unique benefits. EPA supports the heart, immune system, and inflammatory response. DHA supports the brain, eyes, and central nervous system which is why it is uniquely important for pregnant and lactating women."[130] Furthermore, "[i]ncreased intake of EPA and DHA has been shown to prevent pre-term labor and delivery, lower the risk of pre-eclampsia and may increase birth weight" and "[r]esearch has confirmed that adding EPA and DHA to the diet of pregnant women has a positive effect on visual and cognitive development of the baby."[131] Moreover, "[s]tudies have also shown that higher consumption of omega-3s may reduce the risk of allergies in infants."[132] If we want our babies to develop properly and reach their highest potential, omega-3s contain nutrients that help do exactly that. "These nutrients help to maximize the intelligence of your child, and protect your baby from brain injuries such as autism, pervasive developmental delay, and ADHD" says Joseph Mercola, MD.[133] This is all good news.

Our baby relies completely on us for their omega-3s. "[A] fetus must obtain all of its omega-3 fatty acids from mother's diet," says Dr. Mercola. "A mother's dietary intake and plasma concentrations of DHA directly influence the DHA status of the developing fetus."[134] In other words, if we get plenty, our baby does, too.

For best results and a good mix of nutrients, it is advised that pregnant women get their omega-3s from all of the following: fish, seeds, and supplements.[135] According to the International Society for the Study of Fatty Acids and Lipids, and recommended by the American Pregnancy Association, the minimum amount of DHA a pregnant woman should get every day is 300 mg.[136] A study of pregnant North American women showed that the average dietary intake of DHA was only about 80 mg a day; 90 percent of the women consumed less than 300 mg of DHA daily,[137] suggesting supplements may be of particular importance for pregnant women. While a standard hasn't been set for EPA during pregnancy, it doesn't make it any less essential. It is recommended that adults get a combination of at least 500 mg a day of EPA and DHA (a minimum of 220 mg a day of each).[138]

CHAPTER 9

Pregnancy Issues

Scene: Grocery store parking lot on a Tuesday morning

CHARACTERS: Mom (a nine-month pregnant me) and
my one-and-a-half-year-old daughter

PROPS: Shopping cart, recyclables, diaper bag, coat button

The scene opens, and Mom is loading recyclables into the cart. It is raining and the cart is soaked, so very pregnant Mom gets her daughter out of the car and slings her on one shoulder to carry her inside. Mom hefts the diaper bag on the other shoulder, and attempts to get her keys out of her concealed right pocket and lock her car with her free hand. As she does, a strong gust of wind blows and starts to take the filled cart away, so Mom hooks it with her left foot.

Silence.

Then . . .

Tink tink tink . . .

A necessary button on Mom's coat falls to the ground and rolls into the lane. Mom ponders the situation. Hands, arms, and one foot already in use. Remaining right leg is supporting pregnant body and is unable to retrieve button.

Random shopper watching: "Do you need that? And can I help?!"

Mom: "Yes, please."

PROBLEMS IN PREGNANCY

> *"No illness which can be treated by diet should be treated by any other means."*
> —MOSES MAIMONIDES, 12th Century Physician

To increase our ratio of good days to not so good days, and tip the scale in our favor (since goodness knows our new physique is already doing a good job of tilting it the other way), we have to be prepared to make some executive decisions about our health. There is so much we can't do while we are pregnant. (My snowboard is getting dusty.) But we can, and should, focus on our health. We are going to have a new little person soon. This is a wonderful thing. Keeping that in perspective, but putting it gently aside for now, we still don't want to feel like crud.

There are dozens upon dozens of issues that women can be faced with during pregnancy, delivery, and afterwards, either preexisting or due to pregnancy itself. This chapter cannot possibly address them all. What I hope you can take away from here is information about a nutrition-based approach for some of the most common issues pregnant women experience. Always discuss your options with your healthcare provider. However, you will likely find, as I did, that doctors and pregnancy health books alike have a predominately traditional medical—in other words, pharmaceutical—perspective. "Take drugs" or "deal with it" aren't satisfactory solutions. Don't be afraid to keep learning about natural alternatives. We all want the same thing in the end: healthy babies and healthy moms. It would be nice to be comfortable and happy during our pregnancy, too.

Perhaps our greatest concern during pregnancy is the safety of our baby. Each vitamin, and its safety during pregnancy, has been discussed earlier in this book in its dedicated chapter. As you seek out nutritional therapies for common health issues during pregnancy, please refer to those chapters for more information about the importance and safety of each nutrient.

ACID REFLUX

I can't tell you how many tacos I ate during pregnancy. Sometimes it would be hard to tell you how many I ate in one meal. Stuffing myself, and then heading to bed, would invariably result in me trying to sleep vertically, propped up on pillows in an attempt to make gravity keep my stomach contents where they belonged.

Note to self: "Smaller meals, well in advance of bedtime."

I also found digestive enzymes to be a helpful addition to a large meal.

ANEMIA

Getting enough iron during pregnancy is important,[1] because pregnancy demands additional iron. *Absorbing* that iron is the key. It's not enough to just pack your body full of it; you aren't a steel mill. Maximize the impact of the iron you ingest (and the iron available in your supplement) by taking ample amounts of vitamin C along with it. Yes, your prenatal probably contains some C, but that may not be enough. Eating iron-rich meals is great, too, and vitamin C can also help you absorb the iron you get from food sources. Too much iron may constipate you. That extra vitamin C can help keep your bathroom visits comfortable, as can a diet rich in fiber, and supplemental magnesium. (See Constipation, below.)

You can also develop anemia during pregnancy due to lack of folic acid, vitamin B_{12}, manganese, and B_6.[2] Doctors are pretty hip to folic acid these days, so you've probably heard about getting enough of that one. It's safe and important for the prevention of birth defects. B_{12} is also very safe. Both vitamins can be found in a B complex supplement, along with B_6, and it is likely your prenatal contains them as well. (You may wish to read the B vitamin chapter for more about the B vitamins and anemia.) Manganese may or may not be included in your prenatal vitamin.

BACKACHE

First try hot showers, moderate stretching, pregnancy yoga, good posture, regular prenatal massages, chiropractic adjustment, and tossing those high heels in the back of the closet for nine months. If those aren't enough, consider that vitamin C strengthens ligaments and tendons, and magnesium can help relax sore muscles.

BACTERIAL VAGINOSIS (BV)

Antibiotics are the go-to drug for treatment of bacterial vaginosis. However, they have a poor "cure" rate of only about 60 percent.[3] Even if antibiotic treatment for BV is successful, all too often women end up with an opportunistic yeast infection afterward,[4] a side effect of antibiotic use.[5] Swapping out one infection for another seems awfully pointless. Even after antibiotics have blasted away the bad BV bacteria (and your good bacteria, too, as they are not selective) many women suffer recurrent bacterial infections. This is due in part to their body's failure to reestablish normal vaginal flora after treatment.[6] Taking more antibiotics is ineffective at preventing recurrences, even with maintenance therapy.[7] Taking antibiotics and then more antibiotics when the first ones failed is hardly a solution, especially when you are pregnant.

What is truly curative of BV would appear to be something other than a drug. Instead of utilizing antibiotics, build a robust immune system, and you'll find BV won't stand a chance. Skip the side effects of drugs, and seek the side benefits of vitamins and nutrition. To deal with a current infection, consider that when yogurt containing *Lactobacillus acidophilus* was inserted into the vagina it was shown to treat BV and prevent infection in pregnant women by increasing vaginal acidity and normal vaginal flora, creating an environment less hospitable for BV bacteria like *Gardnerella vaginalis*.[8] (Stick with a plain, additive-free, fruitless yogurt, of course.) Don't forget to eat yogurt every day, too. Inserting 250 mg a day of vitamin C vaginally once a day for six days has been shown to cure vaginitis in pregnant women and reduce vaginal pH.[9]

Vitamin D deficiency is linked to higher rates of BV during pregnancy,[10] as is iron deficiency.[11] About half (or more[12]) of pregnant women are deficient in vitamin D,[13] even when taking prenatal vitamins.[14] If your level of vitamin D is less than optimal, you are not alone. More may be in order. (Please see Vitamin D chapter). You can help your body absorb supplemental iron by taking it along with plenty of vitamin C. Personally speaking, if the word "infection" is ever part of my doctor's diagnosis, I take very large doses of vitamin C regularly for several days until the infection is gone. (Please see the chapter on Vitamin C for more about taking therapeutic doses.)

Chronic stress is also associated with BV during pregnancy,[15] suggesting yet another reason to make stress reduction part of your pregnancy routine.

BLEEDING GUMS

It is not uncommon to experience inflamed, bleeding gums during pregnancy. This is usually attributed to pregnancy hormones, and treatment advice basically suggests that you practice good hygiene. However, careful brushing and all the dental floss in the world may not solve the problem. Consider the benefits of extra vitamin C. Bleeding gums and gingivitis are notorious signs of vitamin C deficiency. Capillary walls have to be weakened to bleed. Vitamin C strengthens this bond and holds cells together. If you bleed when you brush, it may be your body's way of indicating your need for more C. James. F. Balch, MD, says, "Increase the intake of vitamin C rich foods as a deficiency in this vitamin can contribute to bleeding gums."[16]

COLDS, FLU, AND MORE: SICKNESS DURING PREGNANCY

"Drugs make a well person sick.
Why would they make a sick person well?"
—ABRAM HOFFER, MD

If you think this section is going to recommend vitamin C, you are way ahead of me. Good for you. Being pregnant is work enough, but getting sick while you are pregnant makes everything even harder. Throw in a busy work schedule and taking care of family and being sick is positively overwhelming.

A trip to the doctor will help you better understand what is you are fighting, but I've found that their protocol is often the same. You'll leave with a prescription for an antibiotic, and perhaps a suggestion to take over-the-counter pain relief or cold medicine. If you are fighting a virus, the antibiotics won't work. If you are fighting bacteria, the antibiotics might work and they might not, thus leading you back to the doc for another variety of the drug.

Some of us may find it difficult to feel comfortable putting medicines into our bodies, whether we are pregnant or not. We have been so careful to do the right thing during pregnancy and avoid any potentially harmful substances, and to start taking medication now because we are sick may be pretty scary. If you are looking for options outside of the medical bag, please read the section "Vitamin C: An Alternative to Antibiotics" in the chapter dedicated to this important nutrient. See that you get enough zinc, between 12–40 milligrams (mg) each day, too. Most pregnant women don't.[17] Your baby needs zinc, and so do you. Divide your dose and take it with meals to avoid stomach upset.

Don't forget all your other vitamins when you are feeling under the weather, especially vitamins A and D. Drink plenty of water and juice fresh, raw (organic, if possible) veggies each day that you are sick. And rest. If you are too busy to rest, then you are too busy. This may be inconvenient, but being sick is more inconvenient. You can stack the deck in your favor and get well sooner.

FLU SHOT DURING PREGNANCY? I SAID, "NO, THANK YOU."

Just yesterday on a morning news program, the flu vaccine was being pushed on pregnant women again. The guest ob-gyn emphasized how critically essential it was for women to get the flu vaccine administered during pregnancy, adding to this that she had known a pregnant woman who had died from the flu. Even the Centers for Disease Control and Prevention (CDC) say "Pregnant? Get a Flu Shot!"[18] (Yes, the exclamation point is included.) Furthermore, the CDC insists it is safe for both mom and baby and that millions of pregnant women have received the vaccine.

Millions of women may get the flu vaccine, but that has nothing to do with whether or not it is safe. It also has nothing to do with whether or not it is effective. It happens to be neither.

First, let's talk safety. Thimerosal is a mercury-based preservative in most flu vaccines.[19] Mercury has NEVER been safe for anyone, let alone a developing baby. It is inherently toxic. If you choose to immunize your children, you'll find that most vaccinations for kids don't contain thimerosal anymore. Why would we go and blast mom and an unborn infant with a dose? "There is a stack of evidence that strongly supports that the mercury used in nearly all flu vaccines is clearly associated with brain injury in children that are born to vaccinated mothers," says Joseph Mercola, MD.[20] There is no safe dose of mercury for your baby. There is also the inherent risk of side effects. "Whatever you may have heard, there is no such thing as a medication without the risk of side effects," says prominent British physician Damien Downing. "In vaccines that risk can also come from the adjuvants. A vaccine is a small dose of an organism plus adjuvants—chemicals that are irritants to the immune system and trigger it to react to the organism part. Without adjuvants vaccines generally won't work. Popular adjuvants include the antibiotic gentamicin (too much of which can make you deaf), aluminum compounds (which probably contribute to Alzheimer's and other neurological diseases), and the mercury antiseptic, thiomersal/thimerosal (long known to be toxic and recently suspected in autism)—after all, they have to be toxic to work as adjuvants. Fluarix, one of the main brands of flu vaccine in the USA and UK, is stated by the manufacturers to contain both gentamicin and thimerosal."[21]

Would getting the vaccine be safer than risking death from the flu? "Death caused directly by the flu virus is very rare," says Dr. Mercola. "The vast majority of so-called "flu deaths" are in fact due to bacterial pneumonia—a potential complication of the flu if your immune system is too weak." [22] Yes, it is possible you could die from the flu, but according to Mercola, it is unlikely that the flu vaccine can prevent that unlikely death.[23]

Let's talk efficacy. "The decision to vaccinate pregnant women was based on two weak studies that in no way support this recommendation" says Mercola.[24] If you are worried about passing the flu on to your baby, don't be. Mercola says, "When you carefully analyze the first [study] you will find that the pregnant moms did not transfer the flu infection to their babies."[25] Pregnant women are led to believe that vaccination will prevent complications from the flu.[26] "The stinker here is that the government used the fact that there were significant differences in complications between vaccinated and unvaccinated pregnant women," says Mercola. But these complications were not potentially fatal illnesses, like pneumonia, but "merely symptoms like chest pain and other minor issues, which could have even been related to a strong immune response providing permanent authentic immunity to the infection."[27] This would appear to make the flu shot less than necessary.

The CDC says, "If you're pregnant, a flu shot is your best protection against serious illness from the flu."[28] But where is the evidence to support this claim? "Study after study comes back showing the same dismal results," says Mercola. "[T]he flu vaccines are not an effective method of prevention of the flu, and they do not save lives."[29]

"Whatever you may have heard, there is no such thing as a medication without the risk of side effects."
—DAMIEN DOWNING, MD

WHAT ABOUT TAMIFLU? (I heard there is a shortage.)

If you get the flu while you are pregnant, you may be urged to take a drug like Tamiflu. Not only can taking this drug be unsafe during pregnancy and lactation,[30] but these medications are "practically useless" says Dr. Downing.[31] Authors of a comprehensive review in *The Lancet* concluded that "the use of antiviral drugs for the treatment of people presenting with symptoms is unlikely to be the most appropriate course of action."[32] This review of Tamiflu (oseltamivir) and Relenza (zanamivir) showed that the overall reduction in flu symptoms when taking these antivirals was *less than a day*.[33] You have to ask yourself this question: Is it worth taking a drug—and risking side effects, especially during pregnancy—when they do such a poor job anyway?

Being sick sucks, but taking Tamiflu isn't the answer for wellness. Many women may put a false sense of hope in medication, when what their body really needs is nutrition.

CONSTIPATION

You may have noticed your "going" habits have changed while you are pregnant, and by that I mean it's harder to go and less frequent, too. One culprit is iron.

Pregnant gals are supposed to make sure they are getting enough iron. With the Recommended Dietary Allowance (RDA) set at 27 mg (and 18 mg for non-pregnant ladies) all that extra iron is helping your body build an additional person. You may find when you are not getting enough iron, you feel fatigued. Sure, if it's the first trimester, you'll be feeling tired anyway, but once your second trimester comes along, you should be feeling more energetic. If you are relying on a prenatal vitamin, it is likely that it comes with the recommended dosage of iron. Iron supplementation may also come with the unpleasant side effect of constipation. Side effects from constipation include hemorrhoids (ouch!) and just not feeling very . . . well . . . clean and empty. But it's important to make sure you are getting enough iron, and it's also important that you are absorbing enough of the iron you get. Taking vitamin C along with iron helps iron absorption. (I take about 6,000–10,000 of vitamin C a day. I make a point to take some of it, 4,000 mg or so, along with my iron supplement.) Taking extra vitamin C along with iron also helps you avoid constipation. This is one of the advantages of taking larger doses of vitamin C. In fact, reaching "bowel tolerance" is when you have taken enough vitamin C that you get loose stools. This is called "saturation" of vitamin C, and it means that your body has absorbed all it can of the vitamin for the moment. Among the many other benefits of vitamin C, it may offer the relief you are looking for if you are constipated. Having prolonged periods of diarrhea is not good, so the goal is to take enough C to get the result you seek (a bowel movement) without an explosive visit to the potty. Knowing your own particular limit takes practice. Keep in mind that there will be days when your body can handle more C (if you are sick or stressed out) and days when less will do the trick. Vitamin C is one natural way to move things along when needed.

I also take supplemental magnesium citrate (an additional 100–200 mg). Magnesium is important and needed for over 300 biochemical reactions in our bodies.[34] In larger doses, magnesium, like vitamin C, has the added advantage of being a natural laxative. Epsom salt baths are also indicated for folks who wish to relieve themselves of minor constipation. Tossing a cup or two of Epsom salt in a warm bath and soaking for fifteen minutes can give you a constipation-relieving dose of magnesium transdermally, and may be more easily absorbed by your body than oral forms of the mineral.

Some foods, like meat and cheese, are notorious for binding up our bowels. Focus on all that fiber we are supposed to be eating. I have yet to drink a glass of fresh, homemade, carrot juice without a regularly scheduled visit to the loo. Other fiber-rich foods include whole wheat, bran, brown rice, fruits (prunes are great for this) and berries, nuts, seeds like flaxseed, veggies, lentils, and beans. And of course, drink plenty of water.

CRAMPS, TIGHT CALVES, AND BODY SORENESS

Painful leg cramps bother many a pregnant gal. There were a couple of nights during my third trimesters when I woke up with tight calves. I would immediately flex my feet (not point my toes) and the sensation of the looming cramp would subside. However, even if I avoided the full-blown cramp, my lower legs would still feel like they were taut rubber bands, just waiting for a chance to spring back and bunch up into a painful little ball and give me a heck of a charley horse. While I was fortunate to experience only one painful leg cramp during my first pregnancy (the kind that has your leg feeling sore for days), I didn't enjoy the tight-calf feeling at all. So I did something about it.

Stretching, walking, exercising, drinking plenty of fluids, and massage were all helpful. So was additional magnesium.

A warm bath was always a welcome activity when I was pregnant. Here's another good reason to get your hands on some Epsom salt, also known as magnesium sulfate. For years folks have known about the benefits of magnesium when it comes to muscle relaxation. Soaking my tight calves (and sore neck and shoulders from carrying my first bundle of joy around all day) in this extra magnesium often made the difference between a restless and restful night's sleep. During my second pregnancy I was able to avoid painful cramping entirely.

Vitamin C, 1,000 mg twice a day, may also help you get rid of pregnancy-induced leg cramps.[35] Calcium supplementation, 1,000 mg a day, was also shown to be as effective as vitamin C for leg cramps.[36] Carolyn Dean, MD, would recommend you balance your intake of calcium with supplemental magnesium. Up to 400 mg a day of supplemental magnesium may help with cramps during pregnancy.[37]

> Melvyn R. Werbach, MD, says, "Magnesium has shown itself in double-blind studies to be an effective treatment for leg cramps."[38]

CRAVINGS

Maybe it occurred to me that I was dealing with pregnancy-related cravings the night I so desperately wanted chocolate mousse that I couldn't think about anything else. I needed cream for the recipe, and had none. My husband was away and the baby was in bed. I nearly woke her and dragged her sleepy self to the store in her pajamas. She was spared when I found the ingredients for chocolate pudding instead, which was a sorry second choice as far as I was concerned. I mixed up a batch, waited impatiently for it to (mostly) cool in the fridge, and after a few warm spoonfuls decided that I was still unsatisfied and what I really wanted was chocolate mousse.

Or maybe it was the next night, when my pregnant belly and I were at the grocery store late in the evening and I noticed the sheer quantity of chocolate from my cart moving determinedly down the conveyor belt toward the grocery store clerk. Double chocolate hot chocolate, dark chocolate chips, a chocolate protein beverage, a decadent chocolate dessert that consisted of a thick layer of chocolate cream, another of chocolate fudge, both sandwiched between two fluffy cake-like chocolate brownies, topped with chocolate icing, chocolate drizzle, and chocolate sprinkles. Oh yes, and a package of emergency chocolate mousse mix.

The next week my doctor looked over his glasses, tapped on my chart, and commented that I gained a bit much for two weeks . . . about five pounds.

Hmm. I can't imagine why.

It's hard to resist treats when you are pregnant. I mean, you're going to be huge anyway. Why not have some sugar? There will be plenty of time post pregnancy to chase the kids and work off that extra weight and regulate the intake of sweets. Perhaps I felt even more justified in my actions since I had shed all the baby weight from my first pregnancy before I became pregnant with my second child. It's okay, I told myself, to have some dessert.

I can't possibly be the only pregnant gal who has convinced herself of this.

But perhaps this was getting a bit out of hand. I was a bit embarrassed at the grocery store that day, as I was with the gentle "tap tap" on the doctor's clipboard and gentle scolding.

So what is *with* these cravings? What can we do about it? I'm sure that exhibiting some level of self control is in order, first and foremost. But when this feels impossible, maybe we can make it easier on ourselves and use a bit of nutrition to take the edge off.

We know we need to keep weight gain under control during pregnancy. And if you are craving dirt or some other non-food substance (a condition known as pica), especially items that could be toxic for you or your baby, you should talk to your doctor about it and see if an underlying cause can be determined. If you are craving odd or abnormal foods, low levels of zinc or iron may be to blame.[39] It's been said, for example, that some women find intense cravings for ice that are due to their need for more iron during pregnancy. (It is also worth considering that perhaps your body needs more help absorbing the iron it is getting. Taking additional vitamin C could be helpful.) And then there are pickles.

Pregnant with our second child, my husband knew the drill. Without being asked, he came home from the grocery store with a jar of pickles he deemed "pregnancy size." Indeed it was. He hefted an enormous jug of marinated cukes onto the counter. It was considerably larger than my head. He had to rearrange the shelves in our refrigerator to compensate for the sheer volume of the vessel. Craving vinegar-laden foods is not uncommon during pregnancy. If you, too, have the pregnancy-pickle hankering, or have eaten mustard straight off a spoon, or poured copious quantities of hot sauce on, well, whatever you can, your current intake of calcium should be considered. Vinegar is a weak acid and helps dissolve calcium. You may find that increasing your calcium intake reduces your craving for foods soaked in vinegar.

DEEP VEIN THROMBOSIS (DVT)

While it is rare, DVT occurs more commonly in pregnancy than in non-pregnant women. It can be serious, and should be treated. If drinking plenty of water, exercising, eating right, and not smoking don't keep you DVT-free, then it is likely your doctor will suggest anticoagulant drugs. It is also just as unlikely that they will discuss vitamin E. Vitamin E can entirely, or in part, substitute for anticoagulant drugs, and do it more safely.[40] There is good reason to consider non-drug alternatives. Here's why:

The blood thinner warfarin should not be taken during pregnancy. Sodium warfarin (Coudamin, Jantoven) is, believe it or not, rat poison. Take too much and you will die from internal bleeding. (Just like the rodents do.) There is good reason right there to not take it while pregnant. And sadly, there is more. According to RxList, "Coumadin exposure during pregnancy causes a recognized pattern of major congenital malformations (warfarin embryopathy and fetotoxicity), fatal fetal hemorrhage, and an increased risk of spontaneous abortion and fetal mortality."[41] These are the *known* problems. This may be hard to imagine but RxList also says, "While Coumadin is contraindicated during pregnancy, the potential benefits of using Coumadin may outweigh the risks for pregnant women with mechanical heart valves at high risk of thromboembolism."[42]

Don't believe it.

Miscarriage, birth defects, and the death of your baby *are too much to risk,* especially when there is a far safer alternative available in vitamin form. We can protect mom and baby at the same time, and do it safely with nutrients.

If they are smart enough to not prescribe warfarin, Heparin sodium (an anticoagulant) is likely to be your doctor's choice for DVT during pregnancy. While it is regarded as a less dangerous alternative to warfarin, heparin still comes with a lengthy list of possible side effects, as drugs often do. Keep in mind, "There are no adequate and well-controlled studies on heparin use in pregnant women," says RxList. If we choose to accept this treatment, we choose to be an experiment as well as a patient. These are strong words, but I feel very strongly about this. When in doubt, say no to drugs.

Vitamin E, however, has an extraordinary safety record and is a nutrient necessary for a healthy pregnancy. Its importance is evident by its very name "tocopherol," which means to bring forth life. No drug carries this kind of credential. Vitamin E's blood-thinning effect is the reason Drs. Evan and Wilfrid Shute (both obstetricians) used 1,000–2,000 international units (IU) a day to treat thrombophlebitis (swelling in a vein caused by a blood clot) and related conditions.[43] You can experiment with your doctor's drugs, or you can learn more about vitamin E and its benefits that have been known by orthomolecular doctors and specialists for decades. (You can read more about dosage and safety in the chapter dedicated to vitamin E.)

DIABETES

It is estimated that 1.85 million women of childbearing age in the United States have diabetes, with an estimated half a million of these women unaware that they even have the condition.[44] If a pregnant woman has pre-existing diabetes, her risk of fetal birth defects is nearly four times that of pregnant women who are not diabetic, increasing her chances of having a baby with a birth defect to about one in fourteen.[45] I don't like those odds, and you probably don't either. It doesn't mean you'll have a baby with a birth defect, but let's do what we can to decrease the possibility.

Ideally, diabetes should be addressed before conception. This can be done by improving our diet, exercising, and working with our doctor to keep blood glucose levels under control. Lifestyle modification is a huge part of the answer. If we are already pregnant, we can do even more. Let's reduce the risk of having a baby with birth defects any way we can. Vitamin supplementation is one way. Pregnancy is no time to ignore the optimal intake of essential nutrients both you and your baby need.

Nutritional deficiencies are very common in diabetics.[46] According to orthopedic surgeon Marc S. Stevens, MD, "Diabetes frequently causes nutritional deficiencies, often initiated by changes in diet or medications. As a result, people with diabetes must use supplements."[47] Deficiencies of vitamin B_{12}, Vitamin D, vitamin E, and magnesium are often found in people with diabetes, he says. Therefore, says Stevens, "It is absolutely critical that people with diabetes not only work closely with their doctor to control their blood sugar, but also pay equally close attention to nutrition and nutritional supplementation."

Antioxidant vitamins like C and E may be helpful for the prevention of birth defects in diabetic moms. In an animal study, administration of vitamin E decreased the rate of embryo malformations and increased their size and maturation.[48] In other animal studies of experimental diabetic pregnancy, vitamin C, along with vitamin E, "decreases fetal malformation rate and diminishes oxygen radical-related tissue damage."[49] Fewer deformities is good news for rodents. It is really good news for us. While lower levels of antioxidants still achieved positive results, specifically "high-dose antioxidant supplementation decreased fetal dysmorphogenesis" (abnormal tissue formation) "to near normal levels."[50] Another animal study, using much higher doses of vitamin C, found even that *extremely* high doses of vitamin C caused *no adverse effects for the offspring* even when their diabetic mothers were getting up to 15 percent of their diet as vitamin C,[51] an incredibly huge amount of vitamin C to be sure. No, we don't need that much. But seeing that something is safe, even in very large quantities, can help us feel better about taking less, even if "less" for us is still more than what's listed on the label of our prenatal vitamin.

Gestational Diabetes

Pregnancy-onset diabetes is gestational diabetes, and if you have it you aren't alone. It is one of the most common health issues during pregnancy. A good diet with plenty of veggies and seeing that you get regular exercise is always important, and is especially important if you have gestational diabetes. Now, for the health of our baby, we may have more motivation than ever to eat right and exercise. It is also important to address nutrient deficiencies.

According to the National Institutes of Health, "Women who have had gestational diabetes are at increased risk for developing diabetes in the future, and their child is also at increased risk for obesity and type 2 diabetes."[52] There is a strong dietary connection here. Not getting enough vitamin C in your diet is linked with an increased risk for gestational diabetes.[53] Higher levels of homocysteine (an amino acid in the blood) are also found in women with gestational diabetes,[54] and "serum homocysteine is significantly associated with vitamin B_{12} and folate levels."[55] Not enough B_{12}, folic acid, and B_6 means more homocysteine, whereas increasing your intake of these vitamins means less homocysteine. Eat your green leafy veggies, keep taking folic acid, and investigate your B_{12} levels. B_{12} deficiency may be an underlying risk factor for gestational diabetes.[56] According to nutrition expert Patrick Holford, supplementing with extra

B[3] (25 mg) and chromium (200 micrograms (mcg)), in addition to your multivitamin, will help manage glucose.[57] There's more. "Women who develop gestational diabetes should be particularly concerned about getting adequate amounts of zinc," says Ian E. Brighthope, MD, author of *The Vitamin Cure for Diabetes.* "In fact," he says, "zinc may help prevent diabetes during pregnancy." [58] In addition to zinc, [59] vitamin D,[60] vitamin E,[61] and selenium[62] are all going to be of special importance, as lower levels of these nutrients are often associated with increased risks for gestational diabetes.

ENDOMETRIOSIS

Antioxidants may help women reduce pain and inflammation due to endometriosis. One study demonstrated that 1,200 IU of vitamin E and 1,000 mg of vitamin C helped women experience significant improvement of their endometriosis pain and inflammation.[63] During the study, five women in the vitamin group became pregnant (versus none in the control group) and were excluded from the rest of the study.[64] (We know endometriosis can make it more difficult to get pregnant. Did vitamin therapy help these women conceive?) Interestingly, no one in the control group got pregnant nor did they experience any improvement in pain or inflammation.[65] James F. Balch, MD, recommends 2,000 mg of vitamin C, three times a day, and 400–1,000 IU of vitamin E for endometriosis.[66] Vitamin C and E are important. But so are all the other nutrients, including vitamin A, zinc, selenium, magnesium, and more. If you suffer with symptoms of endometriosis while you are pregnant, nutrition may be a welcome option for you. Make your body as healthy as possible so it becomes an inhospitable host for illness.

ENDOMETRITIS

Endometritis is one of the more common infections and causes of fever in women after childbirth. Having a C-section increases that risk. Although it may sound similar, endometritis is *different from endometriosis.* Endometritis is when the lining of your uterus becomes inflamed or irritated. In other words, it is an endometrial infection. Symptoms include abnormal vaginal bleeding or discharge, malaise (feeling "blah" all over), fever, abdominal pain, and swelling.[67]

You can get endometritis through sexually transmitted diseases (a good reason to have safe sex), it can be caused by imbalances in your normal vaginal bacteria, an infection that moves up from your lower genital tract, or after miscarriage. While endometritis can occur after vaginal birth, it more commonly occurs after C-section.[68] Besides having protected sex, prevention tactics include not douching, as douching disrupts your normal balance of bacteria and may increase your risk for endometritis,[69] keeping your immune system strong, and taking your vitamins and ingesting probiotics.

Antibiotics will be the go-to drug given to women with endometritis.[70] However, antibiotics may not have all the answers. These drugs do not kill selectively; they target good bacteria right along with the bad. To help avoid creating additional problems from a bacterial imbalance caused by antibiotics, regularly reintroduce probiotics (for example, by eating yogurt everyday) and keep your immune system strong with a great diet (try doing fresh, raw vegetable juicing), and take your vitamins. Whenever "itis" is part of the conversation so should "vitamin C." If you have any infection, take enough C to reach bowel tolerance. Keep the dosage up until your symptoms are gone. Gradually reduce your megadose to a maintenance dose to help keep your immune system strong. Vitamins A and E are excellent immunity builders and infection fighters, too.

FATIGUE

Ladies, you are going to be tired, and the best prescription for fatigue is rest. There is no substitute for sleep. For goodness' sake, you are growing a whole other human being. This is exhausting work. It takes a huge amount of energy to construct a kid. You must make the time to take a load off. When I was teaching middle school during my first pregnancy, I would close the door, turn off the lights, and fall asleep at my desk for fifteen minutes during my lunch break. That little catnap allowed me to get through the rest of my day. Be sure to eat many small meals to keep your energy up. Pregnancy exercise could also improve your sleepy state. Nutrient deficiency could also be to blame for your fatigue. Not getting enough iron could make you sleepy, as could inadequate levels of vitamin C, the B vitamins, and magnesium. Selenium, zinc, and the omega-3 fatty acids are also important. Take your vitamins, and take a nap.

FORGETFULNESS

I started paying more attention to vitamins when I found myself unable to pay attention to little else. I could forget a conversation I had mere seconds before; I could lose my keys while they were in my hands. I would stand outside a store and blink dumbly at a lot full of cars in the hope that inspiration might spark my memory as to where my vehicle might be, or even which vehicle I drove there in the first place. I guess I could always press the car's panic button. . . .

Then came the day I found myself lost in my own city. I should have been able to get home in twenty minutes. Instead, I was on the wrong expressway, going farther and farther away from where I needed to be but unable to determine where I made the wrong turn or where I could even get back to a place I recognized. To make things worse, I took the exit ramp into a maze of side streets where I just made myself even more lost. Unfamiliar surroundings prompted me to stay in my car, and inhibited any common sense that might have led me to a convenience store to ask for directions. This sounds silly, I know. I feel silly writing it down. It seems I *should* have been able to figure out what to do. But I just sat in my car and drove around becoming more confused. Foolish me, I didn't have my GPS on board, and I still have one of those old phones that can't determine my location and attempt to get me home. I made some phone calls, hoping someone might be next to a computer, but of course, folks were unavailable. For over an hour I drove through unknown streets in a direction I thought might lead me toward where I was aiming to be—without success. Finally I got in touch with my husband and he (with Google maps, as even he was confused as to where I ended up that day) was able to get me on the right path.

The existence of "pregnancy brain" may still have the scientists guessing, but not me. I didn't need a study to confirm whether or not what I was experiencing was real. It seemed as if the little life inside my belly was sucking up my last working brain cells along with everything else it required from me to grow.

Enough is enough, I thought. I decided to hit this "pregnancy brain" issue head on. And it turns out lecithin was just what I was looking for. Choline (considered part of the B vitamin group) is found in lecithin as phosphatidyl choline. When pregnant rats were given choline it helped improve the brain function of their young. If taking lecithin could provide, as stated in *Journal of the American College of Nutrition,* "lifelong memory enhancement"[71] for rodent babies, I figured it may just help me find my car in the grocery store parking lot.

When I suffered from "pregnancy brain," I bolstered my lecithin intake and found it to be true: lecithin helped clear my mind and rid me of that fuzzy-brain feeling. I also found my car. Lecithin helped me think more clearly and remember what the heck I was supposed to be doing. It was an added bonus that my baby would likely benefit as well.

GALLSTONES

Gallstones are common during pregnancy and postpartum. The most common gallstones are cholesterol gallstones, and cholesterol levels increase during pregnancy. Studies have shown that higher serum levels of vitamin C are inversely related to incidence of gallstones in women.[72] A vegetarian diet, which is typically high in vitamin C, protects against gallstones.[73] In fact, if you are interested in cutting your risk of stones in half, become a vegetarian.[74] Or if you prefer to be an omnivore, you can add plenty of fruit, vegetables, and fiber to your meals and get the same benefit.[75] More vitamin C in your system means less suffering from stones. Along with vitamin C, a diet to help prevent gallstones or help them dissolve would contain an adequate intake of vitamin E, vitamin A, essential fatty acids (like those found in lecithin), and the B vitamins.[76]

GROUP B STREP

If you are pregnant, it is likely that you have been screened for group b Streptococcus (GBS). About a quarter of all healthy women have it.[77] It naturally exists in the body like many other kinds of bacteria. However, due to the risk of transferring GBS to an infant, which could potentially make them ill, women with GBS will routinely be given preventive intravenous (IV) antibiotics during delivery.[78] If you have GBS, this will be presented to you as a requirement, not a choice. Before "agreeing" to an IV, you may wish to consider this:

How healthy you are impacts how healthy the baby is, or will be. When babies are born they are exposed to trillions of bacteria in mom's vaginal tract.[79] Emerging research shows this exposure (and that obtained through breastfeeding) impacts the lifelong health of the child.[80] If we are giving IV antibiotics to a mother at this crucial time in her baby's life, we have to ask ourselves if reducing the risk of GBS is more important than making sure babies are exposed to plentiful and diverse beneficial bacteria at birth; microorganisms that are essential for building baby's tolerance and immunity.

And just because we aim to prevent exposure at birth does not mean we prevent exposure. "Indeed human milk frequently contains low amounts of non-pathogenic bacteria like Streptococcus, Micrococcus, Lactobacillus, Staphylococcus, Corynebacterium and Bifidobacterium."[81]

Perhaps these microorganisms aren't to be feared, but revered, or at least respected. Bacteria are literally everywhere. This is how immune systems develop. (I like to remember this when my toddler will inadvertently swallow mouthfuls of lake water at the beach.) "Good" and "bad" bacteria are always present; in a healthy body they live together peacefully and in balance with one another. Should we seek to annihilate bacteria with antibiotics, or work to achieve strong immune systems that can effectively manage inevitable exposure to microorganisms? Infections can be serious. But I think it is high time for us to remember words that were attributed long ago to Louis Pasteur: "The germ is nothing. The terrain is everything."

If you are given antibiotics during delivery for GBS, help regain your beneficial bacteria by eating probiotic foods and taking probiotic supplements every day, starting in the hospital, and preferably long before. If your infant has been exposed to antibiotics, you can promote beneficial bacteria by slipping a tiny little bit of watery yogurt into your baby's mouth or by putting it on your nipples before breastfeeding. Keep your immune system strong with good diet and ideal vitamin intake to fend off post-antibiotic opportunistic infections.

HEMORRHOIDS

Applied topically, Vitamin E can provide relief and comfort for this uncomfortable addition to our list of pregnancy woes. And drink more water. You'll also want to buy a juicer or higher-powered blender—and use it. Raw vegetable juicing (or blending) will make bathroom visits more frequent and comfortable, and will reduce the need for straining on the toilet. Homemade vegetable juice contains both soluble and insoluble fiber. Soluble fiber helps keep cholesterol in check and lower your risk of high blood pressure or cardiovascular disease during pregnancy. Insoluble fiber keeps your gastrointestinal tract healthy and constipation-free. Fresh vegetable juice provides extra liquid and is also packed with nutrients straight from the source that both you and your baby will thrive on.

HERPES: COLD SORES AND VAGINAL LESIONS

You don't need to permanently be on antiviral medication to keep herpes lesions or cold sores away. Your immune system can do it for you. Your job is to provide the necessary tools so it can: eat right, exercise, drink fresh, raw veggie juice, rest, and drink plenty of water. But that's not all. Take your vitamins. They are all important, but this is *especially* true for vitamin C, which is great for fighting any infection, including herpes,[82] and is necessary and beneficial for a body under stress, a common precursor to herpes outbreaks. (To find out more about the benefits of vitamin C, see the Vitamin C and Pregnancy chapter.) Vitamin A is also needed to fight infection. (There's a chapter on this vitamin, too.) Do your best to manage stress *and* take your vitamins. Everything listed above will help your body cope with inevitable stress, and also keep your body healthy and free of those uncomfortable and unsightly sores.

And there's even more you can do.

L-lysine, an essential amino acid that is necessary for life, will help minimize, shorten, or prevent a herpes outbreak, naturally. The "beneficial effects" of lysine include "accelerating recovery from herpes simplex infection and suppressing recurrence" in patients taking 312–1,200 mg a day[83] and "decreasing the recurrence rate of herpes simplex attacks" in patients taking 1,248 mg a day.[84] One study (using 1,000 mg of lysine daily) found "significantly more patients were recurrence-free during lysine than during placebo treatment."[85] Another concluded "L-lysine (3,000mg/day) appears to be an effective agent for reduction of occurrence, severity and healing time for recurrent HSV [herpes simplex virus] infection."[86]

Dose matters. Higher concentrations of lysine in the blood mean significantly fewer outbreaks, according to one study.[87] The amount it takes to achieve the optimal level of lysine may vary from person to person.

Taken at the earliest "tingle," several thousand mg (3,000–5,000 a day) can keep lesions away or reduce the severity of an outbreak. To reduce recurrences, consider taking smaller, daily maintenance doses of 500–1,000 mg.

If you are pregnant you should talk to your doctor before taking a supplement. But lysine is very safe. It is naturally present in all sorts of foods like chicken, pork, turkey, potatoes, yogurt, milk, cheese, lentils, and eggs. A three-ounce serving of chicken provides about 2,500 mg of lysine. A cup of yogurt contains nearly 3,000 mg of lysine. Your doctor is probably not telling you to avoid poultry or dairy products while pregnant. Instead, I imagine that he or she would encourage you to eat such foods.

If the only answer your doctor has for herpes is an "antiviral drug" then maybe it is time to see what essential nutrients can do for you. If your doctor says, "Well, there aren't any studies about pregnancy and lysine— better not take it," you can mention that there is also a conspicuous lack of studies about antiviral drugs during pregnancy.

Herpes, like any infection, is opportunistic. But you do not have to depend on drugs to keep you free of sickness. Depend on your immune system instead. But you have to take care of yourself. Prescription drugs are not the easy way out. Not a single cell in your body or your baby's body is made out of a drug. A body that craves nutrients will get no real relief with medications. The only way to achieve a consistently healthy self is through nutrition. Remember, nutrients like vitamins and essential amino acids are vastly safer than drugs. They always will be.

HIGH BLOOD PRESSURE: GESTATIONAL HYPERTENSION

Magnesium and potassium work with sodium to regulate blood pressure.[88] Goodness knows most of us get plenty of sodium in our diets. It's the other two nutrients we have to wonder about. Recommended levels of potassium are 4,700 mg a day during pregnancy and 5,100 mg a day if you are breastfeeding, but the average gal gets only half that, just 2,500 mg a day.[89] The same is true of magnesium. Only about half of us are getting what we need.[90] Consuming plenty of fruits, vegetables, and beans is important during pregnancy, and you can also choose to supplement your diet with extra magnesium, such as magnesium citrate tablets or powder. You may want to pass on supplemental potassium, though. It's just easier (and less expensive) to get potassium from your diet instead. Sure, there are potassium pills out there, but they contain very little of the mineral compared to the amount available in lots of tasty foods, like citrus fruits, beets, beans, yogurt, nuts, spinach, and potatoes. Calcium may also help prevent pregnancy-induced high blood pressure.[91] Getting 1,200–1,500 mg a day should do the trick.[92]

Vitamins C and vitamin E are also helpful, as is vitamin D. "Vitamin C deficiency has been shown to play an integral role in the actual causation and sustaining of high blood pressure," says Thomas Levy, MD. "Vitamin C alone is effective in lowering the blood pressure of hypertensive patients."[93] Studies have shown that vitamin E can normalize blood pressure.[94] "In some hypertensive persons, commencement of very large vitamin E doses may cause a slight temporary increase in blood pressure, although maintained supplementation can then be expected to lower it," says Andrew W. Saul, PhD. "The solution is to increase the vitamin gradually, along with the proper monitoring that hypertensive patients should have anyway." [95] And, as for Vitamin D, it may help decrease your chances of having high-blood pressure.[96]

Staying active and practicing relaxation are very effective stress reducers, a factor which may contribute to higher blood pressure. Lugging around all that extra weight has probably made you feel more like curling up on the couch under a soft blanket with a bowlful of ice cream rather than pulling on stretch pants and busting your butt in a sweaty work out. (We're *relaxing*, right? And . . . getting some calcium?) But really, there's no need for excessive sweating. When you are pregnant, you'll be encouraged to stick to moderate exercises like walking and yoga. Achieve the benefits of activity without all the extra laundry.

INFECTION

Your best defense against serious illness is being healthy. That is not always as self-evident as it may sound. If we aim to have a body with a strong immune system that protects us against infections of all types, we should consider how immunity boosters like vitamins can play a role in our health. Our bodies are under enormous amounts of stress during pregnancy. The baby's demands for nutrients are ever increasing. A healthy diet rich in fruits and vegetables is essential to build our tolerance and immunity and give back to our body what our babies need and use. Getting optimal levels of nutrients through our food is difficult, even when we are paying close attention to what we eat. Vitamin and mineral supplementation over and above what you may be getting in your diet and prenatal multivitamin may be what you need to keep infections away.

When I think of the word infection, the first vitamin that comes to mind is vitamin C. And *lots* of it. By "lots" I mean saturation level doses, or what it takes to reach "bowel tolerance." But that's not all. When faced with any sort of infection during pregnancy, give yourself the advantage by eating well (skipping the sugar and drinking raw vegetable juice), taking all your vitamins and essential nutrients such as vitamin D (especially when you can't get any sunshine), vitamin C, vitamin E, vitamin A, and zinc, all of which are known infection fighters. Don't forget about probiotics. And surely you have heard these before: get adequate rest, reduce stress, exercise, and drink plenty of water. In fact, all of this probably sounds pretty familiar if you've been reading right along. But it's important enough to warrant restating.

We all get sick. How we choose to get better is where we differ. There is a way to heal from illness both safely and naturally. You don't have to do this, or anything thing else in this book for that matter, but this is what I do, pregnant or not, and it always helps me feel better.

INFERTILITY: TROUBLE GETTING PREGNANT

When you want to be pregnant, and aren't, you may find little else occupies your mind. Having trouble getting pregnant is not uncommon, but knowing this doesn't make it any easier when confronted with the possibility that maybe you can't. Sure, there are medical interventions that can help a couple achieve a pregnancy, but there are also nutritional avenues to consider. Things you can do right now to better the odds for that baby. Providing your body with the essential nutrients it needs so it can be in its most baby-ready state makes a whole lot of sense. It may also make you a whole-lotta-pregnant.

Current research suggests antioxidant intake may play an even greater role in combating infertility than we think.[97] Which antioxidants are important? Well, all of them. Nutrients work best together, so it's no surprise that many studies of infertility combine vitamins and minerals to achieve positive results. For example, vitamin E, zinc, selenium, and iron were shown to help increase pregnancy rates in women who had been trying to get pregnant for up to three years.[98] It is a great reason to start taking a multivitamin, if you aren't already. A daily multivitamin lowers the risk of ovulatory infertility[99] and supplementation with a multivitamin that contains folic acid may improve fertility.[100] Other studies have shown that 750 mg a day of vitamin C may help increase pregnancy rates.[101] Vitamin E and A may also help increase fertility potential, as a low concentration of these vitamins are associated with an inability to ovulate.[102] Magnesium (600 mg per day) and selenium (200 mcg per day) may also be helpful,[103] as may a daily intake of 15,000 IU of beta carotene, 400–1,000 IU of vitamin E, 150 mg a day of B_6, and a B complex vitamin.[104]

Don't forget your stud muffin. If he's feeling a bit helpless through all of this, hand him a vitamin bottle. According to researchers, the value of antioxidant treatment for male infertility "cannot be ignored."[105] In a recent review that looked at the effectiveness of oral antioxidants vitamin C, E, A, folate (B9), selenium, and zinc, it was shown that in 82 percent of trials, antioxidant therapy improved either sperm quality or pregnancy rates.[106] On the other hand, insufficient levels of antioxidants may contribute to male infertility.[107] Supplementing his diet with nutrients he needs anyway is a safe, inexpensive, and potentially effective way to help you both make a baby.

There are plenty of other options out there for a couple who wants to have a baby but is having difficulty doing so. Goodness knows your local fertility clinic has many ways to help, and countless families have benefited from their services. It would be great if something as simple, pain-free, and inexpensive as increased vitamin intake helped you have a great pregnancy.

PREGNANT PUTTY TATS

Based on the number of strays that roam through our property (they just love old barns), cats appear to have no trouble reproducing in astounding numbers. They are exposed to severe weather, infections, parasites, cars, and coyotes, but I have yet to see any decline in their population around these parts. (In fact, two of our house guests are former strays, and we have access to many more grateful freeloaders if we so choose.) Apparently, even cat reproduction can be affected by a suboptimal diet. Many, many years ago, Francis M. Pottenger, MD, ran a decade-long nutritional experiment. Yes, with cats. One group of kitties received heat-processed foods; the other felines were given only raw foods. Among their numerous health problems, the cats fed cooked food were infertile by the third generation.[108] Is there a lesson for people here? Carolyn Dean, MD, thinks so. "The Pottenger Cat Study is very instructive on the absolute requirement for good nutrition in pregnancy."[109] Cooking food can destroy nutrients, especially those particularly sensitive to heat, like vitamin C. Many health-conscious pregnant gals will make a point to incorporate lots of fresh fruits and veggies into their meals. A good diet is always a good idea, and the addition of vitamin supplements can be one way to regain nutrients we lose through cooking. Cats make their own vitamin C, and even they were still missing out on important nutrients destroyed when their food was cooked.

INSOMNIA: *See* SLEEPLESSNESS

MIGRAINE HEADACHES

I avoided the use of medications during pregnancy. Oh sure, maybe I *wanted* a drug or ten now and again, but I simply couldn't bring myself to take something that could possibly harm my baby. But when you have a headache ranging anywhere from mildly irritating to downright horrendous, it may be desperately hard to say no to drugs.

Prior to being pregnant and working in a high stress career, I had to battle through many a migraine headache that would have me unable to move. I remember one headache in particular that was so painful, nothing has really compared since. I'm saying this now with full knowledge of just how painful labor contractions can be, but even they were intermittent. Unlike a contraction, a migraine doesn't give you a second to recover. It presses and pounds and drives its way into you and behind your eyes with overwhelming tightening, stabbing pain. Being immobilized by pain is an awful experience. I was literally rescheduling everything around the "I'm probably going to have a migraine" week. I blocked it off on my calendar and made a point to not have any obligations. I could count on the headache coming in just prior to my period showing up, and lasting for a few days beyond. These "menstrual migraines" were predictable. It wasn't a question whether I'd get it or not. It was just a question of how bad it was going to be and how many days it would last. I wasn't interested in taking medication. I wanted a natural way out of this spin cycle. I wasn't going to accept that "hormonal changes" meant inevitable monthly migraines. I was going to be a woman for a long time. A migraine a month was unacceptable. I started looking into lifestyle factors that could be contributing to my pain: stress, lack of sleep, foods, beverages, food additives, etc. I wanted to know what helped, and what hurt—literally.

I found that stress is always a reason behind my pounding temples. Pain is a powerful motivator to change the way you live your life. I loved my job but stress was ruining a week out of every month. It didn't make my relationship any better, either. And I had had enough. My shoulder muscles would tense and tighten sending a cord of pain right up my neck to behind my eyes, where a headache settles in. A stressful experience that causes a rush of adrenaline is a sure sign I'll be getting a migraine within hours. Reducing stress is my first line of effective defense against migraines.

Getting enough rest is the other. But stress and lack of sleep is common, and therefore so, too, were my headaches.

Not everybody can change what they do for a living, but that's exactly what I decided to do. Now I am an author and a stay-at-home mom of two. Stress is still inevitable, but manageable. Once the intense stress I was under was alleviated, the migraines went with it for the most part. As a new mom, lack of sleep was harder to remedy. Occasionally, every so many months, I get a migraine for an afternoon or evening. They don't last nearly as long and they are not nearly as uncomfortable as they used to be, but a headache is still a pain, and never a welcome companion.

Each time I was pregnant, I also experienced a migraine that "set in" for a day. I used the same techniques to ease the pain of these headaches that I used to bypass the pain completely, if I tended to the symptoms of an oncoming migraine immediately. So while I was pregnant, there were the beginnings of a couple of migraines that I was able to overstep entirely, successfully and naturally, because I tended to them right away.

If you get headaches often, you are probably familiar with the signs that one is coming on. Mine always start small and then intensify over time. Left unattended, they can get the best of me. Treated early, I can get the best of them. As soon as I feel a migraine coming on, my migraine-stopping arsenal consists of the following:

1. **Take Niacin.** I take 100–250 mg of niacin (B_3) in the form of nicotinic acid specifically to achieve a flush, a side effect of taking this form of the vitamin. I do this immediately. If I do not experience a niacin flush, I take another 250 mg. My goal is to achieve a flush where my skin reddens and gets a little itchy. Once I am flushing, my headache often goes away—as long as I take the niacin as soon as my migraine begins.

   If the migraine takes hold, I still take the niacin. Once the migraine has "set in" a niacin flush does not take my headache away, but it *does* make it less painful. Steve Hickey, author of *The Vitamin Cure for Migraines,* has a doctorate in medical biophysics. He says, "Niacin is an excellent supplement for fending off a migraine attack—taken at an early stage, niacin can abort a migraine."[110]

   Since my migraines almost always surface after an adrenaline rush from a high-stress situation, I take niacin *immediately* after the rush; enough to achieve a flush. I am especially sensitive to my headache trigger the week before my period; this time of the month doesn't guarantee

I'll have a headache, but if a high-stress moment/adrenaline rush occurs, a headache is practically inevitable if I don't intervene. I make a point to carry niacin with me wherever I go.

2. **Drink Water.** I drink several pint glasses of water, on the spot. Sometimes this is all it takes. Dehydration can make headaches much worse, and I've found that chugging water can also get rid of a migraine that is about to start. I take water with me everywhere, too. "To handle a headache, begin drinking one eight- to twelve-ounce glass of water every five to ten minutes for one hour or until the headache is gone; whichever is less," says Jennifer Daniels, MD, MBA.[111]

3. **Get Magnesium.** I soak in an Epsom salt bath to give my body a large dose of magnesium. I also supplement by ingesting magnesium citrate tablets and/or powder. Stress hangs out in my neck and shoulders and can "pull" at one side of my face or the other. Magnesium relaxes muscles and can alleviate that pulling sensation, and also help lessen my migraine pain. After my bath I'll stand in the shower with my face right in the shower water. The droplets hitting my face allow my face muscles to unclench, and this, too, provides some pain relief. Magnesium is recommended by the European Federation of Neurological Societies for the treatment of migraines during pregnancy.[112] For prevention, I soak once a week, and more often after exercising.

Magnesium is recommended by the European Federation of Neurological Societies for the treatment of migraines during pregnancy.

4. **Take Vitamin C.** I get near to saturation of C. Large doses of vitamin C help relieve pain and help reduce inflammation.[113] I start by taking 3,000–4,000 mg of C, and then again an hour later if the headache persists. You can always start with less.

5. **Take B$_{12}$.** At early onset of a headache, B$_{12}$ may help. Take a sublingual tablet (one that dissolves under the tongue). Dr. Hickey explains, "Vitamin B$_{12}$ inhibits nitric oxide and can lower the inflammation and blood vessel dilation that occurs in a migraine."[114]

6. **Take riboflavin (B$_2$).** Studies have shown 400 mg a day can safely and effectively reduce migraine headache attacks.[115]

7. **Take Coenzyme Q$_{10}$.** In folks that get regular migraine headaches, 100 mg a day of coenzyme Q$_{10}$ reduced the number of migraine headaches and headache days and was found to be well tolerated.[116]

8. **Get some sleep.** When nothing else does it, a good night's sleep often does, as least it did in my case. When you are pregnant or have an infant, you often don't get the rest you need. My husband occasionally took over the baby feeding responsibility for a night on a weekend so I could get some needed shut-eye—you know, five hours at once instead of the usual two to three. Sometimes a night off is all it takes to reset. During the day, meditation or a quick nap while the kids sleep or play in their rooms helps me keep headaches away.

9. **Relax.** Ice or heat packs for my neck and shoulders, homeopathic remedies, fresh air, friends and other distractions away from stress, and therapeutic massages have all found a place in my headache hampering armory. Life does not always afford us such leisure, but we must find time to take care of ourselves if we are to be in any shape to take care of others.

10. **What about caffeine?** Caffeine helped my headaches when I wasn't pregnant, but I didn't want to use it for headache treatment when I was pregnant. We know caffeine is a drug. It is a widely used drug, but a drug nonetheless. The potential problems caffeine can cause for a developing baby[117] kept me away from it while I was pregnant. I felt the same when I was nursing. I didn't want caffeine transmitted into the milk and into my baby. While I avoided caffeine entirely while I was pregnant, when I was nursing my baby (and also the mother of an active child) sometimes a little compromise was necessary. If I needed to, I would drink some regular organic coffee or caffeinated green tea to get a little bit of caffeine into my system. This, in conjunction with everything else I was doing to fight my headache, was often enough to do the trick and ease the pain.

Prevention is always preferable to first-aid treatment. Much of the above can serve in this capacity. For example, I regularly take my vitamins, soak in Epsom salt baths, drink plenty of water, and make a point to rest and relax. Making sure I eat regularly helps, too. For ladies who suspect sensitivity to foods or beverages may be involved, it's worth it to track what you are eating before a migraine sets it. If anything is a modifiable factor, modify! Everyone is different. Do what works for you. Nobody knows you better than you do.

If prevention techniques ever fail you, take care of a headache as soon as you feel it start. Migraine sufferers will tell you this is the best time to fight its full blown effects. Knowing about natural treatments for headache pain is helpful when drugs are not a welcome option. I avoided taking pain pills during pregnancy, but I do not like hurting. "Just deal with it" was not going to work for me. Pregnancy forces us to contend with many aches and pains, and I didn't want headaches to be one of them. As far as I'm concerned, natural alternatives are always preferable, particularly when they work, and nutrients are always safer than drugs.

MISCARRIAGE

The worst possible occurrence during pregnancy is to lose the baby altogether. While the causes of miscarriages or spontaneous abortions may be unclear, we do know nutrition may help prevent them. You may find little comfort in these words, especially if you have suffered the loss of your baby, but knowing that nutrition could be part of solving the mystery of miscarriage may be encouraging.

There is a link between a diet low in antioxidants and recurrent pregnancy loss.[118] Research has shown that women who have experienced recurrent miscarriages have significantly lower levels of antioxidants than their healthy counterparts.[119] Even with careful attention, it may be difficult to achieve optimal levels of antioxidants such as vitamin E, vitamin C, beta-carotene, zinc, and selenium in our diets. Considering as many as 50 to 60 percent of recurrent miscarriages may be attributed to oxidative stress,[120] meaning for some women a higher intake of antioxidants may be needed. Additionally, women with high levels of homocysteine are more likely to experience recurrent miscarriages.[121] Higher levels of homocysteine are caused by deficiencies in certain nutrients like B vitamins (B_6, B_{12}, and folic acid) suggesting that B vitamin supplementation could be helpful.[122]

> As many as 50 to 60 percent of recurrent miscarriages may
> be attributed to oxidative stress, meaning for some women,
> a higher intake of antioxidants may be needed.

Good nutrition is always a good idea. If it helps you hold a pregnancy and give you the baby you have always wanted, it's an even better idea.

MOOD SWINGS AND INTENSE EMOTIONS

Hormones take us on one wild ride while we are pregnant. It's like experiencing the joys and pleasures of premenstrual syndrome (PMS) every day for nine months. Sure, we may not have to deal with our period for a while, but this is hardly a consolation. Month after month of moody mayhem hardly makes us feel lucky to be saving money on tampons, pads, and contraception. At least when we have PMS we know that it will pass in about a week and we can enjoy some time off the emotional rollercoaster.

Pregnancy (and afterward) gets a solid grip on our emotions and can make anything feel weep-worthy. To my great annoyance, I found my eyes moistening while watching home remodeling advertisements. Sure, their bathroom looks better now. But still. (I daresay the only redecorating going on in our house was the layer of eggshells added to our floors that my husband so carefully walked upon.) A fluffy puppy, a cute baby, actors smooching, kids baking cookies; just about anything could bring on a waterfall. It's not easy being pregnant, and the emotional turmoil that accompanies the mile-long list of worries we already have can make this time very difficult.

The B vitamins, like niacin (B_3) and B_6, are going to be especially helpful for mood swings, anxiety, or depression. Eat cashews, foods high in L-tryptophan, take magnesium, vitamin C, vitamin D, the omega-3 fatty acids, and stay as active as pregnant-ly possible. Read about nutritional therapy for postpartum depression in the chapter on post-pregnancy problems.

MORNING SICKNESS (NAUSEA)

Tossing your cookies? Or do you feel like you are about to? I know that morning, noon, and night sickness sucks. I had it. I should have bought company stock in Canada Dry. If you keep saltine crackers by your bedside, nibble on ginger strips you keep in your purse, or sip soda just to try and keep from periodic gagging and worse, adjusting your B_6 intake may help you feel less sick to your stomach. In one study of several hundred women, supplementation with 30 mg of B_6 every day significantly helped women feel less nauseous.[123] For women who experienced severe nausea and vomiting, another study in *Obstetrics and Gynecology* showed significant improvement with 75 mg a day of B_6.[124] The authors note, "At the completion of three days of therapy, only eight of thirty-one patients in the vitamin B_6 group had any vomiting, compared with fifteen of twenty-eight patients in the placebo group."[125] While your prenatal probably contains B_6 (see that it does) you may find more is helpful if your morning sickness is severe. The American College of Obstetrics and Gynecology currently recommends women take 10–25 mg of B_6 three to four times a day for nausea and vomiting during pregnancy, for a total dose of 40–100 mg a day.[126] Nutrition expert Patrick Holford suggests taking 50 mg of B_6 twice a day and a daily dose of 200–500 mg of magnesium for morning sickness.[127]

"Wait. The RDA for pregnant women is a teeny 2 mg a day. Is taking extra B_6 safe?" Yes. And it's a whole lot safer than drugs. (For more about B_6 safety, please see the chapter on B vitamins.)

What about Prescription Puke Pills?

The pharmaceutical industry would be happy to sell you expensive prescription medicines to help you feel less sick. For example, the drug Diclegis advertises that it's the only FDA-approved pill for run-of-the-mill morning sickness.[128] (It has not been approved for hyperemesis gravidarum, that super-awful form of morning sickness that prevents you from eating anything, including air, and lands you in the hospital with IV fluids.) Trials for Diclegis used a tool called the PUQE (I kid you not) score, or the Pregnancy-Unique Quantification of Emesis, to determine if the drug could help pregnant women *PUQE* less. Each Diclegis tablet consists of 10 mg of doxylamine succinate and 10 mg of B_6.[129] While they call the drug a "fixed-dose combination," many women need to take up to four a day to see a benefit.[130] Well, you don't need to take a pricey prescription to get that 10 to 40 mg a day of B_6. Your prenatal vitamin or over-the-counter B_6 (taken along with a B complex) provides more and costs less. It's the other ingredient we need to worry about.

Doxylamine is an antihistamine found in sleeping pills like Unisom SleepTabs. Under Diclegis's "Important Safety Information" it states "[f]atalities have been reported from doxylamine overdose in children. Children appear to be at a high risk for cardiorespiratory arrest" and "the safety and effectiveness of Diclegis in children under 18 years of age have not been established."[131]

Wait a minute. The safety of the drug hasn't been established for kids under eighteen? How old is a fetus?

Diclegis's safety information continues to explain, "Women should not breast-feed while using Diclegis because the antihistamine component (doxylamine succinate) in Diclegis can pass into breast milk. Excitement, irritability, and sedation have been reported in nursing infants presumably exposed to doxylamine succinate. . . . Infants with apnea or other respiratory syndromes may be particularly vulnerable to the sedative effects of Diclegis resulting in worsening of their apnea or respiratory conditions."[132]

Oh, boy. So it's not deemed safe for a nursing baby either. Do we really want to trust that it is okay for a *developing* baby?

I'm not comfortable with the risks of Diclegis or doxylamine. Nor am I comfortable with the risks of other anti-puke meds like Zofran (ondansetron) or Phenergan (promethazine HCI). Statements like "Zofran is not expected to be harmful to an unborn baby"[133] bring me no comfort. "Not expected" means it is unknown. Controlled studies have not been done on pregnant women to find out.[134] In effect, your baby becomes a guinea pig. Must we remember Thalidomide? In the 1950s and '60s, Thalidomide was prescribed for morning sickness and some 10,000 babies were born with severe birth defects.[135] For the mothers, children, and families affected, an apology, even if it took half a century to get one, just isn't good enough.[136] It would seem there is a safer option for the management of morning sickness.

Robert G. Smith, neurophysiologist and Research Associate Professor of Neuroscience at the University of Pennsylvania says, "It seems likely that pyridoxine (vitamin B_6) along with other B vitamins and vitamin C (an antihistamine) might be similarly effective." We can ditch the drugs and take vitamins as an alternative. I didn't want to take chances. I took vitamins instead.

I didn't want to take chances.
I took vitamins instead.

MULTIPLE CHILDREN . . . AT HOME

Is this a problem during pregnancy? It is certainly a complication. And when you are three months pregnant and exhausted, and you have a toddler or two to take care of, it's a *problem*.

Get help. Get help. Get help. Did I mention get help? This can come in many forms. Mine came wearing a monochrome brown shirt, pants, and hat with three little embroidered letters: "UPS." While I'm pretty sure he's a little "judgy" of the contents of all those boxes that he lugs onto our porch, just about everything, and I do mean everything, is shipped to our door. Baby food? Diapers? Wipes? Yes. Batteries? Cat food? Toothpaste? Yep. Vitamins? Shoes? Underwear? You get the idea. I even had our new toilet shipped. Then, I took it one step further and put stuff on auto-ship. Brilliant. Merchandise just *shows up,* without having to be asked, like good little consumables. This is far easier than dragging children to a department store to buy soap. Not only that, but it is actually *cheaper* than if I were to buy the same goods in stores. It also saves time, gas, and effort. The only things I have to leave my house to buy are groceries. I do so willingly, as I really like to see and select my own food. *Let* the UPS guy wonder about all the stuff I buy. I've just made having multiple kids a heck of a lot easier, at least on me.

NAUSEA: *See* MORNING SICKNESS

PREECLAMPSIA: TOXEMIA

You aren't likely to get preeclampsia if you are eating lots of fruits and vegetables and taking your vitamins. It will certainly do no harm to eat right and see to taking optimal levels of antioxidants, and most assuredly they will do some good.

At each visit to the ob-gyn you can count on them strapping a band around your arm and checking your blood pressure. Preeclampsia is defined as high blood pressure (also known as hypertension) and protein in your urine during pregnancy. (Blood pressure is a measurement of the arterial pressure of blood in your circulation system and is indicated by the systolic pressure over the diastolic pressure. High blood pressure is indicated at 140/90 millimeters of mercury (mm Hg) or greater.) Preeclampsia puts a pregnant woman at risk for some pretty serious complications that, although rare, are certainly scary. These include premature separation of the placenta from the uterus, bleeding problems, rupture of the liver, eclampsia (preeclampsia plus seizures), stroke, and possibly even death.[137] The exact cause of preeclampsia is unknown; possible causes include problems with blood vessels and blood flow to the uterus, and your genes. But the cause could also be due to diet or a problem with your immune system.[138] There is good news here, though: two out of the four possible causes can be directly influenced by you—diet and strengthening your immune system. There is no need to wait and see if things get worse. Address your nutrition first. You and your baby are likely to be just fine, but the more severe your preeclampsia, the more risk placed on you and your child.

If you do experience preeclampsia, your doctor is likely to tell you that you need to be on bed rest. This sounds lovely in theory but is not nearly as wonderful when you actually can do nothing but lie around and only get up to eat and pee. Your doctor will also tell you to drink more water and eat less salt, something we should probably all be doing anyway. If your condition is severe, it could mean hospitalization.

But I don't think you should take this lying down. You should work to strengthen your immune system by eating well and taking vitamins. For example, good diets with a high intake of fruits and vegetables decrease your risk of preeclampsia, and eating processed meat, sweet drinks, and salty snacks increase your risk of the condition.[139] Being overweight also increases your risk, as does developing gestational diabetes, and/or a history of conditions like "chronic high blood pressure, migraine headaches, diabetes, kidney disease, rheumatoid arthritis, or lupus," says the Mayo Clinic.[140] Better nutrition can help improve all of these, and decrease the likelihood that you will have to deal with preeclampsia.

Both the serum levels of magnesium and calcium are lower in women with preeclampsia,[141] and selenium supplementation (100 micrograms a day) may also be associated with a lower frequency of preeclampsia,[142] suggesting that close attention should be paid to making sure we get enough of these minerals.

Vitamin D deficiency is also associated with an increased risk for preeclampsia.[143] Even relatively small amounts of vitamin D (just 400–600 IU a day) have been shown to reduce the risk of preeclampsia.[144] However, it is far more likely that we need more than that, especially if we are already deficient in D, and up to half of us are.[145] It would be a good idea to ask your doctor to test your vitamin D levels. Research suggests in order to maintain optimal levels of D in the body, the ideal dosage during pregnancy is closer to 4,000 IU of vitamin D a day.[146] The RDA's recommendation of a mere 400–600 IU[147] has been shown to be inadequate.[148]

Women with preeclampsia have been found to have higher levels of homocysteine.[149] Folic acid and other B vitamins help break down this homocysteine.[150] Higher blood levels of B vitamins are also related to lower concentrations of homocysteine,[151] suggesting that adequate intake of B vitamins may be protective against preeclampsia. One study found that women at increased risk for preeclampsia were over four times more likely to have low riboflavin (B_2) status as compared to those women with adequate levels of the vitamin.[152] Thiamine (B_1) may be of particular interest. According John B. Irwin, MD, 100 mg/day of thiamine was found to be safe in his patients, and virtually 100 percent effective in preventing toxemia of pregnancy.[153] In women with an increased risk of preeclampsia, coenzyme Q_{10} supplementation (200 mg a day) during pregnancy significantly reduced the risk of developing the disorder.[154]

Additionally, probiotics, like those found in yogurt, could offer some protective benefit against preeclampsia, and cause no harm.[155] A study that looked at the dietary habits of over 33,000 women over a seven-year period found that women who consumed five ounces of dairy-based probiotics a day had a 39 percent lower risk of preeclampsia; consuming probiotics only once a week produced a 25 percent lower risk of the condition.[156]

Vitamin C and E for Preeclampsia

The Internet and news magazines were plastered with the findings of a large study published in the *New England Journal of Medicine* that claimed no benefit from taking vitamins C and E in doses of 1,000 mg a day and 400 IU a day respectively for preeclampsia.[157] The study found no significant difference between the rates of preeclampsia or adverse perinatal outcomes between women in the vitamin C and E group and those taking placebo.

Our first instinct may be to take this as the authors and the media wish us to: don't bother taking supplemental vitamins C and E, because they aren't going to do you any good when it comes to preeclampsia. Their advice would be to not recommend these important antioxidants for prevention of gestational hypertension. That's certainly one way to look at it. Here's another:

First, doses given of vitamins C and E far above RDA levels for pregnant women (about 85 mg a day of vitamin C and about 22 IU of vitamin E) did no harm. Second, other studies have had different outcomes. Authors concluded "supplementation with vitamins C and E may be beneficial" in a study published in *Lancet* of nearly 300 women shown to be at increased risk for preeclampsia.[158] In one prospective study of around 58,000 women, increasing dietary vitamin C intake was associated with a reduced risk of severe preeclampsia, eclampsia, or HELLP (the breakdown of red blood cells, elevated liver enzymes, and low platelet count).[159] Another study of over 500 women showed that low-plasma vitamin C was a risk factor for preeclampsia,[160] suggesting increased intake is a good idea. A review looking at seven trials involving over 6,000 women showed the benefits of antioxidant supplementation for reducing the risk of preeclampsia.[161] The results demonstrated that "supplementing women with any antioxidants during pregnancy compared with control or placebo was associated with a 39 percent reduction in the risk of pre-eclampsia."[162] However, when this review was updated, the conclusion drawn by the authors was quite different. They decided antioxidants were not helpful for the reduction of the risk of this disease. Linus Pauling had said researchers can misinterpret their own data.

Are we missing something? A recent study of nearly 700 women showed a food bar that contained the amino acid L-arginine and antioxidant vitamins—yes, including vitamins C and E—"reduced the incidence of pre-eclampsia in a population at high risk of the condition."[163] There was also an "observed benefit" in women who received the antioxidant bar alone, without L-arginine.[164]

We shouldn't rule out the idea that antioxidants are helpful, and that perhaps we need them in combination to reap optimal benefits. There is also another possibility. Consider this study that also showed vitamin C (1,000 mg a day) and vitamin E (400 IU a day) did no better than placebo.[165] The authors' conclusion was, "Vitamins C and E *at the doses used* did not prevent pre-eclampsia in these high-risk women" (emphasis added).[166] Okay, so you can say vitamins didn't help. But you can also say the doses were inadequate. For example, according to Thomas Levy, MD, "adequate vitamin C levels . . . make the development of significantly high blood pressure unlikely."[167] "Adequate" means you need *enough*. This adequate amount may be much higher than the 1,000 mg of vitamin C a day used in the above study, which determined it ineffective. Remember, Dr. Klenner gave four times this amount of vitamin C or more every day to pregnant women. Vitamin C and E are not ineffective. Low doses are ineffective. You can't buy a yacht for $1.98.

Focusing on only two antioxidants in limited dosages for only one condition does not do justice to the overall benefit of vitamins for healthy moms and healthy babies. Doesn't it make sense to address a major portion of possible causes of preeclampsia by focusing on maternal nutrition and all nutrients, including vitamin C and E, which have numerous other benefits during pregnancy and a long history of safety?[168]

Any study can be set up to fail. Antioxidants *are* important during pregnancy. It would be a real shame to turn away from what we know to be right.

PREGOBESITY

Between caring for your current toddler(s), working, and the million other demands made upon a mom, it isn't easy to put yourself first and focus on fitness. It is even harder if you get pregnant soon after you have already had a baby, and well before you had a chance to lose weight from the previous pregnancy. Now, sheer exhaustion and morning sickness may make it almost impossible to think about eating right and exercising. And yet, weight gain during pregnancy can't be taken lightly.

My doctor had no problem giving me a gentle reminder to lay off the bonbons when, sporting baby number two, I gained more than I should have between checkups. I wasn't exactly surprised. I knew why I was being reprimanded, and I confessed. Over the past weeks chocolate had become a food group in my diet. It was obvious to me where I had gone awry, and apparently it was obvious to my doctor, too. (I probably still had some on my face.) My doctor gave it to me straight: at this point in my pregnancy, I should only be gaining about a pound a week. Not five.

Many physicians, however, may not be leveling with their patients. Weight is a *really* sensitive topic. Doctors may not want to broach the issue. Frankly, pregnant patients aren't likely to want to hear about it either. Had my doctor tapped my chart and peered over his glasses on a different day, I may have bitten his head off instead of acquiescing. However, I was in a good mood. His reminder was the one and only one I needed. I shaped up, both figuratively and literally.

Ultimately, we—not our doctors, not our kitchen cupboards, not the unbearably enticing bakery shop displays of confections, not the little growing babe in our womb that makes us look fat even if we eat perfectly, not our loving partners with takeout bags in hand—*we* are responsible for our weight gain during pregnancy. We may give ourselves permission to eat poorly because we feel we have earned it; we deserve it. We may have watched our diet all our life and see pregnancy as a time to not worry about weight. We may have morning sickness that prevents anything but pudding to go down the hatch. We may have many justifiable reasons or understandable excuses for the pounds we put on or have yet to lose. Whatever the reason, we are responsible. This is the hard truth.

Whether we like it or not, getting back to pre-pregnancy weight before getting pregnant with another baby is important. And it's not for our self-image, it's for our, and our baby's health. Excess weight during pregnancy increases our chances of having pregnancy issues such as gestational diabetes, preeclampsia,[169] and infections.[170] Our babies are at increased risk for prematurity, stillbirth, birth defects, overweight at birth, and childhood obesity.[171] Allergies,[172] asthma,[173] and even autism[174] in children may be related to mom's excess weight during pregnancy. It may also increase your chances of having a C-section.[175] None of this is pleasant, but it must be mentioned. We must manage our weight like we manage everything else. It is important. It is a priority. It is one more damn thing to do. And we still must do it.

Here's how:

1. Do not "eat for two." We need only a few extra calories a day (300 or so) to help with that new human we are growing. Make them good calories.

2. If we have junk in the house, it is likely we will consume it. Don't. (Don't have it in the house, that is.) Pack your fridge and pantry with healthy goodies you actually want to eat.

3. Exercise when you can, in moderation. My toddler thinks it's a blast to work out.

Once the baby is born:

1. Remember that breastfeeding burns about 500 calories a day.

2. Join a gym if you can. Many have affordable or free daycare.

3. Drink nutrition-packed fresh, raw veggie juice as often as you can make it.

4. Settle in to a healthy routine. Losing weight takes time. Set a goal and track your progress.

5. Make a small change that you can stick to. Master it. Then take on the next challenge.

6. Seek support. New moms need plenty of support anyway.

7. Fall off the wagon? Get right back on. Life is a journey.

The advice for healthy weight loss post-baby or at any time has pretty much always been the same, and it is still true: eat right to lose weight and exercise to keep it off. And take your vitamins. (See also Weight Gain later in this chapter.)

POLYCYSTIC OVARIAN SYNDROME (PCOS)

Even though it makes it more difficult, you can still get pregnant when you have PCOS, but it increases your chances of complications during pregnancy for both you and your baby, including miscarriage, gestational diabetes, preeclampsia, preterm birth, and the chances you'll have to have a C-section.[176] That's quite a lot to worry about. Around half of women with PCOS are obese. While preventive nutrition is best, it is never too late to start: avoid sugar and simple carbohydrates, exercise in moderation, drink plenty of water, and eat lots of vegetables.

In addition, 200 mcg a day of chromium picolinate has been shown to improve glucose tolerance in women with PCOS.[177] Chromium helps level out the highs and lows of blood sugar, but so does exercising and . . . not eating sugar.

PREMATURE BIRTH: PREVENTING PREEMIES

Magnesium, omega-3 fatty acids, calcium, zinc, and a host of other nutrients may be influential in the prevention of premature and low birth weight babies.[178] Healthy, full-term babies start with healthy moms. Every single cell in a baby's body is made out of nutrients. There is no substitute for good nutrition.

PREMATURE RUPTURE OF MEMBRANES

Lower levels of serum vitamin C "appears to be directly related to the risk of premature rupture of the fetal membranes" explains Melvyn R. Werbach, MD.[179] This is one more good reason to take vitamin C throughout pregnancy. Vitamin C helps prevent ruptured membranes in general. Vitamin C makes collagen, and collagen holds your skin together. Selenium status is also important. In a recent study, women given 100 mcg per day of selenium effectively reduced the incidence of premature rupture of membranes.[180]

SLEEPLESSNESS (INSOMNIA)

Lecithin not only helped me think more clearly during pregnancy, it also improved my rest at night by helping me *stay* asleep. One may have been because of the other, and frankly I didn't care which symptom the lecithin was helping—the sleeplessness or the forgetfulness. Sure, if you are stressed out, busy, or short on sleep (or all three), a side effect could be difficulty remembering things. I was waking up several times a night to pee . . . and pee . . . and pee . . . and then hopefully falling asleep again. I was also in the process of writing my first book and worrying about giving birth to my first baby. Increasing my lecithin intake (and thus my intake of choline) was helping me think more clearly and sleep more soundly, pre- and post-baby. This is good news for many women who find it harder to get some decent shut-eye when they are sporting a baby bump. (Please see the section on choline in The B Vitamins and Pregnancy chapter for more information about the benefits of lecithin for mom and baby.)

Niacin B$_3$ is another asset. Niacin (B$_3$) can help quiet your mind and help you get to sleep.[181] When I was pregnant I would take about 50–100 mg of niacin in the form of nicotinic acid before bed to help bring on sleep. Getting the other B vitamins during the day may also help you snooze. "[A] vitamin B deficiency can often cause insomnia," says James F. Balch, MD. (Read more about the different forms of niacin, and the common side effect of "flushing" in the chapter dedicated to the B vitamins.)

Magnesium intake can also influence restful sleep. Have you ever found yourself lying in bed, trying to sleep, only to start thinking about all the things in your world that stress you out? Instead of feeling calm, relaxed, and drowsy, you get pangs of nervousness, adrenaline rushes and your thoughts race and just won't stop. Carolyn Dean, MD, explains, "Prolonged psychological stress raises adrenaline, the stress hormone, and results in a myriad of metabolic activities, all of which require and therefore deplete magnesium. Magnesium depletion itself stresses the body, which can result in panic attacks, which results in more bursts of adrenaline and creates irritability and nervousness. Not only do our overworked adrenals cause magnesium depletion, but even more adrenaline is released under stress when magnesium levels are low in the body. It's the proverbial catch-22."[182] The solution? See that you get at least the Recommended Dietary Allowance of magnesium every day. This isn't as easy as you may think. Please read the chapter on magnesium for dosing hints.

Eat foods high in L-tryptophan, an amino acid that converts into serotonin, a neurotransmitter that improves mood, to help you get to sleep at night and feel more rested in the morning. Yogurt, cheese, milk, beans, cashews, and chicken (along with carbohydrates like bread and crackers) are all high in L-tryptophan.[183]

STRETCH MARKS

Prevention is the best medicine when it comes to stretch marks. Once you've got 'em, they are pretty much there to stay. Plenty of home remedies are out there that you could try, but these mostly lessen the appearance of your baby battle scars rather than cause them to disappear altogether. Stretch marks are not inevitable. This is going to sound farfetched, but here's something you might really want to know. Stretch marks are, indeed, largely preventable.

Stretch marks were virtually nonexistent on any of Dr. Frederick R. Klenner's vitamin C moms. Over 300 pregnant women were taking, in divided doses, 4 grams of vitamin C a day during their first trimester, 6 grams during their second, and 10 to 15 grams per day during their third.[184] They were healthy. Their babies were healthy. And they had no stretch marks. Awesome.

Fifty years ago, Dr. William J. McCormick said that stretch marks are a result of vitamin C deficiency and that taking more C during pregnancy could prevent them. Specifically, as explained by Drs. Hickey and Saul in *Vitamin C: The Real Story,* "Vitamin C is needed to make collagen and strong connective tissue, and vitamin C supplementation rapidly enhances collagen synthesis."[185] They say:

Dr. McCormick suggested that stretch marks are a result of vitamin C deficiency, affecting the body's production of collagen. Collagen consists of long protein molecules that act like tiny strings, holding the tissue components together. We can think of connective tissues as biological fiber composites, working a similar way to fiberglass or carbon fiber materials. In fiberglass, the plastic matrix is given strength by transferring tension to the glass fibers. Similarly, tissues transfer stress to collagen fibers. Tissues in the body are constructed of cells, supported by a matrix of connective tissue. The cells themselves are relatively delicate and have little intrinsic strength. Connective tissue provides the glue that binds your cells together, just as mortar binds bricks. If collagen is abundant and strong, body cells hold together well. Stretch marks, a relatively minor cosmetic affliction, helped develop Dr. McCormick's ideas. As long ago as 1948, he suggested that these disfiguring lesions might be avoided.[186] During pregnancy, the skin can stretch to several times its original length. If the skin of the abdomen and thighs were stronger and more able to repair itself, stretch marks may be lessened or avoided altogether.[187]

My mother, who followed Klenner's vitamin C protocol, was virtually stretch mark free—she had a single half-inch mark. I've had two kids, and I don't have any.

Vitamin E may also help keep your skin supple and stretchy.[188] James Balch, MD, recommends topical administration of a vitamin E mixture to help prevent stretch marks.[189]

Zinc deficiency may also be a culprit behind those purple zigzag lines.[190] Babies need zinc as they grow and they are going to get it from you. It is recommended that you get at least 15 mg of zinc daily so there is enough to go around and your skin can heal and stretch the way it should.[191]

Do lotions work? I dunno. Like many women, I occasionally smeared ointments on my belly during my first pregnancy. Rather, my husband did, which he found irresistibly entertaining. As my tummy stretched for the first time to accommodate a new life, lotion helped alleviate that feeling of tight, itchy skin. But I didn't keep up with the applications, and then abandoned them altogether after a week or two. I didn't bother with lotion at all during my second pregnancy, much to my husband's dismay. Still, no stretch marks. (Not to rub it in, but I just donned a bikini over the Fourth of July holiday.)

I'm not here to discourage you from adding moisturizer to your no-way-do-I-want-a-stretch-mark-anywhere arsenal, but having used it only occasionally during my first pregnancy, and not at all during my second, it seemed to me that my healthy diet and vitamin intake may have more to do with my blemish-free tum-tum than cocoa butter.

SLEEPLESSNESS: *See* INSOMNIA

SWELLING (EDEMA)

If you want to swell less, eat less salt and eat more potassium, found in all those fruits and veggies we are supposed to be munching on anyway. Focus on good nutrition, take your vitamins, especially a B complex vitamin, a multivitamin and mineral supplement, vitamin C, and vitamin D, drink plenty of water, and stay active.

URINARY TRACT INFECTIONS (UTIs)

Whenever you see the word "infection," think "vitamin C." High-dose vitamin C can be used as a safe antibiotic alternative (to read more, please refer to the chapter on this vitamin). Vitamin E and vitamin A are also known infection fighters. Get out that vegetable juicer you have stashed under your counter and start drinking fresh, raw veggie juice, which is loaded with infection-fighting nutrients including beta-carotene. Drink it every day, twice a day if you can while you experience symptoms, and for a week afterward. You may already know about cranberry juice; seek out a variety that is unsweetened, as most "cocktails" are loaded with excess sugar that you, and your UTI, don't need. Drink lots of water, urinate after sex, eat yogurt or take probiotics, and optimize your intake of vitamins. Let's not complicate pregnancy any further by letting a UTI get the best of us.

VAGINAL ITCH

For those of you pregnant gals who, even at this very moment, are desperately trying to resist the urge to squirm, squiggle, squeeze, and or otherwise just haul off and go at that intense itch you feel between your legs with a rake, let's bring some well-needed relief into your life. Since such public displays of "grooming" are generally frowned upon, we simply have to have an answer for our discomfort that won't land us in someone's picture archive on their camera phone and seconds from being downloaded onto Internet social media pages.

Your doctor may recommend topical treatments like benzocaine (Vagisil) for your itchy parts, or miconazole (Monistat) kits for full-on yeast infections. It is likely that what is causing your nether regions to itch like crazy is the same culprit behind a yeast infection: an overgrowth of *Candida albicans (C. albicans)*. If you are looking for a natural cure, probiotics may be your best friend. The most inexpensive way to get probiotics into your system is via yogurt. I know women who use yogurt topically or intravaginally to restore balance to those itchy areas. By creating a more acidic environment, inserting a small amount of yogurt directly into your vagina will create a habitat unfriendly to *C. albicans*.[192] Even though it may sound a bit strange, you may feel more comfortable trying this than the medication your doctor recommended. You may also find yourself able to keep from scratching inappropriate places. Probiotics are also important for prevention. Taken orally, the *Lactobacillus acidophilus* found in yogurt and probiotic tablets helps build immunity against *C. albicans* and decreases the chances you will get a yeast infection.[193] Some women find that applying natural vitamin E provides relief. Taking extra vitamin C can also help. (For more, see also the information about Yeast Infections in this chapter.)

VARICOSE VEINS

"The secret to avoiding varicose veins is to keep your blood vessels in good shape to minimize the restriction of blood flow," says well-known British nutrition expert and author Patrick Holford.[194] He recommends vitamin C, vitamin E, vitamin B₃, and regular exercise.

WEIGHT GAIN

Gaining weight during pregnancy is expected and normal. Your doctor will probably give you a range for how many pounds you should tack on during pregnancy. This is your guideline. Only one person controls the outcome—you. If you are underweight, you will be advised to gain more. If you are already overweight, you will be advised to gain less. If there is ever a time to eat right, it's now.

Pregnancy isn't a food prison sentence, although it may feel like one. Having a baby is often used as an excuse to eat things we shouldn't. I, too, have succumbed to all things chocolate and sucked down a soda in the a.m. to stave off a bout of pregnancy-induced vomiting. Nobody is perfect. Self-control is not easy. Good health takes effort. You will be faced with food choices every single day. You can choose the best food possible, or you can give up and eat like most Americans do.

If we are strong enough to bear children, by golly we are strong enough to push away an unhealthy meal and reach for something nutritious, for us and our baby. (See also Pregobesity earlier in this chapter.)

YEAST INFECTIONS

Some of us have had the incredible good fortune of never having had a yeast infection—that is, until now. If you have yet to get a yeast infection, the rest of us will really try to be happy for you. But for those of us who have, fortunately there are drug-free ways to treat them.

Right now, your hormones are having a ball, and they haven't really stopped to consider what that means for you; they are far more interested in that child you are growing. In the wake of this hormonal mayhem, conditions change in such a way that makes it harder for your body to resist the overgrowth of *Candida albicans (C. albicans)*, the culprit behind your yeast infection. "If you have a healthy immune system," explains Hyla Cass MD, "these fungi (*candida*) interact symbiotically with your friendly intestinal bacteria such as *Lactobacillus acidophilus* and *Bifidobacteria bifidum*."[195] *C. albicans* naturally exists in our vagina, but being pregnant increases our estrogen levels, a hormone that makes it even harder for our vaginas to naturally inhibit the growth of *C. albicans*.[196] Plus, *candida* thrives in warm, dark, and moist living conditions. We ladies are naturally accommodating because we are all equipped with just such a perfect little habitat.

The Downside of Drugs for Yeast Infections

Some of us are more than a little hesitant to add drugs to a pregnant body, and with reason. When it comes to yeast infections, "for reasons of liability, pregnant women have been largely excluded from controlled clinical treatment studies by the pharmaceutical industry."[197] Still, if you go to the doctor, they will probably recommend you use a topical, over-the-counter drug like miconazole (Monistat) to treat a yeast infection while you are pregnant. Unfortunately, the drugs don't always work. If they do work, results may only be temporary.

Not only is there a higher prevalence of yeast infections in women who are pregnant as opposed to those who are not, but recurrence is more common, and "therapeutic responses are reduced."[198] *C. albicans* is suppressed, not eliminated, with azole-medications like Monistat. Medication may initially stifle your symptoms, but recurrence is possible, and more likely,[199] during pregnancy. Additionally, a growing number of non–*C. albicans* species attributed to recurrent infections are intrinsically resistant to medication.[200]

SUGAR: FRIEND OR FOE?

Sometimes, morning (and noon, and night) sickness makes it so the only food we might possibly consider eating is something that tastes amazing. This can often take the form of a sugar laden snack. At one point, a pregnant friend of mine was unable to keep down anything but vanilla milk shakes for dinner. When I was pregnant and holding down a job as a middle school teacher, there were moments when I was so nauseous that ginger ale was just about the only thing I could ingest that would prevent me from an untimely toss of my cookies. I'd sip a can in the shower before work, or if I was lucky, I'd make it all the way there before I had to crack one open. Class would be proceeding as normal (or as normal as any class can be when you teach a bunch of middle schoolers) but then, without much warning, my eyes would water, my mouth would fill with saliva, and my throat would tighten and ready itself to wretch. To avoid vomiting in front of a whole class of thirteen year olds, I would gingerly sip a can of ginger ale and, occasionally, the urge to upchuck would pass. My students may have suspected I was pregnant but they didn't know for certain. They were suspicious of my often worn sporty fleece athletic jacket, my "pregnancy cloaking device" as I referred to it later, and its inability to fully disguise my midsection. There were rumors circulating, but none confirmed. (Adolescents don't let much get by them.) However, I was sure that puking during second period each day might give me away. So, when necessary, ginger ale came to the rescue. Since not all of my anti-puke plans worked as expected, I was also grateful to have a bathroom sink down the hall just a hop, skip, and a jump away.

Some rules can be modified based on the current situation, but in general, if you aim to be your healthiest for the next nine months, you are going to want to keep away from excess sugar. Try to eat small meals throughout the day and always have a snack handy, one that isn't loaded with sugar. Many women report feeling less morning sickness when they have eaten.

But nobody's perfect, and avoiding sugar isn't easy. I mean, we're huge and pregnant anyway. We aren't exactly worried about maintaining a waistline. We are supposed to gain weight. But if the occasional treat causes you to have days of distress, you have to weigh the advantages of dessert against the disadvantages of discomfort. Consider, for instance, that "yeast overgrowth often leads to sugar cravings" and "sugar literally feeds the yeast and helps it grow even more," says Dr. Cass.[201] If you are suffering from yeast infections during pregnancy or you find yourself constantly itchy and uncomfortable down there, reduce your sugar intake. Basically, whatever is wrong, sugar makes it worse. That goes for artificial sweeteners, too. Sucralose, for example, is capable of killing half of your good gut bacteria, bacteria that is essential to your health.[202] Authors of *Rich Food Poor Food* say, "Your gut is home to 80 percent of your immune system, and these same bacteria can help fight heart disease, reduce cravings, and, best of all, aid in the absorption of your micronutrients."[203]

So here are your sugar basics:

1. If you are going to have sugar, have a little of the real stuff. It's not "better" for you, it is just less worse.

2. Avoid fake sweeteners like aspartame, sucralose, saccharin, and acesulfame potassium. A quick Internet search will list more for you, including brand names.

3. Avoid high-fructose corn syrup.

4. Read labels. At a quick glance, "Sucrose" (sugar) and "sucralose" (an artificial sweetener) look similar.

5. Remember, sugar is often harvested from genetically modified sugar beets. Go organic and look for "pure cane" sugar.

PROMOTING PREGNANCY PANTSLESSNESS

Everything increases during pregnancy: your waist, your hormones, your appetite (eventually), and, unfortunately, your vaginal discharge. Switching out panty liners all day isn't really a big deal, but sometimes those vaginal secretions can make already-sensitive skin feel irritated and itchy. Yeast, a common culprit behind a not-so-comfy-crotch, loves environments that are warm and moist. Cutting back on sugar, eating yogurt and/or taking probiotics, taking your vitamins, and keeping the area (relatively) dry may help. Do yourself a favor and go commando at bedtime. Pregnancy pantslessness is quite liberating and it also helps keep the area aired out. If you need to wear a panty liner, consider lining those cotton panties with a 100 percent cotton product. Your typical panty shield often contains plastics. There's no point in avoiding synthetic undergarments if we basically end up lining our cotton undies with a plastic bag.

Natural Treatment Options for Yeast Infections

Research suggests tolerance and immunity are the "only relevant defensive factors" against yeast infections,[204] not drugs and more drugs. Using medicines to treat symptoms does not keep yeast from growing. Medication attempts to manage out-of- control yeast overgrowth, but it does not prevent yeast from flaring up again. It does not address the reason behind *why* you are suffering from a yeast infection in the first place. Address the underlying factor of the infection—other than the one factor you can't control: your pregnancy.

Eat plenty of plain, unsweetened yogurt: "Probiotics such as *acidophilus* and *bifidius* are natural, 'friendly' bacteria that restore balance to your digestive system," says Dr. Cass. "The best prevention (of yeast overgrowth) is to continue taking probiotics daily or every other day and avoid sugar and other offending foods."[205] Are probiotics safe during pregnancy? Yes. Yogurt surely is, and that's a great way to introduce probiotics cheaply and effectively. Probiotic supplements are also safe during pregnancy and lactation.[206] There may be other side benefits, too. A recent study showed that taking probiotics while pregnant may decrease the risk of later allergies in children.[207]

Drink raw vegetable juice or veggie smoothies, drink plenty of water, eat lots of garlic (a natural antifungal), and take time to de-stress. All help keep yeast at bay and are safe for a developing baby. Reduce your sugar intake to cut down both the incidence and severity of yeast infections.[208] Nutrients helpful for the treatment of infection include beta-carotene,[209] as women with yeast infections have low levels of beta-carotene.[210] Zinc (15 mg a day is recommended for pregnant gals) and vitamin C are also effective infection fighters. When I was pregnant with my daughter, I, too, got a yeast infection. At the first moment I would feel that tell-tale itch, I would load up on vitamin C. Maintaining a high level of C helped heal my infection and it alleviated my symptoms—the burning and itching that made it hard to even go to sleep at night. It was relief I could count on within half an hour of taking a large dose. If I felt any discomfort come back, I'd take more vitamin C. After about two days of extra C, my symptoms were gone completely. I felt far more comfortable taking high doses of vitamin C (as well as eating yogurt, avoiding sugar, and drinking raw vegetable juice) than I did using drugs.

YAY PREGNANCY! SORT OF . . .

Pregnancy was definitely a love-hate experience for me. I was thrilled to have the opportunity to bring little lives into this world. My children bring me such joy. I can't imagine being without them. However, I found plenty to complain about during pregnancy despite how happy I was to be pregnant. I was puking. I was tired. I was huge. I was slow. I was sore. I looked forward to the end result, the baby, but I've never been real keen on the process to get there. Oh, except for all the romping good times in the sack with my husband. That part was all just fine.

Throughout my first and second pregnancy, I steered clear of pharmaceutical medicines and over-the-counter drugs and sought out the benefits of vitamins and minerals. I wanted little to do with a broken "health" system intent on medicating darn near everyone. I wanted to address root causes of health issues, not symptoms. (And by addressing the root causes, we also address the symptoms.) Nutrition helped my body do what it was designed to do. It will help yours, too.

CHAPTER 10

Postpartum Problems

"If you don't make time to take care of yourself, who will?"
—CONNIE PODESTA

Perhaps one of the greatest battles we have postpartum is that the world keeps right on moving at the same breakneck pace it did before you gave birth. Appliances wear out, pipes spring leaks, the lawn needs mowing, and any number of small, medium, or large tasks take their place on an ever growing to-do list that exists merely out of principle, and not because it represents things that will actually get done.

We are in constant demand. We are exhausted and overwhelmed. Health issues are always unwelcome, but now it may feel as if they are downright impossible to manage. When is there time to be sick if there is a baby that needs you? When is there time for rest?

I can't take away all the work for you, but what I can do is provide you with some options. When faced with postpartum health issues, we don't have to resign ourselves to only the doctor's orders. We have some nutritional choices we can make instead of springing for medication and before we give up. Having options is a good thing. Choice can help alleviate fear. Having a newborn is enough to worry about.

ANOTHER (FURRY) BABY

Evidently I was not nearly busy enough, so we adopted a kitten. I don't know if you have ever had a kitten, but if you have you will know what I am saying when I tell you that they are insane. There is not an object in the house a kitten won't climb, claw, or chew. I am well aware of kitten behavior, and there is no way I would have one, except that someone left her by the side of the road to perish. I was out for a stroll with my two babies, there was no way in the world the mother in me could walk past a frightened, mewling, desperate eight-week-old kitten and not help her. I brought the kitten home and proceeded to call everyone I knew to see if anyone wanted a pet.

And now, for the next seventeen years or so, I have a cat.

The day the kitten came into our house, I packed her and my two children up to go to the veterinarian. It seemed like a good idea to have a proper checkup done before I let a stray take up residence with my babies. We were about to walk into our appointment—with my toddler asking me every two seconds, "Meow okay? Meow okay?" and a howling kitty in a carrier in my trunk—when, of course, my squirmy baby boy decides to throw up his dinner all over his outfit and have a blowout, leaving me no choice but to change his clothes and diaper in the parking lot in the back of our car. A million mothers before me have done the same. (Knowing this doesn't make it any easier.) Someone driving by starts beeping frantically at me. The stroller, set up and ready but empty at the time, is rolling away from us through the parking lot. The beeping driver, unable to see that the stroller contained no baby, was worried my child was careening toward rush hour traffic.

Mid-diaper and elbow deep in baby byproducts, I just let it go.

Eventually, I somehow managed to wrangle my toddler, the stray kitten, a much cleaner baby, and the renegade stroller (long before it hit the highway) into the veterinarian's office.

I confirmed at that moment that I would never want a third child. Two hands were simply not enough for three babies. This third, furry feline baby was enough, thank you very much.

BEGINNING AT HOME OR IN THE HOSPITAL

"Postpartum" starts when the baby is delivered. Whether you are at home or in the hospital, you can start taking care of yourself right now to make things that much easier later. For me, this took the form of a large bottle of vitamin C on my side table, plenty of water, and a big glass of carrot juice right in the recovery room.

You may feel subject to your healthcare provider's rules and apparent authority. When I was going to give birth to my first child, one nurse looked at me and suspiciously said, "We keep track of what goes in and what comes out." I wasn't exactly sure what she was trying to tell me (was she worried my hubby was going to slip me a submarine sandwich or something?) but I remember feeling a little "under the microscope" when I continued to do what I knew to be right and take my vitamins.

Hospitals can be intimidating. But never forget *you* are in charge of your own health. This includes your choice to take vitamins. The hospital staff cannot take them from you. If anyone does, tell them they are your personal property and you want them returned. Having someone with you in the hospital at all times is ideal. They can be your advocate when you cannot. Overall, our birthing experience at the hospital was a positive one, but I noticed that the more visitors we had in the room, the more the management would stop by and smile and see how we were faring. It is possible this was merely coincidence. It is also possible it is exactly what it seems: greater attention is paid to patients who have others looking out for them. This all may sound a bit paranoid, but patients must protect themselves. Those of you who have ever dealt with managing the care for a loved one in the hospital know this all too well.

For more about how to reduce the risks associated with any hospital stay, how to be your own healthcare advocate, and how to choose the best hospital, doctors, nurses, and surgeons, you may want to read *Hospitals and Health: Your Orthomolecular Guide to a Shorter, Safer Hospital Stay* by Abram Hoffer, MD, Andrew W. Saul, PhD, and Steve Hickey, PhD.

HEALING AFTER BIRTH

Our bodies have been through so much already, but the challenges are far from over. Vitamins can help speed your recovery post-delivery, so you can focus your time on your newest and most important challenge: your newborn.

Healing after Cesarean Section (C-Section)

A C-section is major surgery, no matter how you cut it. (Yes, sorry. That's a bad pun.) Recovery takes a great deal of time. Added to the immense task of caring for a newborn, it is a wonder to me that moms who undergo a C-section get only eight weeks of maternity leave as opposed to the standard six. Surgery is stressful, planned or otherwise. Vitamin C can help many new moms that have undergone a C-section. (This goes for moms who delivered vaginally, too.) Here's why:

According to Melvyn R. Werbach, MD, "Supplementation with mega-doses of vitamin C has been shown to reduce pain."[1] Vitamin C is also needed for the healing of wounds.[2] According to Linus Pauling, "With a low intake of ascorbic acid, wounds heal only slowly and the scar tissue is weak, so that the wounds break open again easily. Increase in the intake of ascorbic acid leads to rapid healing and the formation of strong scar tissue."[3] In addition, vitamin C can prevent and treat infection,[4] and reduce inflammation and swelling.[5]

While vitamin C may be of special importance, please do not underestimate the value of getting ideal amounts of *all* vitamins after any surgical procedure including vitamins A, D, E, and the B's.

Healing from Episiotomy, Rips, or Tears

For topical relief, spreading the contents of a natural vitamin E capsule right on the affected area several times a day will help it feel better. (This could be done after each bathroom visit.) You may find, as my mother and I both did, that vitamin E works even better than those ointments the nurse has given you for relieving your sore, dry skin. Vitamin E oil feels extremely soothing and alleviates that tight, pulling sensation you may have after getting stitches. You don't have to touch the wound. Just puncture the capsule and drip it on.

Vitamin C is necessary for wound healing. It will also help prevent infection, reduce pain and swelling, and help you heal faster after vaginal birth.[6] Along with vitamin C, keep your body stocked with all essential vitamins to help speed recovery and keep you in the best possible health.

BENEFITS OF LACTATION AND BREASTFEEDING

"There are three reasons for breast-feeding:
the milk is always at the right temperature; it comes
in attractive containers; and the cat can't get it."
—IRENA CHALMERS

Fortunately, there is little argument now about the breast being best. It just is. There are numerous benefits for your baby, including protection from numerous illnesses, a reduced risk for obesity, and a lower risk for Sudden

Infant Death Syndrome (SIDS). Breastfed babies may even be smarter than their formula fed classmates.[7]

"One of the best-kept secrets about breastfeeding is that it's as healthy for mothers as for babies," says Alicia Dermer, MD.[8] Breastfeeding lowers your risk for postpartum depression, certain forms of cancer, and helps burn oodles of calories every day, helping you get back to your before-baby body even faster. And formula is expensive. Just think of the money you'll save.

If you decide to formula feed or wean your baby from the breast before twelve months of age, there are organic formulas available that cost nearly the same as nonorganic varieties. This makes choosing organic a no-brainer. But breastfed or bottle fed, vitamins are important.

Vitamins and Breast Milk

"Are those vitamins that I've been taking going to get into my milk and into my baby when she breastfeeds?"

I sure hope so! With a whole brand-new world exposing our little one to millions of new microbes, both those naturally encountered and those found in the dozens of vaccinations our baby gets before she even turns two, there is a great need for vitamins to pass through our milk to our infant.

Mom's level of nutrients determines the nursing baby's access to nutrition. Optimal levels of vitamins for mom mean optimal access to vitamins for baby. Growing a baby, both inside and outside your body, takes a whole lot of work. It is no surprise that nursing mothers need to take additional vitamins and minerals. This is especially important for moms as their body's demand for nutrients increases in order to heal from vaginal delivery or C-section or to fend off post-birth complications such as infections. For more information about dosage and the safety of taking vitamins while lactating, you may wish to refer to the lactation sections in each vitamin chapter.

Vitamins and Formula

Your child's pediatrician might tell you that your formula-fed baby has plenty of vitamins and minerals in her formula mixture. Well, that's what they say about an adult's diet, too: "Just eat a well-balanced diet and you will get all the vitamins and minerals you need."

Uh-huh. I don't buy that for a second.

I believe there is even more reason, not less, to make sure a formula-fed infant gets optimal levels of vitamins. Nutrients found in breast milk are not always in formula. For example, many babies were fed formula in the 1950s, when breastfeeding was actively discouraged. In those days there was no vitamin E or biotin in formula. They were added over a decade later when studies showed they were needed. But these nutrients were always in breast milk from the beginning.

LACTATION AND BREASTFEEDING ISSUES

Let's take a closer look at how vitamins can help some common issues we face during lactation and breastfeeding.

Sore Nipples

While many moms find it's worth it, breastfeeding is not without its challenges. One is dry, cracked nipples. There are products out there to help you manage this discomfort, but my mother and I both found that a little vitamin E goes a long way—and worked better. After feedings, you could try applying a little natural vitamin E oil to your sore nipples to help relieve sensitive, dry skin. Before your baby eats, simply wipe off any excess. Vitamin E is very safe. To read more, please see the chapter on Vitamin E. If your sore nipples are due to yeast overgrowth, please read the section in this chapter on the topic.

Plugged Ducts

Plugged ducts can be very uncomfortable. You can tell you have one because a small, pea-sized lump that is tender to the touch will show up in your breast. The goal is to get rid of these lumps early to decrease the likelihood of a subsequent infection. Even if it becomes infected, have your baby nurse on the breast with the plugged duct first, with her chin toward the blocked area, advises the breastfeeding experts at La Leche League International.[9] The swelling and inflammation can be reduced when your baby nurses and frees the blockage. Nursing on the infected breast will not harm your baby[10] and it will help you feel better. You may also find it helpful to gently massage the blockage toward to the nipple and hand-express some milk, especially after a warm shower.[11] Reducing stress and getting as must rest as possible are key factors in reducing plugged ducts.[12] Healing occurs when your body is strong and capable, and it cannot possibly do its best job without rest. Left unnoticed or untreated, plugged ducts can lead to mastitis, a painful breast infection.[13]

Lecithin supplementation is another safe and helpful nutrient to combat plugged ducts. Lecithin granules are cheaper, but capsules are convenient. Many women swear by lecithin. Read more about it in the chapter on B vitamins.

Mastitis

Mastitis is a painful breast infection. If words like "mastitis" (inflammation) or "infection" apply to you, this is an opportunity to address the needs of your immune system. High dose vitamin C is known to reduce inflammation and fight infection.[14] My dad always says, "Take enough C to be symptom free, whatever the amount may be." The body absorbs and utilizes extraordinary quantities of vitamin C when it is under stress or fighting infection.[15] To learn more about therapeutic dosages of vitamin C, please read the Vitamin C and Pregnancy chapter.

You have the option to treat mastitis with antibiotics. That is what your doctor will give you for a breast infection. You also have the option to use vitamins instead.

A woman I know had suffered with a bout of mastitis and was miserable to find out she had it again only a short time later.

She said:

> My first delivery was uncomplicated and yet still very stressful for me. My baby boy was colicky and nursed many times a night. I was really low on sleep and low on time and motivation to eat right. One day I developed what I thought was the flu: fever, chills, and extreme fatigue. Being a new mom just got a lot harder. I was so sick, and I noticed warm, red patches and streaks on one of my breasts. The doctor told me I had mastitis and I took an antibiotic to get rid of it. To keep from getting a yeast infection, which I often get with antibiotic treatment, I ate yogurt and I put a little unsweetened, plain yogurt onto my fingertip and in my baby's mouth before feedings to promote balanced bacteria and prevent thrush. I got

better, but I got mastitis again the following month. I didn't want to keep taking antibiotics, so I tried vitamins instead. This time I let my immune system do the work, and I took very large, saturation levels of vitamin C to help it along. This was in addition to drinking raw vegetable juice and taking my other vitamins as well. I paid extra attention to clearing plugged ducts, and if I had one I'd increase my dosages of antioxidants accordingly. It worked. The infection went away.

Yeast Overgrowth

Yeast overgrowth can cause sore, painful nipples for you during breast-feeding. Your baby can be affected, too: thrush is the overgrowth of yeast (*candida albicans*) in baby's mouth. *Candida* thrives in dark, moist environments. Diaper rash is also commonly due to yeast overgrowth.

Fungi, bacteria, and viruses are found in every body and everybody's baby's body inside and out. Always have been, always will be. But when "bad" microorganisms overtake good microorganisms, yeast overgrowth and infection may result.

Candida is opportunistic. Don't give it a fighting chance. If you or your baby have been exposed to antibiotics, be sure that you eat yogurt or take probiotics that include acidophilus. This goes for baby, too. Place a small amount of yogurt on your finger tip and wipe it on the inside of your baby's mouth prior to each feeding to introduce beneficial bacteria directly where thrush is present. This will also allow some to be ingested. Yogurt (store-bought or your homemade) can also be spread directly on the afflicted areas to treat a diaper rash or yeast infected nipples. Keep affected areas clean: change diapers often, as you probably are doing already.

If your baby is sensitive to lactose, you may find they still can eat yogurt. If not, a "formula" of crushed probiotic tablets and a smidge of water makes a runny paste that can also do the trick. Avoid excess sugar; yeast thrives on it. The goal is to achieve bacterial balance. Strong immune systems that get plenty of antioxidants and have exposure to beneficial bacteria are less likely to suffer *candida* overgrowth. Good nutrition and vitamins will help keep an immune system strong, which in turn will keep the body protected from infection.

POSTPARTUM DEPRESSION

The baby blues is very common. Most of us will feel anxious, upset, tired, moody, and forgetful after our baby is born. It's hard to handle, but apparently, it's normal. If it lasts beyond the first few weeks, it falls into the category of postpartum depression. It may not even hit you right away. There are a "substantial number" of women who develop depressive symptoms in the first year after childbirth, for example, nine months after the baby is born.[16]

However you want to define it, it stinks. The weight and responsibility of being a new mother, compounded with the complete change in lifestyle, the relentless demands on our body, and the uncertainty and fear that comes along with the incredible task of raising a child is enough. Top it off with a bout of depression, and it's a rough combination indeed.

Maybe you just thought how you felt was part of "being a mom." You might even be sufficiently depressed to not know you are. Here's a checklist of postpartum depression symptoms from the U.S. Department of Health and Human Services Office on Women's Health:

- Feeling restless or moody

- Feeling sad, hopeless, and overwhelmed

- Crying a lot

- Having no energy or motivation

- Eating too little or too much

- Sleeping too little or too much

- Having trouble focusing or making decisions

- Having memory problems

- Feeling worthless and guilty

- Losing interest or pleasure in activities you used to enjoy

- Withdrawing from friends and family

- Having headaches, aches and pains, or stomach problems that don't go away

Tick off any of the above? You are not alone. It seems that some 5 to 20 percent of us have to battle through depression after having a baby.[17]

Post-baby mood disorders aren't limited to depression. Anxiety or panic ("Can I even take care of this baby?"), obsessive-compulsive disorder (making every visitor bathe in hand sanitizer before even laying their eyes on your child), postpartum psychosis ("I'm going to do something horrible to my baby"), and post-traumatic stress disorder (flashbacks and panic about delivery—I'm surprised more women aren't diagnosed with this one). Any of these can affect new moms and repeat moms alike. I am talking about this in a lighthearted way, but these are heavy concerns. Mood disorders can be very serious, and should not be ignored. The only question, then, is how to best treat them.

A friend of mine went through a very serious bout of postpartum depression. She could barely remove herself from under her bedcovers; truly it was a blessing that Grandma was able to be there. Grandma was no stranger to the "baby blues" as she herself had suffered a powerful down after giving birth to each of her children. For many weeks, Grandma basically moved in. She cared for her daughter's new baby, and cared for her own baby, too.

It was some time into her depression that I was asked what might help. I mentioned she might want to read up on the B vitamins, consider the benefits of a B complex, and then adjust her intake of certain B vitamins like niacin, B_3, on an as-needed basis. For example, on an especially rough morning extra B_3 might help get her out of bed.

Later, I asked how she was doing.

She said simply, "I feel better."

Postpartum depression doesn't necessarily show up immediately or knock you flat on your back. It can creep in months later. Your get-up-and-go, your enthusiasm, your desire for intimacy, your willpower to eat right, or even shower all take the back burner. Yeah, you may feel that you don't have the time to take care of yourself. But even more, you don't have the motivation. You may not feel like "you" anymore. And with this loss of self comes feelings of anxiety, sadness, guilt, confusion, or even anger. You still manage daily tasks, responding to one demand after another, but it's all a struggle.

At this point you find yourself especially sympathetic of all those moms with dirty hair wearing sweatpants who still manage to make it to the grocery store on a weekday *with* the kids and *without* help. If they also have a job outside the home, it's a downright miracle. Even for moms without depression it's a momentous accomplishment to have the time and energy to get a lightbulb changed or a load of laundry done, folded, *and* put away. Each new task may seem like an impossible obstacle to overcome. For those with the burden of postpartum depression it is just that much harder.

Getting support, whether it is help around the house; a shoulder to lean on or someone you can vent to on the phone; sharing the night shift so you can get more rest; trying to exercise even if it is just a little (mine consisted, in part, of carrying my toddler upstairs for time-out several times a day); and setting small obtainable goals so you can feel like you have accomplished something (even if it is as simple as "Today my children will be fed and safe—clothing optional") can help, too. Exercise is awesome for improving mood and, says Harvard Medical School, "for those who need or wish to avoid drugs, exercise might be an acceptable substitute for antidepressants."[18]

You can also get a babysitter or help from a trusted friend. If you can't find any friends, you'll just have to settle for relatives. Time away from responsibility can be uplifting. Nourish your body. Nourish your mind.

Food That Helps Treat Depression

> *"Bad nutrition never cured anything."*
> —ANDREW W. SAUL, PhD

With a cuddly little newborn that needs our constant attention, it is no surprise that new moms are likely to eat the wrong foods or avoid meals altogether. Who has time? It seems there isn't time for an uninterrupted trip to the potty, let alone the time to prepare a healthy meal for ourselves. The babies are fed and happy, but some of their mothers just survived half the day on a handful of Junior Mints from last Halloween. Our blood sugar crashes, we reach for anything in sight, and we end up feeling even worse.

Eating healthy while we are pregnant is associated with less depression after the baby is born.[19] Let's keep it going. Healthy eating is *always* a good idea. Eating too much of the wrong thing, eating poorly, or not eating enough is clearly going to make us feel wretched. Our bodies have given so much to grow, give birth, and take care of a baby. We can give back by feeding ourselves right.

First, do yourself a favor and get the junk out of the house. If you reach for a handful of food, let it be cheese cubes or cherry tomatoes rather than gummy bears. If there isn't time for meals, keep your blood sugar in check by making yourself snack throughout the day. You can keep your protein intake up by munching on hardboiled eggs or a bowl of yogurt. Have bite-size veggies around to nibble on. With my first child, a container of nuts and a water bottle sat with me on the couch while I nursed her (for what seemed like every second of every day).

Eat foods high in L-tryptophan, like cashews. Foods containing tryptophan can help you feel much better, says Bo H. Jonsson, MD, coauthor of *The Vitamin Cure for Depression*. "Tryptophan is made into serotonin, one of your body's most potent neurotransmitters. Serotonin is responsible for feelings of well-being and mellowness. Serotonin has such a profound effect that Prozac, Paxil and similar antidepressants artificially keep the body's own serotonin levels high. You can do the same thing naturally through diet by eating high-tryptophan foods," says Dr. Jonsson. "Five servings of beans, a few portions of cheese or peanut butter, or several handfuls of cashews provide 1,000 to 2,000 milligrams (mg) of tryptophan. This will work as well as prescription antidepressants."[20]

We know what we should eat: plenty of fruits and vegetables, healthy fats, probiotic foods, good sources of protein, complex carbohydrates, and plenty of fiber. We know what we shouldn't eat: processed food, unhealthy fats, refined carbohydrates, red meat (except the occasional serving of grass-fed organic), additives, artificial colors, alcohol, and especially refined or artificial sugars. We still want to enjoy a drink once in a while (not while pregnant) or a good ol' steak. (At least I do). This is probably okay for most folks. One meal isn't a problem; it's the hundreds of others we are also eating that need to be evaluated. If you are suffering with depression, what you consume is the first thing to look at.

We know what to do, but we also have to do it. If you feel depressed, frankly, it's hard to even care. We may not be paying close attention to our diet all the time. Supplementation can help fill some nutritional gaps. Optimal dosages of vitamins and minerals can help ease depression. There is no single magic bullet nutrient. They are all important.

Breastfeeding significantly lowers your risk for postpartum depression.
A study of nearly 14,000 mothers that planned to breastfeed, and did so,
were about 50 percent less likely to become depressed than mothers
who planned not to, and didn't breastfeed.[21]

Vitamins and Minerals and Mood Disorders

"If you are depressed, vitamin C is worth considering," says Hugh Riordan, MD.[22] In healthy folks, 3,000 mg a day of vitamin C helped improve
mood.[23]

The B vitamins need each other. If you are depressed, you need them,
too. They work together, so they should be taken together. In other words,
if you want to take extra niacin (B_3) to help battle your depression, you
will also want to take a B complex vitamin each day. B_6 and B_{12} help your
body make feel-good serotonin. Low levels of folate may be associated
with feeling depressed,[24] either on its own or in combination with B_6, B_{12},
and vitamin C deficiency.[25] Folic acid and the other B vitamins can actually help antidepressants work better,[26] and not enough folic acid could
reduce the effectiveness of antidepressants.[27]

Niacin (B_3) is effective for treating mood disorders, including depression. (To read in much more detail about niacin's beneficial properties for
the treatment of depression, see the section on niacin in the chapter on B
vitamins.) Lack of B_{12} can cause feelings of depression and supplementation can be helpful, especially for those deficient in the vitamin.[28] If you
are a vegan and eat no animal products whatsoever, you are virtually
dependent on B_{12} synthesis from your friendly colon bacteria. It may be a
good idea to get your B_{12} status evaluated by your doctor. If your levels
are fine, you are all set, but not everybody has healthy bacterial flora. For
example, if you have ever had an antibiotic, there is a really good chance
your bacteria flora has been compromised. For vegetarians who typically
have yogurt, cheese, or eggs, these are all good sources of B_{12}.

If you have heard of the "winter blues," or Seasonal Affective Disorder
(SAD), then you know that a lack of sunshine can be directly related to
your moods. It is recommended that pregnant and lactating women get
4,000 international units (IU) of vitamin D a day.[29] You can have your
vitamin D levels checked by your doctor.

If you need a little extra assistance with those pangs of sheer hunger
that have you about to lose your mind and resort to chewing on your own

arm, the mineral chromium can come in handy. Chromium helps even out the highs and lows of blood sugar levels, and thus reduce our urge to stuff our face with junk. Specifically, chromium can help with carbohydrate cravings,[30] reduce overeating, and reverse the feelings of depression.[31] Many of us are not getting nearly enough chromium in our diets.[32] If you are depressed, this may be yet another helpful nutrient to consider taking. Malcolm N. McLeod, MD, author of *Lifting Depression: The Chromium Connection,* recommends taking anywhere from 400–1,000 micrograms (mcg) of chromium picolinate daily, or about 4 mcg per pound of body weight. [33] Other minerals can affect depression, including copper, which in excess may predispose women to postpartum depression,[34] while a low intake of zinc, selenium, and magnesium may also contribute to feeling depressed.[35]

Deficiency in omega-3 fatty acids increases a mother's risk of depression, but you aren't likely to hear anything about the importance of omega-3s during pregnancy (and postpartum) from your doctor.[36] According to the American Pregnancy Association, "This may explain why postpartum mood disorders may become worse and begin earlier with subsequent pregnancies."[37] Omega-3 fats can help prevent depression during pregnancy and after your baby is born,[38] and they are essential to your baby's development, too.[39] Want to cut your chances of being depressed in half? In a study of over 11,000 women, those who ate more seafood during their third trimester, and therefore acquired more essential fatty acids and zinc, were about half as likely to suffer postpartum depression for up to eight months after birth as compared to women with the lowest intakes of seafood.[40]

The cure doesn't have to be perfect. You can either: 1. Be depressed; 2. Take medication; or 3. Take vitamins. Remember, the standard is not perfection. The standard is the alternative. And supplements are a whole lot safer to take than pharmaceuticals. Please refer to the chapters dedicated to each nutrient to read about their remarkable safety in both pregnancy and lactation.

If you have suffered with postpartum depression in the past, your doctor may suggest you wait many years before attempting to have another child. You know your body better than anyone. Perhaps your depression can be managed successfully with vitamins and nutrition. Restock your body with essential nutrients and be baby-ready sooner.

DEALING WITH SLEEP DEPRIVATION

A Short Illustrative Play

SCENE OPENS: Monday night. Dinner is set on the table for our family.

CHARACTERS: Dad, Mom, and baby daughter

PROP: Full glass bottle of dark-brown, sticky, sesame stir-fry sauce

Script as follows:

BABY: (Fusses and points.)

DAD (SLEEPY): "You want this?"

BABY: (Nods yes. Daddy reaches to hand her the bottle of sauce.)

MOM TO DAD: "Honey. You are ridiculous. Give that to me. And I'm putting this on Facebook."

When you are a new mom, or a mom with a new baby and other little ones who already demand so much of your time, lack of sleep alone is enough to trigger depression, tumultuous emotions, and forgetfulness.

I was downright loopy. Existing in a dreamlike lack-of-sleep-haze, I would forget what I was saying mid sentence. I would forget why I was holding something in my hand. I would forget what day of the week it was. I was on the phone with my father and I forgot I was talking to him. If something wasn't written down, it wouldn't be done, and if I forgot what to write down, oh well.

We have an enclosed, unheated mudroom, much like a covered porch. Occasionally our cat, with her size-appropriate name of "Little Kitty," runs out there when an opportunity presents itself. It's usually a good idea to remember to let her back into the main house, as the small mudroom doesn't contain her food dish, water bowl, or litter box. Once or twice she experienced what my husband calls "Mommy and Daddy Appreciation Nights" when she was accidentally left out there on a frigid winter evening. After my second child was born, I would try to note when she got out there and remind myself to let her back into the house. I would, of course, promptly forget. Hours later if I happened to be heading out, a furry blur would race back inside, convinced I had forgotten about her this time. Well, I had. With far more important things (babies!) getting my attention,

I wasn't sympathetic in the slightest. Anyway, you would think she would have known better by then.

There is no substitute for sleep. "Sleep when they sleep" is great advice, until you have more than one child, anyway. If you are lucky, your kids will have similar schedules. If you are lucky, you have a helpful spouse that can ease the burden and help provide the time for you to get a few minutes of rest. If you aren't so lucky, and even if you are, sleep deprivation always sets in. There is nothing quite like adequate amounts of rest to help you feel like a normal human being, but this can be next to impossible with babies in the house. You'll make a point to rest when you can, you'll seek out help when and where you can, you'll try to eat right and take of yourself when there is a moment to spare, but this is none too easy when you are a mom, and your mind and body are under constant demand. I am not overstating this. This is literally the case. And dads are exhausted, too.

I found it very difficult to sleep on a schedule, or a lack thereof, really. Sometimes it's hard to say "Body, sleep *now*!" It's stressful knowing you need more than a half hour nap, anyway. You may lie there the entire time knowing full well that *something* will wake you. Between cats, toddlers, visitors, phone calls, baby monitors, and noises from outside, I was just about ready to invest in a sensory deprivation sleep tank. How *do* you shut off the world when you are a mom? You are always a mom. Moments to yourself are just borrowed time. And yet that makes them all the more important.

It's not uncommon to feel like you are losing it. As a mom with a three-month-old baby and a toddler running around the house as I write this very sentence, my body is constantly called upon to do something physically challenging. This is draining and tiresome. A nursing mom has little escape; newborns require the food you are manufacturing, they desire the warmth and comfort that your touch provides. They only have one mom. It seems no other will do but you. This is wonderful, and overwhelming, at the same time. It is the rule, not the exception, that both kids need diapers at the same time, attention at the same time, food at the same time. I marvel that anyone has more than two.

Sleeping Next to Baby: More Rest for You or Less?

As infants, there was no place my children loved to be more than stuffed into my armpit. I found I got more sleep next to them than I did if I put them in a crib or bassinet. Their grunts, groans, and constant movements settled only when they were snuggled right next to me. They were calm, quiet, safe, and warm. I'm pretty sure having their food source immediately available was a huge motivating factor. But I found it comforting, too.

Once they each were a few months old and stronger, their fidgeting by my side woke me frequently throughout the night. Now that I wasn't sleeping as well, I felt it was time for them to have their own space. Transitioning the babies to their cribs took about a week (of even less sleep) to be accomplished, but both became comfortable in their cribs and I regained those precious few hours of rest.

Like every important parenting decision, you are going to have to decide this one for yourself. Sleeping next to my infant children seemed to be the best option at the time. I trusted my instincts. When my sleep was compromised, I made the necessary adjustments, keeping in mind that it was important that I get as much rest as possible so I could better attend to them during the day.

When I used to wake to feed the children in the middle of the night, I would go lay in the guest bed upstairs. If I fell asleep while they nursed, so what. Sleep was good. If I stayed awake enough to get back into my own bed, however, that was even better; I would be woken by cries of hunger rather than jabs to the ribs. But in order to be woken, I had to be asleep first. It wasn't so hard to get up and stay up with them. What was hard was getting *back* to sleep. This is where B$_3$ (niacin) came in very handy, as did lecithin. Magnesium also helped me feel more calm and relaxed so I could get some needed shut-eye.

THOSE OTHER POSTPARTUM ISSUES

Millions of women just like us have struggled with the same issues we have as we recover from our pregnancy and learn to handle our new (or additional) baby. This may be a little comforting—not that it makes it any easier. Here are a few tips for managing some other post-pregnancy issues on many a mom's mind: weight loss and post-pregnancy sex.

Losing the Baby Weight

We were traveling; this is always an immense task with children. With limited dressier clothing options in my own suitcase and my mounting frustration that I couldn't fit comfortably into any of them, my husband said to me, with the kindest of intentions (but the most maleness of approaches), "We could always go to Walmart and buy you some stretch pants."

I stared at him and blinked.

That wasn't exactly the "answer" I was looking for. I don't think he got it, but my friends on Facebook did.

The weeks following the birth of a new baby are a dizzying, intense, twenty-four-seven cycle of feedings, diaper changes, and brief naps for both mom and baby. There isn't much time to eat or shower, let alone pack a travel bag with flattering outfits. (The kids always seem better dressed than we do, don't they?) Figuring out how we are going to shed the baby pounds has very little room in our top priority list, but it is there in our minds nonetheless. Will we ever look the same again? Does the sacrifice that comes with being a mother also include carrying extra pounds for the rest of our lives? It may seem petty to worry about how we look when it seems like there are more important tasks to attend to, but I'm here to tell you it is okay to want to regain your figure.

My advice is to not feel guilty because you want to trim down. It is okay to be vain, ladies. It is okay to care about your appearance. It is okay to take the time to eat right and exercise. Yes, we are going to have to be a little creative to figure out just how to get that done, but it is worth it. A happy mom means a happy baby, and a happy family.

What You Already Know

We can't expect instant gratification. Growing a baby took months. It is natural and normal for us to gain weight during pregnancy, and it is natural and normal for it to take some time to lose the weight afterward.

The same tricks that can help you lose weight whether or not you are a mom still apply. It's no secret: diet and exercise are what it takes. There are lots of videos, books, and online references to read for quick mom friendly exercises, like yoga with your baby (while your toddler skips around the room), or five-minute workout routines that you can slip in between naps, and instead of showering. But what we eat will be even more important than the exercise we can occasionally squeeze in.

What I Did

I gained thirty-five pounds during my first pregnancy, and nearly forty with my second. It took approximately six months to get back to my regular size, and a year before I was able to reshape and tone my body into its pre-baby state. For some women it will take longer. Others may bounce back more quickly. But it can be done. Before each child was conceived, I ran a half marathon with my hubby. I was in the best shape possible prior to each pregnancy, and I feel that gave me a leg up when it came to shedding pounds post-pregnancy.

I knew that breastfeeding is a great way to burn calories once the baby is born, about 500 extra calories a day. I also drank lots of fresh, raw vegetable juice, stayed active by chasing after a toddler and getting out for stroller walks and doing brief workouts when I had a few minutes. I kept processed foods out of the house. I kept satisfying snacks at hand, like nuts, cheese, and fruit. I prepared and froze healthy meals before the baby was born, and after we ate them all, my husband and I would cook on weekends to provide easy meal options during the week.

Community Commentary, Weight Gain, and Weight Loss

Get ready for people to comment about your weight. When you are pregnant, it'll be "Wow, you're *huge!*" Hopefully, they will keep their mouth shut after the kid emerges.

Weight gain is a natural part of being pregnant, but folks tend to fixate on it and offer up their comments. Often. Moms tend to talk about it a lot, too. Telling others how much you've gained and or lost post-baby is like telling a war story. If you are still trying to lose weight after your child is born, any comment about your weight (even if it is nice) can make you feel overly aware of the weight you have still to lose. On the other hand, for those who have already shed their baby pounds, a "Wow, you are thin!" still may leave you feeling awkward. I guess I'd rather the conversation focus on how cute babies are than talk about how much we all weigh.

Make your goal to be fit. "Thin" can still be unhealthy, and "heavy" is never healthy. "Fit" carries the added elements of good diet and exercise. We know it takes time and effort to achieve a lean body. We have seen the impact of healthy food and lifestyle choices. It is hard to maintain a fit physique, but it's worth it.

Do your best to get near your healthy pre-pregnancy size before baby number two or three. Women sometimes say that it can be harder to get back to your pre-baby weight after each additional child. Many women never will, but it is worth doing. Additionally, problems for you caused by weight gain, such as increased cholesterol and elevated blood sugar and blood pressure go away when the extra weight does. Keeping your weight in check benefits your health. It will also benefit the health of your next baby.

Sex

People have multiple children. We know, then, that after the first baby we will have sex at least once or twice more.

Give yourself time to heal. (With a new baby around, you probably won't have any time for lovemaking anyway.) You'll literally have to "ease into it" when you do get the thumbs up from your doc that's it is okay to have sex again. It will be less uncomfortable each time you try. A healthy body will heal more rapidly, so continue doing all the things you know to be right: eat as well as you can and take your vitamins, especially vitamin C which aids in the healing process. Applying topical, natural, vitamin E can help dry skin feel soft and supple and help sooth soreness.

It may feel like sex is just one more physical demand on your body. You had to grow a baby, carry it, give birth, and then breastfeed (and continue to carry) the child for months. Sex may be at the very end of a long list of things that need to be done.

"Do I eat, shower, sleep, or have sex?" Eating or sleeping will win almost every time.

Cut yourself some slack. You aren't Superwoman. The crazy newborn stage will pass. Before you know it, the kids will be borrowing the car. There will be time to be together; you'll make the time, just like you do with everything else. When there is time to be close, you'll find sex makes life a whole lot better.

You love your spouse. Be good to each other. (Sex is just *one* way to do that.) A loving relationship can make raising children a whole lot easier. Remember, there's at least seventeen years of parenting left to go.

CHAPTER 11

Healthy Babies and Healthy Kids

*"The thing that's nice about pregnancy is that
in the end, you have a baby."*
—ANN ROMNEY

You've kept them healthy and safe in your womb; why stop now? You've spent your entire pregnancy being über careful about what you eat, about exercise, about vitamins, about everything, really. Now there is this separate little person to take care of, too. If you are a nursing mother, your body will still be doing plenty of work to sustain your child. Continuing to provide your body and your baby's growing body with ideal nutrition just makes sense.

For those of you interested, here are some tips to help you through some of the challenges we face as parents, once our little ones are finally in our arms. This includes tips on how to feed them the best foods possible; giving your kids vitamins; getting your kids to drink fresh, raw vegetable juice; choosing a pediatrician; and managing sickness and vaccine side effects with optimal doses of vitamin C.

VITAMINS AND BABIES

Our child's pediatrician recommended that, in addition to breast milk, our baby be given liquid vitamins. Had she been on formula, he said, she would get all those extra vitamins she needed. I happen to disagree, but breast milk or no breast milk, I was planning on giving my child vitamins. Breast milk is as close to a perfect food as it gets, and yet additional vitamins are still important for a growing baby.

219

Our pediatrician recommended Tri-Vi-Sol. After reading the package label, I immediately put it back onto the store shelf. I find it quite contradictory and extremely unnecessary, not to mention nauseating, to put artificial color and artificial flavor into any health supplement. I avoid taking vitamins that come formulated with food paint and artificial additives; I was certainly going to avoid giving my baby anything of the like. (Recently, my husband picked up a bottle of chewable vitamin C and was surprised to find that the tablets also contained FD&C yellow #6 and aspartame. Yuck. This is a reminder to always read labels.)

Tri-Vi-Sol contained vitamins A, C, and D. All important to be sure, but I was also sure there were a few more nutrients that were important as well. Seeking a more complete formula, I checked out other adaptations of Enfamil's vitamin complexes for infants. I put them back on the shelf, too. Tri-Vi-Sol with Iron, and its cousin Poly-Vi-Sol with Iron, not only contained artificial ingredients, they also contained ferrous sulfate, a form of iron known to cause stomach upset. Right—let's give our babies vitamins that make them feel bad. *That* makes sense. Well, of course it doesn't. And neither does giving our children vitamins with artificial ingredients, especially when so many other good infant vitamins are out there. (In case you are wondering, I have no financial connection whatsoever with the health products industry. This means I won't recommend brands, but I do occasionally talk about the ones I don't like.)

At our child's one-year wellness visit, the pediatrician sounded a lot like he had a year ago. Since our baby was now weaned, he said to us, "You don't need to give her vitamins anymore." He said that the baby needed extra vitamins when breast milk was the only source of nutrition, but now that she was eating solids, she would get all the vitamins she needed through her food. He had said the same thing about formula all those months ago.

"And you can stop taking your prenatal vitamin, too, now that you are done breastfeeding."

Interesting, I thought, and pretty optimistic.

We chose a different path and it has served the family well: we take our vitamins anyway.

Giving Babies and Toddlers Vitamins

As you may have guessed, both of my kids have been getting supplemental vitamins from the first few days of their lives: a multivitamin and extra vitamin C. The easiest way to get the vitamins down is to offer them to an infant in liquid form. If you have had varying success giving your child vitamins, you know how important it is that they also be tasty.

Knowing that vitamin C in solution loses its potency over time, we took our own vitamin C powder and every few days or so we fortified the liquid C vitamin bottle with an additional 1–2 grams of calcium ascorbate and ascorbic acid powder. Our children have done well with a mixture of about 80% ascorbic acid crystals buffered with 20% calcium ascorbate powder. It wasn't an exact science, but it didn't need to be. If we saw the dropper was packed with vitamin C crystals, we'd only give the baby about one-quarter teaspoon of the liquid at a time. We'd give him or her much more before, during, and after immunizations, and when he or she came down with a cold. Our vitamin routine was as follows: they each would get a dropper of multivitamin (also fortified with extra vitamin C powder) with a meal in the morning, liquid C at lunch and snack time, and more C later in the afternoon. We estimated that they were getting about 50–100 mg of vitamin C in each dose.

We kept it up when they were kids. Our children still get a multivitamin and extra vitamin C every day. As kids get older, they can take relatively more vitamin C. Our three-year-old would get 500 mg of chewable vitamin C three to four times daily. At age four, she took about 4,000 mg a day. If there is a need to give larger doses, like when the kids get sick, we give them powdered vitamin C mixed in liquid or fruit juice, about 1,000 mg at a time.

We will also give them more vitamin C more frequently before and after vaccinations. Our goal is to avoid vaccine reactions and side effects by getting them to near saturation of vitamin C. After immunizations, their immune system needs all the help it can get. They will get C as often as every hour until they get gassy, a telltale sign that they are getting adequate amounts. The goal is to get them to the point just before "bowel tolerance," or loose bowels. We don't allow the kids to get diarrhea and dehydrate, but we do want them to have the vitamin C their bodies require when tackling sickness or immunization side effects. Since gassiness comes before loose bowels, it's a helpful indicator. If bowel tolerance is reached and stools become frequent, liquid, or, as was the case for my breastfed three-month-old, frequent and greenish in color (since they are always liquid-like), we reduced the frequency and dose but continued to give it regularly, ramping the frequency and dose up and down as the situation requires. This takes a little practice, but we know we're not hurting our children with extra C. It is a very, very safe vitamin. (In fact, you might be surprised how much a three-month-old can hold after a couple of vaccinations. I was.) To read more about why we give so much vitamin C before, during, and after vaccinations please read the section entitled Vitamin C and Vaccinations.

I've watched extra vitamin C bring down a fever, reduce pain from teething, reduce inflammation, and relieve congestion and coughing. We are far more comfortable giving our kids large doses of vitamin C than we will ever be giving them an antibiotic or any other drug. And we know with some childhood illnesses, especially if they are viral in nature, antibiotics don't work anyway.

Our kids have yet to need baby Tylenol or any antibiotics. They both come right to the kitchen when it is time to take their vitamins. When she was three, my daughter referred to herself and her brother as "vitamin C babies." You may find, as our family did, that healthy kids keep your pediatrician happy. Healthy kids are, after all, what we are all working for.

In *The Vitamin Cure for Children's Health Problems,* pediatrician Ralph Campbell, MD, stresses the importance of a strong immune system. He recommends "immune boosters," including vitamin C, sleep, multivitamins, vitamin E, the carotenes, and the importance of knowing about alternative therapies like the "antitoxic, antibiotic, and antiviral properties of megadoses of vitamin C."[1] Good diet alone may not be enough for our kids. Investing in "nutritional insurance," a phrase coined by Roger J. Williams, PhD, discoverer of pantothenic acid (vitamin B_5), by giving your children vitamins, helps make up for those gaps that at some point or another will appear in their diet. This is powerful and comforting knowledge for a parent to have.

MOVING ON TO SOLIDS AND LIQUIDS: KEEP GOOD NUTRITION GOING

Once your baby is older and done nursing, he is his own independent person. It is both scary and liberating. Breast milk is such a perfect food. It might be hard for you to imagine him surviving without it. Formula babies have had their sustenance provided in a bottle for so many months. Now, they all get to transition into eating what the rest of us do, maybe better.

Our kids watch what we eat. They watch what we put in our shopping cart. Instilling healthy eating habits now will last a lifetime. What is good for you is good for them: eating plenty of fruit and veggies, drinking plenty of water, staying active, and taking your vitamins.

When you really focus on buying the very best foods for your little one, it becomes all the more apparent how much junk is for sale. You can make a point to buy unprocessed, low sugar, preservative free, natural, organic, GMO-free, fresh food, but sooner or later every kid is going to eat stuff that isn't good for him.

You have a choice. You can let them fend for themselves, or you can boost their immune systems so their bodies can fight back when exposed to non-ideal situations. This is how you can continue to fight for the health of your little one, even when they're not at your side.

Children and Vegetables

My daughter was a little over one when we pulled up to the cashier at our local grocery store and among all the other items, I handed the cashier a half-empty container of cherry tomatoes.

Upon noting the container was almost empty and seeing me, obviously semi-frazzled, largely pregnant, and a mom of a toddler, the cashier kindly said, "Oh, you dropped these! You don't have to pay for them. It happens."

A bit confused I replied, "No I want to pay for them. She ate them."

Now the cashier was confused. "She ate them? Tomatoes? Really? My son is fourteen and he won't eat them!" Kids are funny, you know. You never know what they are going to like.

When I was younger, my parents often made fresh raw vegetable juice for us. I wasn't exactly fond of it. A combination of food bribery (afterward we could have whatever we wanted to eat "within reason") and parental authority provided reasonable assurance that it would go down the hatch.

The easiest way to get veggie juice down was to do it quickly. I learned to chug a pint in about four seconds. It wasn't that the juice tasted bad. I just thought other food just tasted *better*, and I wanted to eat it, and soon.

I drink the stuff now not so much because I like the flavor, but more because I like how it makes me feel. Knowing full well this habit is an integral part of our health and well-being, my husband and I decided to juice for our kids, too. I wasn't sure my children would take to it, but I have learned to withhold judgment about healthy foods they might like to eat. One day my one-year-old son decided he liked raw mushrooms. Cool.

Not only did our baby girl drink raw vegetable juice, but she asked for it. This was common when we were drinking it right in front of her. She didn't want to be left out. Still doesn't.

"Would you like some juice?" my husband would ask so many, many months ago when she was very little and having a variety of beverages was still a new concept for her. She nodded yes. He got her some orange juice, half water. She took a sip, set down the cup, and then asked for juice again.

"Oh, do you want *carrot* juice?" looking at the contents of the glass in his own hand.

She nodded yes. He handed her a sippy cup of carrot juice, and down it went.

"Juice" in this household is defined by my daughter and son as fresh, raw veggie juice. When they ask for juice, it is not from a container in the refrigerator, nor is it orange or apple or grape. They know juice is the product of what that large machine on our counter produces. Our daughter and our son both love to help make it, and we have the smiling photos and videos to prove it. Daddy will sit them up on the counter with all sorts of wonderful veggies strewn about. Cucumbers, kale, carrots, beets, cilantro, cabbage, cilantro . . . they will grab a carrot and put it in the juicer, and then push the plunger down. Before Daddy and I drink our glassfuls, they are offered some with a brightly colored straw. Yum.

It's fun to see kids get excited about good food. I know it is only a matter of time before they realize we have been holding out on them, but we will cross that bridge when we get to it. For now, we'll just keep right on doing what's working.

Our one-year-old son likes homemade veggie juice so much, he chugs the stuff.

That's my boy.

HAND, FOOT, AND MOUTH DISEASE

Low vitamin A status may be to blame. A study of 450 children with the disease (and another 113 who did not have it) found "[m]ost of the children with hand, foot and mouth disease presented Vitamin A insufficiency, which was associated with their reduced immunity and more severe illness."[2]

Hey, let's juice some carrots!

You may be wondering, will my kid drink it? You bet. Start them young. Let them help. Parents may prepare all sorts of foods for their babies. Why not make them juice, too, and have some ourselves?

My dad and I teamed up and wrote *Vegetable Juicing for Everyone. How to Get Your Family Healthier and Happier, Faster!* If you'd like to learn more about juicing, why to do it, how to do it, and be entertained with stories about our off-kilter family while being motivated at the same time, you may want to give it a read.

Choose Your Title: "A Convenient Schedule for Baby" or "Confessions of an Obsessed Mother"

It's hard not to be at least a *little* obsessed with your kids' health. Mostly I'm just writing that so I can feel better about the "schedules" I used to leave for my children's caregivers. It listed emergency contacts, mealtimes, foods they would eat (and were allowed to eat) and where they were located, activities they like, naptime, bedtime, the sign language they used, things he or she was likely to get into, bath time and bedtime routines, the most likely portion of each day to expect a full diaper, and even the location and description of "inside shoes" versus "outside shoes," as the sheer number of feral cats in the area almost guaranteed the mingling of their byproducts with my wool area rug if such distinctions were not made clear, and whatever else fit into three color-coded pages. Typed. Single-spaced. With an appendix.

In my defense, the schedule was typed mainly because my handwriting is atrocious. It was color coded for easy reference and easy maneuverability. It was three pages long because it was thorough. Or, perhaps, it was a bit obsessive.

Still, it was important to me that the information be there, accessible, whether or not his or her caregiver read it line for line and followed every instruction. It showed "how we do things around here." Maybe that extra bit of obsessiveness helped folks be just that much more in tune with our preferences. They were our kids, after all. When we would get home they would often mention how our son or daughter would remind them of anything they missed. This always made us smile.

I did mellow out a bit with the second child, but not much. We are still overly clear about the foods we want our kids to eat, and we still have a lengthy typed guide for reference. We kept it easier by not having any junk in our own house. It is hard to eat stuff that is bad for you if it's not there.

It also didn't hurt to increase other people's awareness of our dietary and health preferences. It comes in handy at family events, especially when we stick to our guns and say "no sugar before bed" or "no artificial foods." It is kind of expected that we'll say this. In fact, before each and every meal that we have away from home, my husband and I have a brief tête-à-tête to decide which foods being offered we will let the kids eat. Therefore, our responses to the children, or to anyone else, are consistent. We don't get mad at each other later and say, "Hey, why did you let her eat that!?" (That doesn't mean we haven't done exactly that in the past. We just know better now.) We are clear, to each other first. We speak out to others when necessary, usually before the meal even begins by simply saying out loud what the kids can eat. It's easier to say what they can have in advance of the meal than to scold Grandma or Grandpa for offering the child food we don't allow. For example, before a meal of green beans, sweet potatoes, ham, and watermelon, we say, "She can have some potatoes, beans, and watermelon." We just leave out the ham. We don't say anything bad about why, like the fact that it is heavily processed, loaded with nitrates, and doesn't fit into our idea of a plant-based diet. (Our kids aren't vegetarian, but we choose to give them only modest amounts of grass-fed, organic meat that is free of processing chemicals.) But now is not the time for a food lesson, and, I feel as others may, too, it would be downright rude. Positive phrasing goes a lot better than giving the impression that we are "turning our noses up" and putting down others' choice of food.

When a child is too young to eat what is put on the table for adults, we simply bring the baby food with us. For example, if we wanted him or her to have a certain kind of yogurt (unsweetened whole-milk organic), we didn't leave it up to chance, we brought it. We can't always expect that folks are going to wash produce with soap and water. We won't be able to stand by our children's side at all times and insist they eat only organic, grass-fed meat if they are to have any at all. We won't be able to control every morsel that goes in each mouth. There are lots of kids that have special dietary needs for one reason or another. Packing a lunch may be one way of making this conversation with others a little easier. It's not always comfortable to speak up. But my level of comfort is less important than my children's good health. Folks don't have to agree with us, and often they don't. But my husband and I know we are upholding the values we've had all along, and over time, acceptance by others may follow.

Whoever said it was easy to be a parent anyway?

SMART KIDS EAT THEIR VEGETABLES

Kids that have a high intake of folic acid in their diet get better grades at school, a recent study in *Pediatrics* shows.[3] There's another good reason to eat those leafy greens.

The Cost of Good Food

Some people will say that eating right costs more. And they may be right, at least for now. The "cost" of eating unhealthy foods is revealed in other ways. A very healthy diet loaded with fruits and vegetables may cost another $550 a year.[4] Averaged out, that is the cost of standard cable television or that monthly data plan you may have tacked onto your cell phone service. In our household we do without cable and I have yet to get a smart phone with a data plan. We choose to spend our money on better food instead. What is an extra buck fifty a day, really? Consider the cost of health care. If you are thinking, "Well, if I get sick health insurance will pay," think again. Deductibles are thousands of dollars a year. You will find yourself paying for those extra doctor's visits, medications, and tests right out of your pocket. Even healthy folks getting routine exams pay plenty. Being sick is all that more expensive. Paying for good food now prevents the costs of chronic illness in the future. Paying for good food now means you also get to feel better now, not just reduce healthcare costs later.

I know firsthand that feeding a family of four the best food possible is more expensive. We do what we can. We weigh the costs and the benefits. We may pay extra for organic celery, lettuce, and carrots, but when it's apple season, we buy less expensive non-organic apples in bulk and wash all produce with soap and water to reduce pesticide exposure. Quality is important, but so is quantity.

We should always strive to move up the "food continuum," as it were. For example, yogurt is good. Yogurt free of dyes, fake sugars, and fillers is a big improvement. Organic yogurt is better, and organic yogurt made from the milk of grass-fed free-range cows is best. The step from "yogurt" to "yogurt free of junk" is not an expensive one. Taking the next step to organic yogurt will cost more, but buying organic quarts instead of those nonorganic mini cups will be about the same cost.

This is doable. We can always afford to eat *better*. I don't think we can afford not to.

Did you know that, according to the *European Journal of Clinical Nutrition,* kids who consume probiotics have a lower risk for infection?[5] Pass the yogurt please!

"Example isn't another way to teach, it is the only way to teach."
—ALBERT EINSTEIN

Good Food on the Go

It's pretty nice being a parent these days, especially when it comes to the availability of organic convenience foods. They even come ready-to-eat, straight from the pouch. They are great for traveling or when someone else watches our child. In a perfect world, I would chop and blend and cook and puree my own baby food right from the source. But when I can't, at least there are some good, easy options out there. When I buy prepackaged items, I tend to stick with combinations that include vegetables and fruit rather than fruits alone. Kids have no trouble eating sweet, yummy fruit. It is harder to get down spinach, peas, or broccoli.

YOUR BABY'S DOCTOR

"Jim, you've got to let me go in there! Don't leave him in the hands of twentieth century medicine."
—DR. LEONARD "BONES" McCOY, *STAR TREK: ENTERPRISE*

As you and your baby move more into the natural health world, you may find you are met with a surprising amount of resistance, especially at the doctor's office. While the next section is not about pregnancy, I wanted to share some personal experiences we've had with our children's physicians. Knowledge is power, and there are times I wish I had known more—sooner. I may seem very much the "mother bear" in these next few sections. It's hard not to be. Protecting our children is instinctual. We just do it. Sometimes we must even be on the defensive with those whom we would like to trust most: their pediatricians.

Pediatricians: The Good the Bad and the . . .

Today I fired my pediatrician. I want to take my children to a doctor who will inform, discuss, suggest, reassure, and support. I chose to leave a practice where I felt the doctors dictate, prescribe, lecture, threaten, and scare.

When you are overwhelmed being the parent of a new human being amidst the whirlwind of responsibilities that have suddenly descended upon your shoulders, it is natural to want to believe that your doctors, especially the doctors of your babies, have your very best interests at heart. You want to trust their knowledge. You want to rely on their judgment. You may feel that when it comes to your children's health, this is one area at least where you can let the professionals take over.

Don't.

No matter how amazing your doctor is, your family is more so. You must approach each visit with the trained eye of a veteran health advocate. You must be careful and clear. You must be in tune with the subtle ebb and flow of the appointment. Are you being pressured or supported? Are you being made to feel unimportant or empowered? You must be prepared at all times to question, verify, and challenge. What follows in this section of the book are just some of the reasons why.

RSV and Bronchiolitis

Our six-week-old son came down with a cold. With no fever, no trouble nursing or breathing, and an avid appetite, our son's congestion and cough were still enough reason for me to check in with our doctor. He was very, very young, after all. We wanted to make sure he was okay. And we wanted some reassurance. This is exactly why I like having doctors around. I find comfort in diagnosis.

Instead, the pediatrician scared the living daylights out of us.

Our son's doctor called it bronchiolitis due to RSV (respiratory syncytial virus). Given a title and more recently a new vaccine—advertised in a popular office table baby magazine, showing a happy, brightly lit nursery next to the gloom and doom of a hospital room, suggesting that's where your baby is heading if you don't get the shot—a mention of RSV and a quick Internet search is enough to terrify any parent.

Perhaps our baby's doctor would simply share with me that "the vast majority of cases of bronchiolitis can be cared for at home with supportive care. Make sure your child is getting adequate liquids. Consider saline nose drops or suctioning with a bulb to relieve nasal congestion. Be alert for changes in breathing difficulty. Expect the condition to last for a week to a month,"[6] like the Mayo Clinic says. Perhaps she'd say, "He has a cold, a common one at that." Nope. Or, "Because he is so young, you will want to keep a watchful eye, but otherwise, he'll probably be just fine with home care." She didn't. So I didn't have this information either. (She certainly wasn't going to say anything about giving him large quantities of vitamin C. But I didn't need to hear that to know that's what I needed to do.)

A little doohickey was strapped to his big toe. I shouldn't have had to, but I asked what they were doing exactly.

"Measuring his oxygen level."

"Oh, okay."

I watched as a number on the screen jumped up to a 94 on a couple of occasions, but mostly the reading hovered around 92 or 93. This was only when it registered anything even remotely consistent, though. Most of the time, the strap kept falling off his toe or needed constant readjustment. The device failed to give a steady reading. This seemingly sloppy method of measurement didn't instill much confidence in me in their evaluation system. But I still didn't know what they were looking for. What did those numbers mean?

After some time I finally asked, "What number needs to show up on the screen?" They obviously weren't satisfied with what they were seeing.

The doctor indicated that she wanted to see a 95 or higher. Lower than that was a problem, she said. Nervously, I asked why. I was told that he might need to go to the hospital and receive oxygen!

I was alarmed. I truly was. I felt my blood pumping hard. This was sounding so much worse that I had imagined. She continued on and said a bronchodilator would be the next step, and if that didn't help, then perhaps hospitalization if his numbers didn't improve.

Hospital? Drug? Wait a second. If *what* didn't help? She wants to give him a drug that might not work? I needed her to slow down.

I paused, and first asked about the side effects of the bronchodilator drug treatment. She indicated that side effects included fussiness, rapid heartbeat, and shakiness. And I repeated when she finished, "and it still might not work."

"Right."

"The best doctor gives the least medicines."
— BENJAMIN FRANKLIN

I told her I was uncomfortable giving any drug to a tiny baby, unless it was absolutely necessary. She said it wasn't but held me there in conversation for some time trying to convince me it was important, even sharing a story about her own son and how he had been given that drug when he was sick. I can't say I cared. This is a tad heartless, I know, but I wanted her to pay attention to *my* questions and *my* child. And to be really blunt about it, isn't that what I was paying for?

But now I felt like a pretty awful parent. I want to help my baby feel better. Why was I hesitating to accept this treatment? I said I'd need to talk it over with my husband who was home with our other child, so I gave him a call. After sharing information obtained from his quick Internet search about the drug, the listed side effects alone had us both refusing any such medication for our baby. Our little boy was breathing comfortably. He was nursing without any trouble. For goodness' sake, he was smiling on the examination table. My instinct kicked in. This medication wasn't necessary. Some congestion is normal when you have a cold.

Unsatisfied with my answer, the doctor continued to hold me there. The staff monitored his oxygen levels. I felt like we couldn't leave until the doctor said the appointment was over.

"Look," I said. "I'll bring him back tomorrow, or every two hours if you like, but I'm not giving him any drugs or taking him to the hospital unless it is absolutely necessary."

Apparently, it wasn't necessary. They let us go home with the understanding that we'd make another appointment for the morning, and I did. I came back armed and ready.

At home I did some research of my own. Bronchiolitis due to RSV sounds pretty rough. But RSV is basically a cold, and a common one. According to the American Academy of Pediatrics concerning the management of bronchiolitis in infants,[7] unless the oxygen reader consistently reads below 90, supplemental oxygen would not be needed. Once 90 or better was reached, oxygen treatment would cease. Our pediatrician never said that.

LOW VITAMIN D AND RSV

Low levels of vitamin D may increase the risk of RSV in infants.[8] Jack Challem of *The Nutrition Reporter* says, "Infants with low levels of vitamin D are more likely to contract a serious lower respiratory infection called respiratory syncytial virus (RSV). The research, conducted in the Netherlands, found that infants were six times more likely to develop RSV during their first year of life if they had low levels of vitamin D."[9]

I also learned more about bronchodilators. A bronchodilator helps open up the bronchial tubes, or airways, by relaxing the bronchial muscles. I read in a review from *Cochrane Summaries* that "some infants treated as outpatients showed a short-term improvement in respiratory scores, but infants hospitalized for bronchiolitis showed no significant benefit of bronchodilator treatment" and "bronchodilators do not reduce the need for hospitalization, do not shorten the length of stay in hospital or shorten illness duration at home."[10] Further, this review surmised that "given these side effects and little evidence that they are effective, bronchodilators are not helpful in the management of bronchiolitis."[11]

I kept reading. It turns out, bronchiolitis is "inflammation of the small branches of the bronchial tree in which there are *no muscles* [emphasis added] around them that might respond to bronchodilating medicines," says pediatrician Ralph Campbell, MD.[12]

There it was. The drugs weren't likely to be helpful, and potential side effects made them downright risky. I felt our doctor wasn't being transparent. I felt this along with what I perceived to be an undertone that was both paternalistic and accusatory: "we-know-better-than-you-and-why-don't-you-want-to-help-your-child." I was glad I had followed my instincts and refused drug treatment.

I headed back to the doctor's office as they had wanted, co-pay in hand, and they must have heard me coming. A different doctor checked on my son and decided that with close observation, he would likely be just fine. We headed home somewhat relieved. If our first visit to the doctor had resembled the second, I probably wouldn't be writing this.

I'm not suggesting that RSV isn't serious for some children. It can be. I'm not suggesting you should say no to recommended treatments or avoid going to doctors. What I am saying is that you need to be informed because your physician may not be sharing the whole story. Don't just nod and say "Okay, doc." Slow them down. Ask questions. Make a phone call. Take the time to learn, so you can advocate for the health of your children before being pressured into any situation.

And, when they are sick, consider giving your child large doses of vitamin C. I didn't sit idly by and let my son suffer through sickness on his own. While I worked with his doctor, and researched my behind off, I took extra vitamin C, until I reached bowel tolerance (the step just before loose stools) so C would be available in breast milk as he nursed. I also gave my son liquid vitamin C every two hours while symptoms persisted and then every three to four hours when they waned. How did I know he was getting enough vitamin C? He would be noticeably better: less congestion, no cough, alert, cheery, and seemingly comfortable. When he and I both had lots of vitamin C, his symptoms improved. As the C "wore off" at night, his symptoms would become more prominent toward morning. His cough and congestion would return, and he'd be fussy. I would ramp up both his and my C intake accordingly. I continued this until he was visibly better, which he was again by the end of the each day. By the end of the week, he was symptom free, and back to his regular vitamin C intake. We avoided the hospital. We avoided drugs. I used vitamin C and *watched* him get better.

There are parents who need to leave a doctor's office with something, and doctors who feel they must have something to offer. I like to limit this exchange to "information." Maybe some parents like to be told what to do and have a sense of relief when the doctor has pills, potions, and prescriptions to dole out. Consider that perhaps what modern medicine has to offer isn't always in the best interests of your child. But I imagine that if you are the kind of person that reads a book like this, you do a lot of thinking for yourself.

There are many good doctors out there. But there are many that will make you feel like you are a bad parent in one way or another if you don't follow their advice. Maybe I am a bad parent. Or rather, maybe I'm a *badass* parent. I'm not going to be told what to do when it comes to my kids. I will listen, I will learn, I will discuss. Then, I, and my husband, will decide.

Vaccinations

I never received a single vaccination until I was nearly thirty. I was raised with alternative ways to battle sickness, and those methods also kept me from ever needing an antibiotic until I went to college. Not one.

That being said, my husband and I chose to have our children vaccinated. We think some immunizations are worthwhile.

However, we are not in favor of others, but the law is not set up in such a way where doctors and parents can make decisions together about which particular vaccines children receive. Parents can choose to be in compliance with the law, or they can choose to be completely, religiously exempt. You don't get any, or you get all that are required; there is no "buffet" approach here. Each state has its own regulations, and they may differ based on whether the child will be attending daycare or pre-kindergarten (pre-k), or just going right to kindergarten.

Whether you agree with vaccinations or not, I believe pediatricians have an obligation to explain to the parents of their patients what shots are required under law unless they otherwise have an exemption, and under what circumstances shots are not required. For example, there are several shots required in New York State (NYS) for entrance into daycare or pre-k that are not required for entrance into kindergarten. While I have yet to hear the word escape the mouth of a pediatrician that means they are *optional* in NYS as long as your child does not attend pre-k or daycare. I also believe doctors should talk to their patients about the benefits and risks of each shot, discuss what is required and what is optional, and not just assume the child will receive everything. They should give the parent time to read the literature that their office is required to distribute about each vaccine *well in advance* of administration. Possible side effects should be discussed and so, too, should the likeliness that a child will experience said side effects based on the doctor's experience, not just the stats in the handout. This has not happened in my experience.

As my father has said, you may find soon after your baby is born your physician has the child in one hand and a needle in the other. This is not an exaggeration. For example, the first dose of hepatitis B vaccine is often given at birth. My husband and I have learned from experience it is best to be prepared in advance with information for every visit to the doctor, even on baby's birthday.

Vaccine Reactions

"When it happens to your child, the risks are 100 percent."
—BARBARA LOE FISHER, Co-Founder and President of the
National Vaccine Information Center (NVIC)

Our daughter is four. When she was one-and-a-half, she shocked her pediatrician who looked her chart and said, "Wow. She's only in here for wellness visits and vaccines!"

It was true. She was (and is) a healthy kid. She has had a couple of colds, as has her younger brother, but we manage them at home.

What you know with your second child, you don't always know with your first. This was certainly true for us.

I understand the role vaccines play in the prevention of disease. But I believe in administering shots that are as safe as possible, on a schedule that accommodates the child and their developing immune system. Even done this way, things can go wrong. By fifteen months, our daughter had received sixteen inoculations over the course of nine appointments, with a total of twenty-nine separate exposures to individual diseases, many in repetition. Only with our insistence did the doctor separate the administration of the shots. Otherwise she would have been exposed to as many as seven diseases at a clip. During brief visits, they told us what immunizations she would get, moved us quickly through the paperwork and proceeded to give her several shots at one time. Side effects were presented as rare and unlikely. Previous vaccinations had gone all right; at worst she had been a little fussy a few days afterward.

I had never been a parent before. I had much to learn. If I had been more careful about the pediatrician I chose for my daughter and all the information about immunizations I needed to know before I ever entered the doctor's office, I could have saved her, and our family, a great deal of stress, anxiety, misinformation, and even harm.

At fifteen months, hours after she received two shots for four diseases, DPT (Diphtheria, Pertussis, and Tetanus) and Hib (Haemophilus influenzae type b), my baby girl was screaming, falling over and uncoordinated, and spiked a fever that registered as high as 103.5 degrees on our temporal thermometer. My husband was at work; I was going to have to handle this on my own. Knowing that in large doses, vitamin C is an antipyretic (fever reducer) in addition to being an antibiotic, antiviral, and antitoxin,[13] I acted fast and got the fever under control with very large doses of ascorbic acid and calcium ascorbate, or buffered vitamin C, to bowel tolerance, and a tepid bath. At bowel tolerance of vitamin C, she was no longer screaming and falling over. Within the first hour her fever was down by a degree; in the second hour, another degree. For the remainder of the evening her fever hovered around 100.5.

CHILDREN INJURED FROM VACCINES...WHO PAYS? WE DO.

In 1986, the National Childhood Vaccine Injury Compensation Program (NVICP) was enacted to promote vaccine production. How do you encourage production? Make it attractive for manufacturers. One way to do this is to protect them from costly lawsuits. The NVICP does exactly that, as it is the vehicle through which any vaccine lawsuit must first travel.[14] This provides vaccine manufacturers with a legal shield, protecting them from liability. It is the NVICP, not vaccine manufacturers, that pays for damages to children injured or killed by shots, if their families have the needed perseverance to navigate the "highly adversarial, time-consuming, traumatic, and expensive" process, Barbara Loe Fisher, leading vaccine expert, explains.[15] "[T]wo out of three individuals applying for federal vaccine injury compensation have been turned away empty-handed,"[16] she says. This in light of the $2.6 billion that has been paid to over 3,400 plaintiffs as of 2013.[17]

Vaccine manufacturers don't even have to pay for their own legal defense fees. Joseph Mercola, MD, is not anti-vaccine, but he is pro-vaccine safety and for vaccine choice. He explains, "This program has boosted vaccine sales growth immensely—by 2015 it's estimated that vaccinations will morph into a $21.5-billion industry—largely because they have ZERO liability for the products they produce. If a child becomes seriously injured or even dies after receiving a vaccine, the vaccine makers are completely shielded—and IF they are ever awarded compensation through NVICP, it is the taxpayers who pay, not the vaccine makers."[18] Wait, how did we end up with the bill? NVICP is funded through surcharges from each vaccine sold. "So not only are the vaccine manufacturers shielded from potential lawsuits, they are not even responsible for paying one cent of the claims filed against them—the consumers of their products are," says Dr. Mercola.[19]

We pay for the shot, we pay for NVICP, we pay for the consequences of vaccine injury to our own children, and we pay for the consequences of vaccine injury to others, all while the vaccine manufacturers enjoy "total liability protection for injuries and deaths caused by government mandated vaccines" *even if manufactures could have made a safer vaccine.*[20] Drug companies absorb profits, and we absorb problems and pay for the privilege. Somehow, this doesn't seem fair.

I called the pediatrician to report her severe reaction. They recommended that I give her children's Tylenol, especially if her fever went above 101 degrees. Seeing as the fever was under control at the time, I put her to bed and continued to monitor her temperature each hour. Her fever fluctuated inversely with her intake of vitamin C, so I continued to give regular doses, (250–500 mg every two hours or so), keeping the Tylenol handy just in case. By the next morning, she registered normal.

When I asked for the paperwork to see what had been actually written down the evening I dialed her doctor, it simply said, "Called service last pm withh fever"—misspelling and all. It didn't mention any of the other symptoms. Even if they did report this information to Vaccine Adverse Effect Reporting System (VAERS) as they are legally required to do, the report would have been incomplete. This troubled me. Shouldn't all reported symptoms be documented? Did they not believe me? So began our search for a new, more diligent pediatrician.

It would be years later before we knew which vaccine was to blame for our daughter's severe vaccine reaction at 15 months. Her third, and hopefully last, pediatrician determined based on my detailed written record of side effects (the only record we had) that the Pertussis component of the DPT shot had caused her reaction. He said it was medically contraindicated for her to receive any future doses of the Pertussis vaccine and wrote us a letter to that effect. We are relieved, but we are not out of the woods. There are more vaccines to be given before she can attend school, and still more to come after that. Will she react poorly to any of those shots? What about the ones she has never had before?

There is very little room in the pediatrician's office to "discuss" vaccines. Parents are expected to simply do as the physician says. Take a stand and spread out immunizations, or refuse to vaccinate, and the atmosphere in the exam room becomes tense if not hostile. These days, my husband and I go to each pediatric appointment together, dressed professionally, two-inch thick file folder of documents in hand. We always hope for a smooth visit, but invariably we must battle our way through, sticking to our ground and by the sides of our children. On the plus side, we seem to have finally found a pediatrician that will work with us and treat us with respect.

You would think that choosing to get the shots required by law would have satisfied our children's former pediatricians. Instead they told us why we were wrong to not to get all of the other ones. Choosing to give shots spread out over time instead of in large chunks would seem to make sense, and vaccines actually work better that way. But every time we postponed a shot for our children, their doctors told us why we shouldn't. Choose to bring down a fever with vitamin C instead of Tylenol: more dissonance.

When it comes to immunizations, I think most parents go with the flow, until they have reason otherwise. Our daughter's shot reaction gave us reason otherwise. We are far more careful now. I know exactly which shots are required in NYS, and exactly which ones are not. And "required" does not mean "safe." All vaccines carry with them a risk of side effects. All we can do it try to minimize that risk. Moving forward, we not only expect diligence from our doctors but we have become more diligent, too. For example, we decrease the possibility of vaccine side effects by giving vastly more vitamin C to our children before and after shots. To read more about how we do it and why vitamin C works, please see the section on Vitamin C and Vaccinations.

WHAT ABOUT TYLENOL?

Just in case you are concerned, we have a bottle of Children's Tylenol in our kitchen cabinet. We always have it on hand; it just happens to be unopened. While a mild fever indicates the body's normal, natural *immune response* is in good working order combating vaccines, a high fever that spikes during a *vaccine reaction* is very serious and must be brought down right away. Tylenol can do this, but so can high-dose vitamin C.

Our second pediatrician was very concerned when she learned I didn't give my daughter Children's Tylenol to bring down her high fever during her vaccine reaction. She wrote about me on my daughter's record, "She does not really believe in Tylenol."

You're right, doctor. I don't. As you might expect, I avoided acetaminophen during pregnancy. I am of the mind that what may harm a developing fetus may harm a developing child, and the research suggests as much.

Tylenol (acetaminophen) is not the safe substance we are led to believe it is. Current research suggests "that the marked increase in the rate of autism, asthma, and attention deficit with hyperactivity throughout much of the world may be largely caused by the marked increase in the use of acetaminophen in genetically and/or metabolically susceptible children, and the use of acetaminophen by pregnant women."[21] Acetaminophen overdose kills hundreds of people a year, occurring more often by accident rather than intention, and liver damage can occur even when acetaminophen is taken in recommended doses.[22] You can always check out the current stats online at the American Association of Poison Control Centers (AAPCC) for yourself. I choose not to give Tylenol to my children unless absolutely necessary. So far, it has not been absolutely necessary.

My concern and my doctor's concern was the same: my daughter's fever needed to be reduced. I assured the doctor that my baby's fever *was* coming down, one way or another. Had I not seen a decrease in her temperature within half an hour or so with vitamin C, I would have given her Children's Tylenol. But while Tylenol has numerous proven side effects of its own, vitamin C strengthens the immune system, reduces shot side effects, and actually makes the shot work better.[23]

My daughter's high fever wasn't due to lack of Tylenol; it was due to the vaccinations she received that day. Instead of merely suppressing a fever and symptoms of a vaccine reaction with Tylenol, I brought down her fever with a safe, natural vitamin, strengthening her immune system at the same time, so it could do its job the best it could. Shots take a dreadful toll on our kids. Our job is damage control, and there is nothing easy about it, but it can be done without drugs.

Vaccine Exemptions

Unless your child has a sound medical reason not to get a particular shot, such as a known allergy to certain vaccine ingredients or he or she has a compromised immune system, it is unlikely a doctor will allow a medical exemption. So in many cases a reaction must occur first, and only *then* might a child be excused from further dosages of a particular vaccine. That's like putting up a traffic light at a dangerous intersection only after people are seriously hurt. Additionally, a medical exemption requires the doctor's approval. Will the physician trace the adverse effect back to the immunization? Our child's first pediatrician didn't even *write down* the severity of our daughter's reaction when I called it in that evening. They did not record it as a vaccination reaction. I know this because I asked for the medical records and saw the report with my own eyes. Evidence of just how severe her reaction had been omitted. Even if it had been included, the doctor would have had to take my word for it. It might have read something like: "*Mother states* child has fever of 103 and is uncoordinated, falling down, and screaming." That sure would have been an upgrade from the original report. But would it be enough to get her pediatrician to write an exemption?

We reported her vaccine reaction to VAERS. We strongly suspect her pediatrician did not. I find it terrifying to never know which shot it will be that will cause my child to react. It is an unfair situation. As parents, we are backed into a corner because we have to let our child get the vaccine *before* we find out if it hurts her or not. It is no surprise to me that some parents are saying "no" to vaccines, several or all. Many states allow exemptions due to religious beliefs, and others due to personal beliefs. Two allow only medical exemptions.

Vitamin C and Vaccinations

Giving vaccines to children: Right now, it's a ready, fire, aim approach. Will we know in advance what a little baby, only a few months old, is allergic to? When multiple vaccines are often given at one time, will we know which vaccine caused the reaction? It feels like a game of trial and error—of wait and see. That's simply not good enough, and that's why I give my kids vitamin C, and lots of it.

Vitamin C administration before and after vaccination reduces the likelihood of side effects and increases the effectiveness of the immunization. My kids take vitamin C every day, and always have. Now, in preparation for shots, they receive numerous, regular doses of vitamin C before, during (yes right at the doctor's office), and for weeks after administered immunizations. This is what experience and our daughter's vaccine reaction has taught us. While we had given her vitamin C all along, we weren't nearly as diligent about frequent, timely dosing at vaccination time. We thought we were doing enough. As many folks come to find out, what they think is "a lot" of vitamin C isn't always enough vitamin C. You take enough to get the job done.

I agree with Dr. Levy. I believe every doctor should be telling parents to give kids vitamin C when they get vaccinations. According to Levy, in addition to vitamin C's antitoxin properties (for example, its ability for "neutralizing the toxic nature of mercury in all of its chemical forms") he says "there is another compelling reason to make vitamin C an integral part of any vaccination protocol: Vitamin C has been documented to augment the antibody response of the immune system. As the goal of any vaccination is to stimulate a maximal antibody response to the antigens of the vaccine while causing minimal to no toxic damage to the most sensitive of vaccine recipients, there would appear to be no medically sound reason not to make vitamin C a part of all vaccination protocols."[24]

Parents who want to know how much vitamin C to give their children may find this next section useful. Dr. Levy recommends, "Infants under ten pounds can take 500 mg daily in some fruit juice, while babies between ten and twenty pounds could take anywhere from 500 mg to 1,000 mg total per day, in divided doses. Older children can take 1,000 mg daily per year of life (5,000 mg for a five year-old child, for example, in divided doses)."[25] Ideally, the vitamin C would be given prior to vaccination and continue afterward, says Levy. "For optimal antibody stimulation and toxin protection, it would be best to dose for three to five days before the shot(s) and to continue for at least two to three days following the shot. . . . Even taking a one-time dose of vitamin C in the dosage range suggested above directly before the injections can still have a significant toxin-neutralizing and antibody-stimulating effect. It's just that an even better likelihood of having a positive outcome results from extending the pre- and post-dosing periods of time."[26] As for the kind of vitamin C to give little ones, our children have done well with calcium ascorbate and ascorbic acid in either liquid or, as they got older, chewable form as I mentioned earlier in this chapter. Mixing vitamin C powder into juice to reduce bitterness also works well. We have also had success giving them the liposomal form of vitamin C, although it is rather expensive.

Fear is a powerful motivator. Many parents are understandably worried about vaccinating their children because of the risk of side effects. Our daughter suffered a severe reaction before. Will she again? We don't like to wait and see. We give vitamin C instead. Days before, the day of, and for days after vaccination, we give our children enough vitamin C to get them just to the point of saturation. For example, when our daughter was four, we started her with a relatively large loading dose, 2,000 mg or so, then gave her 1,000–2,000 mg every couple of hours throughout the day. We wait until there is a rumbling tummy or softened or loose stool indicating saturation of C. Once that point is reached, we throttle back the dose. We continue to give C, but give less. The next day, we do it again.

Amazingly, the day of and for several days after our four-year-old daughter's last vaccination, the first shot she had received since her severe reaction years before, she comfortably held fifteen to twenty grams, that's 15,000 to 20,000 milligrams, of vitamin C each day. She had no reaction whatsoever to the vaccination. No swelling. No fever. No redness. Nothing. She was happy. We were happy. That may sound like a lot of C for a child who only weighed about 33 pounds, but it got the job done. Perhaps your child won't need that much.

Vitamin C is incredibly safe and effective. We are very comfortable giving both of our kids high doses of C. Older, bigger children may hold more C, and younger ones not as much. Saturation becomes a helpful indicator of how much your child can hold. When our baby boy was not yet one, he received small, regular doses of vitamin C (about 100–150 mg) every three to four hours during the days prior to his shots, and for a week afterward. The day of the shot he got C (about 150–200 mg) every two hours, or just to the point before he reached bowel tolerance. The only side effects he experienced from his vaccinations were redness at the injection site, a small amount of swelling, and some fussiness. Now that he is older, we have upped the dose of vitamin C, just as Thomas Levy, MD, recommends.

Imagine if more parents could help prevent their children from suffering vaccine reactions and side effects by giving high dose vitamin C. As states continue to pass legislature that removes personal exemptions to vaccinations, many parents will be given no choice about which shots their kids receive.

I don't believe it is fair to let children get vaccines without vitamin C, nor do I believe it is fair to let them acquire natural immunity through exposure to disease without vitamin C. When in doubt, give C. As to the quantity of C to give, my father would likely add, "When in doubt, give more." Dr. Levy is convinced of vitamin C's safety. He says, "Except in individuals with established, significant renal insufficiency, vitamin C is arguably the safest of all nutrients that can be given."[27]

For any parent worried about vaccines, knowing about vitamin C should provide some real comfort. It sure does for us.

FLUORIDATED WATER FOR BABIES

Babies are particularly vulnerable to fluoride toxicity. "Due to their small size, infants receive up to 400% more fluoride (per pound of body weight) than adults consuming the same level of fluoride in water," says the Fluoride Action Network, a group committed to broadening awareness about the toxicity of fluoride. "Not only do infants receive a larger dose, they have an impaired ability to excrete fluoride through their kidneys."[28] Fluoride literally builds up in a baby's body, and this may be why formula-fed babies are more likely to get dental fluorosis.[29]

And that's not all. "Over 30 studies have associated elevated fluoride expo-sure with neurological impairment in children, which may, in part, result from fluoride's affect[sic] on the thyroid gland," says The Fluoride Action Network.[30] "When most people hear the word fluoride, they generally think of their teeth and their dentist. Fluoride, after all, is added to some public water systems and many dental products for the purpose of preventing cavities. Less well known is that fluoride is a highly toxic compound, a major industrial air pollutant, a key ingredient in some pesticides and fumigants, the cause of a tooth defect that currently impacts over 40% of American teenagers, and the cause of a devastat-ing bone disease that impacts millions of people throughout the world."[31]

While the American Dental Association, the American Academy of Pediatrics, and American Academy of Pediatric Dentistry no longer recommend fluoride supplements for newborns, there has been no recommendation saying babies should avoid fluoridated water altogether, "a practice that exposes infants to nearly 4 times more fluoride than supplements," says the Fluoride Action Network.[32]

Does your pediatrician still recommend fluoride? Mine does. Each of the three pediatricians my kids have been to have either verbally recommended "nursery water" (fluoridated water) or fluoride drops for my children. Or, they have given me a handout stating the same. I have simply told them "No, thank you."

Unfortunately, many water supplies are fluoridated. I was able to limit my children's exposure by breastfeeding them when they were infants, and now by avoiding fluoride toothpaste, which small children will inevitably swallow. On average, children under six swallow a third of the toothpaste on their brush and can inadvertently swallow as much as 80 percent or more, according to the United States Centers for Disease Control.[33]

Fluoride is always toxic if enough of it is ingested. Vitamin C can lesson or eliminate the toxicity of fluoride, and may in itself provide some protection from tooth decay.[34] A combination of vitamin C, vitamin D, and calcium has been shown to reverse the earliest grade dental fluorosis in children and significantly improve more advanced stages.[35] "Especially noteworthy was that the vitamin C protocol 'markedly reduced' the fluoride levels in the blood, serum, and urine," says Thomas Levy, MD, author of *Curing the Incurable: Vitamin C, Infectious Diseases, and Toxins.* "It appears that "vitamin C supplementation would have some protective effect against dental decay" and "would be an excellent alter-native to the existing water fluoridation programs already in place in so many communities."[36]

Learning as We Go

"God could not be everywhere, so he created mothers."
—JEWISH PROVERB

We learn from our children, and we learn "on" our children. They are our adorable, pudgy little guinea pigs. We try to do what is right and what works, and it feels like much of the time it is by trial and error.

I often feel like going to the doctor is like going into battle. You must be armed and ready. I was hoping for a happier ending here. I was hoping I could report to you that our children's second doctor was the ideal one I had in mind: someone who would discuss, suggest, reassure, and support. Instead, I found it was still as difficult to get what I wanted for my kids. After two visits and all the work that goes into transferring records, filling out paperwork, and getting a new doctor's office up to speed about our children's health and progress, they dropped us. In a letter stating "we disagree with the protocol for immunizing your children" they told us they would "no longer be providing care" for our kids and that we should find another physician. Apparently, when it came to immunizations, they were unhappy with our decision to "only get what New York State required," as was stated in our medical record. Well in advance of transferring my children to her office, I had made this preference very clear to the physician herself. She agreed to it in our phone conversation, but she *changed her mind*. And my kids were left without a doctor. Evidently, following the law, as a citizen of New York State, was unacceptable to her and evidence of poor parenting.

After a subscription to Angie's List, numerous phone calls, and more in-depth conversations with potential healthcare providers, making it as clear as possible what we were seeking in our children's doctor and asking if they would be willing to work with us, we are now moving on to our third pediatrician.

Anyone who has advocated for the health care of another can probably relate, whether the person they have cared for is a child, a spouse, a parent, or a relative. All I can tell you is that based on my experience and what I have heard from others, there will always be work to do. There will always be a fight. You can *never* let your guard down. If you are fortunate enough to get a doctor who will work with you, that should be considered, in and of itself, a success, no matter how hard it was to achieve it. Board certified pediatrician Robert S. Mendelsohn, MD, wrote an excellent book entitled *How to Raise a Healthy Child in Spite of Your Doctor.* My husband and I have learned that that title is not an overstatement.

> *"Never put your trust into anything but your own intellect.*
> *The world progresses, year by year, century by century,*
> *as the members of the younger generation find out*
> *what was wrong among the things that their elders said.*
> *So you must always be skeptical—always think for yourself."*
> —LINUS PAULING

ONE LAST STORY

New moms don't get out much. Some days we stare blankly at the small being crawling around our floor and dream of things we used to do BC (before children); if only we could remember what those things were. Our new baby seems unaware of our glazed over, bleary, tired eyes. The baby seems fond of her schedule. She sleeps just fine. Mom, however, can't even put a proper speaking sentence together. It is a miracle indeed when a mom finds herself with that rare burst of energy that gets her off her couch and out of her living room and outside to shovel a half-foot of snow in her "I-really-should-have-hired-someone-to-plow-this-" sized driveway.

And there I was. Resourceful. Determined. Motivated. I was a Good Mom. I was going to take my child Outside. Not just to play in the snow. Oh no. It was time to *work*. I was going to shovel that entire driveway with her perched in a satchel on my back.

It took half an hour to get a down coat zipped and snapped, boots laced, hood fastened, and gloves pulled on. And then I had to get my eight-month-old baby girl dressed, too. I hefted her insulated body into the baby backpack with her arms and legs outstretched and, her little face peeking under her hood, we ventured outdoors, shovel in my hand.

It was snowing—that beautiful, soft, downy snow that adds several inches of fluff to the ground in no time. This was no deterrent. We had made it Outside. I started to shovel. It felt good to move. It felt good to breathe fresh air. On my back, my baby girl cooed her happy sounds. She was enjoying this, too. I was feeling rather proud of myself. Cars drove by and people stared at us. I was sure they must be thinking, "Look at that mom shoveling her driveway with her baby on her back. What an amazing mom. What energy!" They kept staring. I kept shoveling. Car after car went by. They all looked. My ego puffed right up.

A good forty-five minutes later, the driveway was finished. With a healthy glow of satisfaction and accomplishment on my cheeks, we headed for the warm indoors. As I reached to undo the buckles of the carrier to let out my baby girl, I caught a glimpse of her in the mirror. On top of her poor little head, her hood having obviously fallen down some time ago, stood a mound of some two inches of snow.

Suddenly all those glances from folks driving by made a whole lot more sense. They weren't in awe of my incredible capabilities as a mother. They were in shock that my tiny baby was outside without a hat in the freezing cold weather with a pile of snow her head.

This won't be the only time my children are exposed to the elements. While I try to do my best to protect them, the wind, weather, and cold will be there again when they take off their coats on the playground at school in January and throw snowballs with their bare hands. We can count on them coming into contact with a seemingly endless list of things that will challenge their little immune systems such as illness and stress and junk food and environmental toxins.

All we can really ever do is stack the deck in their favor. We can reduce the chance of trips to the doctor, sick days, and sleepless nights by instilling healthy habits early (now), and by giving them the best food possible with optimal doses of vitamins. We can give their bodies the tools necessary to survive our parenting and the rest of the world. Here's to being happy and healthy.

Appendix

"The germe is nothing; the terrain is everything."
—LOUIS PASTEUR

The following articles written for the *Orthomolecular Medicine News Service* (OMNS) may be of interest for anyone interested in better health for themselves and their families. The peer-reviewed *Orthomolecular Medicine News Service* is a nonprofit and noncommercial informational resource. Subscribe (free of charge) to receive the latest OMNS articles at: http://www.orthomolecular.org/subscribe.html. You can also read past issues in the online archive at http://orthomolecular.org/resources/omns/.

To locate an orthomolecular physician near you, go to: http://orthomolecular.org/resources/omns/v06n09.shtml.

Pass the Mustard, or Just Pass on the Hot Dog?

COMMENTARY BY ANDREW W. SAUL

(OMNS July 2, 2010) More hot dogs are eaten at the 4th of July holiday than at any other time of the year. The National Hot Dog and Sausage Council (yes, an all-too-real trade organization) says that "during the Independence Day weekend, 155 million will be gobbled up" and that Americans will consume more than seven billion hot dogs over the summer. "Every year," they proudly proclaim, "Americans eat an average of 60 hot dogs each."[1]

That looks to be a modest average of just over one hot dog per week per American. But there are at least 7 million vegetarians in the U.S., and another 20 million who would be inclined to avoid meat.[2]

This means that even if you do not eat any hot dogs at all, someone else is eating your share.

But a hot dog or two a week? Big deal!

Maybe it is. Children who eat one hot dog a week double their risk of a brain tumor; two per week triples the risk. Kids eating more than twelve hot dogs a month (three a week) have nearly ten times the risk of leukemia as children who eat none.[3]

And it is not just about kids. Of 190,000 adults studied for seven years, those eating the most processed meat such as deli meats and hot dogs had a 68 percent greater risk of pancreatic cancer than those who ate the least.[4] Pancreatic cancer is especially difficult to treat.

Think twice before you serve up your next tube steak. If your family is going to eat hot dogs, at least take your vitamins. Hot dog eating children taking supplemental vitamins were shown to have a reduced risk of cancer.[5] Vitamins C and E prevent the formation of nitrosamines.[6]

It is curious that, while busy theorizing many "potential" dangers of vitamins, the news media have largely ignored this clear-cut cancer-prevention benefit from supplementation.

May I also suggest that you have your kids chew their hot dogs extra thoroughly. In landfills, "Whole hot dogs have been found, some of them in strata suggesting an age upwards of several decades."[7]

Bon appétit.

References

1. National Hot Dog and Sausage Council Home Page. "Get Your Fill of Hot Dog and Sausage Facts, Culture and History. http://www.hot-dog.org (accessed Nov 2014).

2. Vegetarian Times. "Vegetarinaism in America." http://www.vegetariantimes.com/features/archive_of_editorial/667 (accessed Nov 2014).

3. Peters, J.M., S. Preston-Martin, S.J. London, et al. "Processed Meats and Risk of Childhood Leukemia." *Cancer Causes Control* 5(2) (Mar 1994): 195–202.

4. Nothlings, U., L.R. Wilkens, S.P. Murphy, et al. "Meat and Fat Intake as Risk Factors for Pancreatic Cancer: The Multiethnic Cohort Study." *J Nat Cancer Inst* 97 (2005): 1458–65.

5. Sarasua, S., D.A. Savitz. "Cured and Broiled Meat Consumption in Relation to Childhood Cancer: Denver, Colorado (United States)." *Cancer Causes Control* 5(2) (Mar 1994): 141–8.

6. Scanlan, R.A. "Nitrosamines and cancer." The Linus Pauling Institute. http://lpi.oregon state.edu/f-w00/nitrosamine.html (accessd Nov 2014). Cass, H.J. English. *User's Guide to Vitamin C.* Laguna Beach, CA: Basic Health Publications, 2002, p 64–67.

7. *Smithsonian,* July 1992, p 5.

Steps to Better Health:
Are You Sick of Sickness?

BY HELEN SAUL CASE

(OMNS Oct 19, 2013) Better health? It takes effort. You have got to want it, and then you have got to work for it. There is no one-step solution. We need to eat right, *and* drink plenty of water, *and* take our vitamins, *and* drink fresh, raw, vegetable juice, *and* exercise, *and* reduce stress. All of these things make your immune system stronger, and your body inhospitable to sickness. This isn't easy. But isn't suffering from illness harder?

Know Your Options

I was raised in a household where instead of drugs we used vitamins. They are far safer and often more effective. When I went off to college, I thought I'd give mainstream medicine a try. Not only did drugs not cure my own "feminine ailments," they actually made things worse. I went back to what I knew: vitamins and nutrition work. I'm not a doctor, but I believe you don't have to be a doctor to help yourself. My father explained that medical doctors are trained to practice medicine and prescribe medications. Natural, vitamin alternatives just aren't visible in the medical tool bag. I sought out nutritional cures because I needed to. I go to my doctor, but I don't always get the drugs she recommends. Using vitamins and nutrition to prevent and cure illness works better for me. Sure, we can always go to our doctors with our health problems. But wouldn't it be nice to not *need* to go?

Ditch the Drugs

Adding a chemical to your body doesn't address the underlying cause of illness. No cell in the human body is made out of a drug. You have a real choice: medication or nutrition. One of these two choices is remarkably safer, cheaper, and, in many cases, more effective than the other. Guess which one that is? People put their faith in pharmaceuticals because they are sick and they want to get well. But when drugs don't work, which is surprisingly often, we have to make a decision. We can choose to keep returning to the disease-medicate-disease-medicate spin cycle or we can choose to get onto excellent nutrition and a healthy life style. You may find that your doctor agrees, but simply needs some education about the benefits of vitamin supplements.

Take Your Vitamins

I sure do. There is no single magic bullet in the list of essential nutrients. They are all important. The right dose is crucial. High doses help the body get adequate amounts of essential nutrients when it needs them. Many people do know the value of great nutrition, but knowing how to use high-doses of vitamins to treat our health issues is another story. Which vitamins should we take? How much? (Really, *that* much?) Do they work? Yes. Vitamins do work, and you don't have to take my word for it. Experienced physicians Abram Hoffer, MD, Thomas Levy, MD, Carolyn Dean, MD, Ian Brighthope, MD, Ralph Campbell, MD, Michael Janson, MD, and many others have shown time and time again the safety and efficacy of nutritional therapy. Clinical evidence is strong. Vitamins and nutrition can prevent and arrest chronic disease.

Know You Can Do This

Learn about your options, especially those you aren't likely to hear about in the doctor's office. Read studies on effective vitamin therapy, and then check the references. If you don't have time for all of that, orthomolecular books can help. You don't need to be reliant on a drug-based medical system.

Pharmaceutical Drug Marketing to Our Children: Bordering on Criminal

By Helen Saul Case

(OMNS June 11, 2013) I can't be the only one noticing. In fact I'm pretty sure I'm not. Drugs are being marketed directly to our children. If you don't believe me, just take a closer look at the commercials plastered about our TV shows at an estimated and alarming 80 an hour,[1] many targeting our little ones with images of animals and cartoons. Everywhere in the world, except the United States and New Zealand, direct-to-consumer pharmaceutical drug advertising is prohibited.[2] Perhaps it's time to think about why it should be banned here, too.

TV ads are designed to make an impact. They are meant to foster brand familiarity and loyalty. They appeal to our emotions. They often emphasize our shortcomings as fathers, mothers, friends, and spouses. Commercials influence us into thinking that using a particular product is a normal, ordinary, good idea: an everyday thing to do that everybody is doing.

I remember being shocked the first time I saw a pharmaceutical drug ad on TV. I couldn't believe that anyone would take a medication with a list of side effects that seemed so much worse than the disease it supposedly helped treat. Now, it is easy to become numb to them. The sheer volume of drug advertisements we are inundated with on a regular basis practically ensures we accept them as a natural part of life. Now that their presence isn't as shocking, it is easy to pay more attention to the beautiful imagery on the screen rather than the described dangers of the drug. I can rattle off brand name after brand name, and I'm not even paying attention, nor do I have any interest in them.

Until recently. When my baby girl starting pointing at cartoons and animals in pharmaceutical ads, I had had enough.

Profits and Preschoolers

There is no money in selling something nobody believes in. Drug companies want their commercials to be appealing. When I was little, I once asked my dad why they called a certain candy a "Thin Mint." He said because no one would buy them if they called them "Fat Mints."

Drug ads are alluring, especially to young eyes. The commercial for the drug Abilify, a buddy for your antidepressant, has a friendly little cartoon "A" coming to the rescue of a happy little Rx pill and a lovely cartoon woman. Variants of their commercial showcase a childish depression cloud and a rainy cartoon umbrella. A quick glance would have you believing you are watching children's programming meant to teach about the alphabet or the weather.

The antidepressant Zoloft bouncing cartoon ball can't be described as anything but cute (who doesn't love a cowlick?) and even more "adult" commercials like those for the inhaler Spiriva have real live elephants capturing the attention of my toddler.

How about those positively mesmerizing Lunesta commercials with the peaceful glowing butterflies? (She loves those.) An entire nation appears to be on drugs as the butterflies, indicated with thousands of illuminated specks, glow across a map of the United States. They capture your attention as a voice softly coos, "Join us." This particular ad doesn't even tell you the name of the drug, and therefore doesn't have to tell you what is wrong with the drug, either. The commercial advises you to seek out their website, ProjectLuna.com, which dons a name rather similar to their "unnamed" product. Of course, they've already made you familiar with their drug in numerous other broadcasts, so they don't even *need* to tell you what it's for. It's kind of like the Nike Swoosh. We all know what it means.

Do adults really need cartoons to understand what a drug can do? Or is there a more sinister plot afoot?

Drugs for the Whole Family

Some of you are telling me to turn my TV off. What business has a toddler watching "Let's Make a Deal" anyway? And while I hear you, I can tell you that unless I leave the TV off all the time, she's going to see a drug ad sooner or later. She does love books and magazines, especially ones with animals. Maybe we will just stick to those. Of course, the most recent publication we received wasn't any better.

My cat receives a magazine in the mail from her veterinarian. It encourages her to come in for her checkups. She can't read very well, but if she could, she'd see the pages are dotted with drug ads appealing to the emotions of her owner.

Drugging pets is big business. For example, Pfizer Animal Health is now Zoetis, a multi-billion dollar company, just one in a multi-billion dollar industry. There is real money to be made medicating our "companion animals." And unless you have some sort of animal prescription drug coverage, which is highly unlikely, you will be paying for those meds out of pocket. And we are. A *New York Times* article about our "Pill-Popping Pets" indicated that "surveys by the American Pet Products Manufacturers Association found that 77 percent of dog owners and 52 percent of cat owners gave their animals some sort of medication in 2006."[3] That means half to three-quarters of our furry friends are being drugged. By us. (Apparently, there is even a pill for all that puking my cat has been doing.[4] Who knew?)

A Lesson to Be Learned, Again

Have we forgotten about Joe? Perhaps we should take a step back in time and consider the R.J. Reynolds Tobacco Company. Joe Camel, the cartoon promotion for Camel cigarettes, "which the Federal Trade Commission (FTC) alleges was successful in appealing to many children and adolescents under 18, induced many young people to begin smoking or to continue smoking cigarettes and as a result caused significant injury to their health and safety." R.J. Reynolds was accused of promoting a "dangerous" product through "a campaign that was attractive to those too young to purchase cigarettes legally." Joe Camel was "as recognizable to kids as Mickey Mouse." After the campaign started, the FTC claimed "the percentage of kids who smoked Camels became larger than the percentage of adults who smoked Camels."[5] Were kids starting to smoke, and continuing to smoke, because of good ol' Joe? Were they too young to know what hit 'em?

> *"As to 'medicine,' I used to use very little of this stuff for infants. Now, I categorically state: just say no to drugs."*
> —Pediatrician Ralph K. Campbell, MD

We're Asking for It

Maybe kids can't get their own prescription, but they know someone who can get it for them. We lead by example. We are going to our doctors and *asking* for drugs for ourselves and for our children. Our doctors are all too happy to dole them out. They'll even throw in some free samples to get you started. There are billions of dollars spent every year advertising drugs directly to us, and it is working. The most heavily advertised pharmaceuticals see the largest increase in prescriptions and purchases.[6]

A Slippery Slope

I believe advertising drugs in a child-friendly way is dangerous. For example, what kid doesn't have a bad day? Or a ton of them? Being moody is part of being human, and it is certainly part of being an adolescent. Putting the idea in a young mind that being upset is an emotion that should be medicated is tricky territory. Critics of the pharmaceutical industry agree that "a lot of money can be made from healthy people who believe they are sick."[7]

Kids want to be happy. Parents want to help their children feel better. They may see minimized risk due to the positive associations drawn from drug commercials. We may be overconfident in drugs and in the doctors that prescribe them. We may think, "Well, if my physician gave it to me, it must be okay."

Making drugs a common and everyday part of life: it appears that's what pharmaceutical companies are trying to do. I think back to school trips I took with my middle school students. We are required to carry their medications when we travel, and each year, over the course of many, the hefty Ziploc bags I lugged around filled with medications grew and grew until I practically had my backpack overflowing with them. Eight to twelve kids, and a backpack full of meds. What was happening? I was surprised, but perhaps I shouldn't be: one out of every two people in America is taking prescription medications.[8] And so, too, is their cat.

It took twenty-three years before Joe Camel was taken out. How long before we pop the Zoloft bubble and squash the Nasonex bumblebee?

Safety of Supplements versus the Dangers of Drugs

I believe drug treatment for disease should be last on the list, and nutrition should be first. Are there folks that need medicines? Yes. But what about natural, effective, and safe ways we can combat allergies, depression, and trouble sleeping? I haven't seen any commercials about niacin (B_3) for mental disorders. Or about the importance of high-dose vitamin C. Or the health benefits of optimal doses of vitamin D. We often turn away from nutrition and toward medication. This, ladies, gentlemen, and children, is wrong.

Just Say No

Drugs are dangerous.[9] The front page of Zoloft's own website states "Antidepressant medicines may increase suicidal thoughts or actions in some children, teenagers, and young adults especially within the first few months of treatment."[10] *With over a hundred thousand deaths every year due to pharmaceuticals taken as directed,*[11] I really don't want my kid to be among them.

The old adage is true: just say no to drugs. And if the results of the "Say No to Drugs" campaign[12] are any indication of how well it works to do so, it will be a sorry success indeed.

References

1. Spiegel, Alix. "Selling Sickness: How Drug Ads Changed Health Care." October 13, 2009. Accessed June 2013 from http://www.npr.org/templates/story/story.php?storyId =113675737

2. Woodward, L. D. "Pharmaceutical Ads: Good or Bad for Consumers?" ABC News, February 24, 2010. Accessed June 2013from http://abcnews.go.com/Business/Wellness/ pharmaceutical-ads-good-bad-consumers/story?id=9925198

3. Vlahos, James. "Pill-Popping Pets." July 13, 2008. Accessed June 2013 from http:// www.nytimes.com/2008/07/13/magazine/13pets-t.html?pagewanted=all&_r=0

4. Cerenia. Accessed June 2013 from http://online.zoetis.com/US/EN/Products/Pages/ cerenia_home.aspx

5. Federal Trade Commission. "Joe Camel Advertising Campaign Violates Federal Law, FTC Says. Agency Charges R.J. Reynolds With Causing Substantial Injury to the Health and Safety of Children and Adolescents Under 18." May 28, 1997. Accessed June 2013 from http://www.ftc.gov/opa/1997/05/joecamel.shtm

6. Findlay, S. "Research Brief: Prescription Drugs and Mass Media Advertising." National Institute for Health Care Management Foundation (NIHCM Foundation), September 2000. Accessed June 2013 from http://www.nihcm.org/pdf/DTCbrief.pdf

7. Ibid.

8. Carroll, J. "Half of Americans Currently Taking Prescription Medication." Gallup News Service, December 9, 2005. Accessed June 2013 from http://www.gallup.com/poll/ 20365/halfamericans-currently-taking-prescription-medica-tion.aspx

9. Mercola, Joseph. "Pharmaceutical Drugs are 62,000 Times More Likely to Kill You than Supplements." July 24, 2012. Accessed June 2013 from http://articles.mercola.com/ sites/articles/archive/2012/07/24/pharmaceutical-drugs-vs-nutritional-supplements.aspx

10. Zoloft. Accessed June 2013 from http://www.zoloft.com/

11. Starfield, B. "Is US Health Really the Best in the World?" *JAMA* 284(4) (Jul 26, 2000):483–485.

12. Reaves, Jessica. "Just Say No to DARE." Thursday, Feb. 15, 2001. Accessed June 2013 from http://www.time.com/time/nation/article/0,8599,99564,00.html#ixzz2Va6a9TK7.

Not Taking Supplements Causes Miscarriage, Birthing Problems, Infant Mortality

BY ANDREW W. SAUL, EDITOR

(OMNS Jan 27, 2014) It is simply incredible what people have been told about vitamins. Now the press is trying to scare women away from prenatal supplements.[1,2] Didn't see that one coming, now, did you?

Several friends who work as missionaries asked me if vitamin C supplementation would help the indigenous peoples they work with in South American rainforests. Since I think supplemental C is valuable for all humans, I said "yes." They took it from there, and for years now have been giving multi-thousand-milligram doses of ascorbic acid powder to the natives daily. The result is that miscarriage and infant mortality rates have plummeted.

Vitamin C Protects Mother and Baby

Far from being an abortifacient, vitamin C in fact helps hold a healthy pregnancy right from the start. Pediatrician Lendon Smith, MD, known to TV audiences nationwide as "The Children's Doctor," had this to say: "Vitamin C is our best defense and everyone should be on this one *even before birth.* Three thousand mgs daily for the pregnant woman is a start. The baby should get 100 mg per day per month of age."

For centuries, postpartum hemorrhage was a leading cause of death in childbed. Hemorrhage very often occurs in scorbutic (vitamin C deficient) patients.[3] Optimum dosing with vitamin C prevents hemorrhage and saves women's lives. One way it may do this is by strengthening the walls of the body's large and small blood vessels.

"Harmful effects have been mistakenly attributed to vitamin C, including hypoglycemia, rebound scurvy, infertility, mutagenesis, and destruction of vitamin B(12). Health professionals should recognize that vitamin C does not produce these effects." (Levine, M., et al, *Journal of the American Medical Association,* April 21, 1999. Vol 281, No 15, p 1419)

Dr. Frederick R. Klenner, MD, gave very large doses of vitamin C to over 300 pregnant women and reported virtually no complications in any of the pregnancies or deliveries.[4] Indeed, the hospital nurses around Reidsville, North Carolina, noted that the infants who were healthiest and happiest were the "Vitamin C babies." Abram Hoffer, MD, has similarly reported that he has observed a complete absence of birth defects in babies born to his vitamin-C-taking mothers-to-be.

Specifically, Klenner gave:

1. 4,000 mg each day during the first trimester (first three months of pregnancy)

2. 6,000 mg each day during the second trimester

3. 8,000 to 10,000 mg each day during the third trimester

Some women got 15,000 mg daily during the third trimester. *There were no miscarriages in this entire group of 300 women.*

Klenner gave "booster" injections of vitamin C to 80% of the women upon admission to the hospital for childbirth. But just with oral supplemental vitamin C, the results were wonderful. First, labor was shorter and less painful. (My children's mother, with her 2 hr 45 min and 1 hr 45 min labor times, can confirm this.) Second, stretch marks were seldom to be seen. (Yes, I can vouch for this, too.) Third, there were no postpartum hemorrhages at all. And, there were no toxic manifestations and no cardiac distress. Among Klenner's patients were the Fultz quadruplets, which at the time were the only quads in the southeastern U.S. to have survived.

Vitamin C even helps with conception. Vitamin C supplementation increases sperm production. More sperm, stronger sperm and better swimming sperm all manifested within only *four days,* at 1,000 mg daily C doses, in a University of Texas study. And this has been known now for over 30 years; it was first reported in *Medical Tribune,* May 11, 1983.[5]

Sex: Another Reason to Take Vitamin C Supplements?

A randomized, double-blind, placebo-controlled 14 day trial of 3,000 mg per day of vitamin C reported greater frequency of sexual intercourse. The vitamin C group (but not the placebo group) also experienced a decrease in Beck Depression scores. This is probably due to the fact that vitamin C "modulates catecholaminergic activity, decreases stress reactivity, approach anxiety and prolactin release, improves vascular function, and increases oxytocin release. These processes are relevant to sexual behavior and mood."[6]

Supplemental vitamin C is also good for rapidly reproducing rabbits and fabulously fertile fish.[7,8] And the odd thing here is that fish and rabbits make their own vitamin C, inside their bodies, 24/7. Humans don't, and can't. If animals that make vitamin C benefit from more of it, then people who cannot make C (and that is all of us) will benefit more.

Vitamin E Supplementation Prevents Miscarriage

This has been well known for nearly 80 years.

> *"1922 was the year the USSR was formed and Alexander Graham Bell died. And it was the year that vitamin E was discovered by H. M. Evans and K. S. Bishop. In 1936, Evans' team had isolated alpha tocopherol from wheat germ oil and vitamin E was beginning to be widely appreciated, and the consequences of deficiency better known. Health Culture Magazine for January, 1936 said, "The fertility food factor is now called vitamin E. The expectant mother requires vitamin E to insure the carriage of her charge to a complete and natural term. If her diet is deficient in vitamin E, the woman is very apt to abort. It is more difficult to insure a liberal vitamin E supply in the daily average diet than to insure an adequate supply of any other known vitamin."*
>
> *"As early as 1931, Vogt-Moller of Denmark successfully treated habitual abortion in human females with wheat germ oil vitamin E. By 1939 he had treated several hundred women with a success rate of about 80%. In 1937, both Young in England and the Shutes in Canada reported success in combating threatened abortion and pregnancy toxemias as well. A. L. Bacharach's 1940 statistical analysis of published clinical results "show quite definitely that vitamin E is of value in recurrent abortions."*
>
> *"Yet when the MDR's (Minimum Daily Requirements) first came out in 1941, there was no mention of vitamin E. It was not until 1959 that vitamin E was recognized by the U.S. Food and Drug Administration as necessary for human existence, and not until 1968 that any government recommendation for vitamin E would be issued."*[9]

Taking supplemental vitamin E (at least 200 IU and perhaps 400 IU daily) greatly reduces the chance of miscarriage. By the end of WW II, there were already dozens of medical studies confirming this.[10]

Vitamins Vital for Pregnancy

Vitamins deliver healthier babies. The first few weeks of pregnancy are especially crucial to the developing embryo. Yet many women only begin to eat right and take necessary vitamin supplements once they know they are pregnant. This is weeks or even months too late. Nutrition needs rise during pregnancy. Even the RDA's are higher. This may be obvious to you, but many women eat really poor diets in general. Then, in a vain attempt to "get all the nutrition they need from a balanced diet" while "eating for two," they tend to eat more of that same poor diet. Telling them to not take prenatal supplements is a genuine tragedy, for which the media and the medical professions cannot easily be excused.

One can only wonder why the media continually, repeatedly fails to even mention how vitamin supplementation benefits mother and baby. Here is what they missed:

- If you *really* want to avoid miscarriages and birth defects, avoid drugs of all kinds, prescription and over-the-counter. Avoid alcohol, cigarettes, and all but the most essential medications.

- Vitamins are safer, vastly safer, than any drug. A really good diet, properly supplemented with a daily multivitamin plus appropriate quantities of other vitamins, will go a very long way to protect mother and baby.

(Andrew W. Saul founded the Orthomolecular Medicine News Service at the request of Drs. Abram Hoffer and Hugh Riordan. OMNS is celebrating its 10th year of continuous, free access, peer-reviewed publication. Some of the text of this article has previously appeared in Andrew W. Saul's books Doctor Yourself *and* Fire Your Doctor! *That copyrighted material is reprinted here with permission of the author and Basic Health Publications, Inc.)*

References

1. http://www.dailymail.co.uk/health/article-2546477/Taking-multivitamins-raise-risk-miscarriage-Mothers-likely-lose-baby-taking-supplements-six-weeks-conception.html

2. http://ije.oxfordjournals.org/content/early/2014/01/21/ije.dyt214.abstract

3. http://www.doctoryourself.com/mccormick.html

4. http://www.doctoryourself.com/klennerpaper.html See also: Stone, I. (1972) *The Healing Factor.* New York: Grosset and Dunlap. Chapter 28. http://vitamincfoundation.org/stone/

5. http://jama.jamanetwork.com/article.aspx?articleid=386823 See also: Dawson, E.B., W.A. Harris, W.E. Rankin, et al. "Effect of Ascorbic Acid on Male Fertility." *Ann NY Acad Sci* 498 (1987): 312–23. PMID: 3476000 http://www.ncbi.nlm.nih.gov/pubmed/3476000; and: Dawson, E,B., W.A. Harris, M.C. Teter, et al.. "Effect of Ascorbic Acid Supplementation on the Sperm Quality of Smokers." *Fertil Steril* 58(5) Nov 1992): 1034–9. http://www.ncbi.nlm.nih.gov/pubmed/1426355.

6. Brody, S. "High-Dose Ascorbic Acid Increases Intercourse Frequency and Improves

Mood: A Randomized Controlled Clinical Trial." *Biol Psychiatry* 52(4) (Aug 15, 2002): 371–4 http://www.ncbi.nlm.nih.gov/pubmed/12208645.

7. Yousef, M.I., G.A. Abdallah, K.I. Kamel. "Effect of Ascorbic Acid and Vitamin E Supplementation on Semen Quality and Biochemical Parameters of Male Rabbits." *Anim   Reprod   Sci   (2003).   PMID:12559724 http://www.ncbi.nlm.nih.gov/pubmed/12559724.

8. Ciereszko, A., K. Dabrowski. "Sperm Quality and Ascorbic Acid Concentration in Rainbow Trout Semen are Affected by Dietary Vitamin C: An Across-Season Study." *Biol Reprod* (1995). PMID:7626724. http://www.ncbi.nlm.nih.gov/pubmed/7626724.

9. Saul, A.W. "Vitamin E: A Cure in Search of Recognition." Reprinted with permission from the *Journal of Orthomolecular Medicine,* 18(3–4) (2003): 205–12. http://ortho-molecular .org/library/jom/2003/pdf/2003-v18n0304-p205.pdf

10. Bicknell, F., F. Prescott. *The Vitamins in Medicine.* Third Edition. William Heine-mann Medical Books Ltd., 1953. http://www.worldcat.org/title/vitamins-in-medicine/oclc/ 8581908/editions?referer=di&editionsView=true

More about the history of vitamin supplementation during pregnancy:

Dr. F. R. Klenner's megavitamin vitamin C therapy: http://www.doctoryourself.com/klennerpaper.html and http://www.doctoryourself.com/klenner_table.html

Case, H.S. *Vitamins and Pregnancy: The Real Story.* Basic Health Publications, CA.

Hillemann, H.H. "The Spectrum of Congenital Defect, Experimental and Clinical." *Journal of Applied Nutrition* 14 (1961): 1,2.

Smith, L., ed. (1988) *Clinical Guide to the Use of Vitamin C: The Clinical Experiences of Frederick R. Klenner, M.D.* Tacoma, WA: Life Sciences Press. http://www.whale.to/a/smith_b.html and http://www.seanet.com/~alexs/ascorbate/198x/smith-lh-clinical_guide _1988.htm.

Vitamins: It's Dose That Does It

(OMNS, February 2, 2009) There is a spin to most media reporting on vitamin research. The recent anti-vitamin media blitz, led by the *Associated Press* and *USA Today,* provides yet another demonstration. ("Vitamins C and E Don't Prevent Heart Disease." *The Associated Press* Nov. 9, 2008. Also: *USA Today* http://www.usatoday.com/news/health/2008-11-09-supplements-study_N.htm) With a paternalistic pat on the head, the media once again seeks to send you off to play with the reassurance that, well, vitamin therapy HAS been tested, and it just does not work.

Nonsense. Thousands upon thousands of nutritional research studies provide evidence that vitamins do help prevent and treat serious diseases, including cancer and heart disease, when the nutrients are supplied in sufficiently high doses. High doses are required. Low doses fail. Says cardiologist Thomas Levy, MD: "The three most important considerations in effective vitamin C therapy are dose, dose, and dose. If you don't take enough, you won't get the desired effects."

Effective doses are high doses, often hundreds of times more than the US Recommended Dietary Allowance (RDA) or Daily Reference Intake (DRI). Abram Hoffer, MD, PhD, comments: "Drs. Wilfrid Shute and Evan Shute recommended doses from 400 IU to 8,000 IU of vitamin E daily. The usual dose range was 800 to 1600 IU but they report that they had given 8,000 IU without seeing any toxicity." The Shutes successfully treated over 35,000 patients with vitamin E.

All the recent, much touted JAMA study does is confirm what we already know: low doses do not work. The doses given were 400 IU of vitamin E every OTHER day and 500 milligrams of vitamin C/day. Try that same study with 2,000 to 4,000 IU of vitamin E every other day (1,000 to 2,000 IU/day) and 15,000–30,000 mg/day of vitamin C and the difference would be unmistakable. We know this because investigators using vitamins E and C in high doses have consistently reported success.

Low doses do not get clinical results. Any physician, nurse, or parent knows that a dose of antibiotics that is one tenth, or one-hundredth, of the known effective dose will not work. Indeed, it is a cornerstone of medical science that dose affects outcome. This premise is accepted with pharmaceutical drug therapy, but not with vitamin therapy. Most of the best-publicized vitamin E and C research has used inadequate, low doses, and this JAMA study falls right into line.

High doses of vitamins are deliberately not used. Writes Robert F. Cathcart III, MD: "I have been consulted by many researchers who proposed bold studies of the effects of massive doses of ascorbate (vitamin C). Every time the university center, the ethics committee, or the pharmacy committee deny permission for the use of massive doses of ascorbate and render the study almost useless. Seasoned researchers depending upon government grants do not even try to study adequate doses."

The most frequently proffered reason is the allegation that "high doses of vitamins are not safe." That is a myth. 25 years of national poison control statistics show that there is not even one death per year from vitamins. Check the research literature and see for yourself exactly who is being harmed by vitamins. Aside from the pharmaceutical industry, virtually nobody. Half of Americans take vitamin supplements every day. So where are the bodies?

Decades of physicians' reports and controlled research studies support the use of large doses of vitamins. Yet to hear the media (and JAMA) tell it, vitamins are a Granny's folk remedy: a buggy- and barrel-stave technology that just doesn't make it.

In the broadcast and print media, vitamin therapy is marginalized at best and derided at worst. Is this merely laughable, or is there method to it? One may start by asking, who does this serve? Could it possibly be the media's huge advertising-cash providers, the pharmaceutical industry? Pharmaceutical advertising money buys authors, ad space, influence, and complicity. Unfortunately, this is as true in the newspapers as it is in the medical journals.

Let the news media begin by disclosing exactly where their advertising revenue comes from. It may explain where the spin on their articles comes from, too.

Additional Reading

"An education should make you want to learn more."
—MY GRANDMOTHER

To learn more about nutritional (orthomolecular) medicine and healthful living both now and after your baby is born, here is a short list of some titles you may wish to look into.

Brighthope, I.E., A.W. Saul. *The Vitamin Cure for Diabetes: Prevent and Treat Diabetes Using Nutrition and Vitamin Supplementation.* Laguna Beach, CA: Basic Health Publications, 2012.
Written by Australian physician Ian Brighthope, MD, who has tremendous experience in the area of nutrition, this book will help women (or men) who struggle with diabetes and want to know more about natural treatment approaches.

Calton, J., M. Calton. *Rich Food Poor Food: The Ultimate Grocery Purchasing System (GPS).* Malibu, CA: Primal Nutrition, 2013.
A guide for navigating the grocery store and helping work your way up the food continuum to the best food possible, this is a useful resource for any pregnant gal or new parent—or just anyone, period.

Campbell, R., A.W. Saul. *The Vitamin Cure for Children's Health Problems: Prevent and Treat Children's Health Problems Using Nutrition and Vitamin C Supplementation.* Laguna Beach, CA: Basic Health Publications, 2011.

Campbell, R., A.W. Saul. *The Vitamin Cure for Infant and Toddler Health Problems: Prevent and Treat Young Children's Health Problems Using Nutrition and Vitamin C Supplementation.* Laguna Beach, CA: Basic Health Publications, 2013.

Board certified pediatrician Ralph Campbell, MD, and my father, Andrew Saul, wrote these books to help parents conquer health issues common to many children, and to do so safely and effectively with nutrition. My husband and I don't go to our pediatrician without checking these books first.

Case, H.S. *The Vitamin Cure for Women's Health Problems.* Laguna Beach, CA: Basic Health Publications, 2012.

My first book, aimed at helping women successfully treat common health problems like premenstrual syndrome, yeast infections, stress, anxiety, depression, urinary tract infections, and menopause, and more with vitamins and without pharmaceuticals.

Cass, H., K. Barnes. *8 Weeks to Vibrant Health: A Take-Charge Plan for Women to Correct Imbalances, Reclaim Energy and Restore Well-Being.* New York, NY: McGraw Hill, 2011.

Written by Hyla Cass, MD, this book takes a balanced approach looking at both prescription drugs and nutrients for the treatment of disease with a focus on doing the least invasive, safest option first. It is easy to read and packed with valuable information by a nationally recognized expert in the field of integrative medicine.

Challem, J. *The Food Mood Solution: All-Natural Ways to Banish Anxiety, Depression, Anger, Stress, Overeating, and Alcohol and Drug Problems—and Feel Good Again.* Hoboken, NJ: Wiley, 2008.

Nutrition expert Jack Challem has written numerous books and articles. Known as "The Nutrition Reporter," he demystifies research by clearly explaining scientific studies. Here he shows you how food can work for you.

Crook, W.G., C. Dean, E. Crook. *The Yeast Connection and Women's Health.* 2nd edition. Jackson, TN: Professional Books, 2005.

Here is a book that should be on every woman's bookshelf. Yeast overgrowth is more common than most people think, and we aren't just talking about localized yeast infections.

Dean, C. *The Magnesium Miracle.* Revised and updated. New York: Ballantine Books, 2007.

That title is not a typo. You may be amazed at just how much this mineral plays a role in your health and the prevention of illness. Carolyn Dean is both a medical doctor and a naturopath and has written over two dozen books on natural health.

Downing, D. *The Vitamin Cure for Allergies*. Laguna Beach, CA: Basic Health Publications, 2010.

This one is often borrowed off my bookshelf. Damien Downing, MD has written a very real and engaging book about how to manage (and prevent) allergies naturally.

Hickey, S. *The Vitamin Cure for Migraines: How to Prevent and Treat Migraine Headaches Using Nutrition and Vitamin Supplementation*. Laguna Beach, CA: Basic Health Publications, 2010.

If you suffer from migraines, you know you need all the help you can get. Written by Steven Hickey, who has a doctorate in medical biophysics, this book shows you why nutrition should be your first choice when it comes to the treatment of migraine headaches.

Hickey, S., A.W. Saul. *Vitamin C: The Real Story, the Remarkable and Controversial Healing Factor,* Laguna Beach, CA: Basic Health Publications, 2008.

If you want to know more about vitamin C this is the book to read. I've been taking C my whole life, but for those getting started, or those who want to know more, this book is an incredible resource.

Hoffer, A., A.W. Saul. *Orthomolecular Medicine for Everyone: Megavitamin Therapeutics for Families and Physicians*. Laguna Beach, CA: Basic Health Publications, 2008.

My go-to guide. Those interested in orthomolecular medicine may want to read this first. Written in part by Abram Hoffer, MD, a pioneer of orthomolecular medicine, this book is truly for everyone.

Hoffer A., A.W. Saul, H. D. Foster. *Niacin: The Real Story*. Laguna Beach, CA: Basic Health Publications, 2012.

For women who must discontinue antidepressants or similar drugs prior to pregnancy, this book will be of special interest. This is an excellent resource for those who want to learn more about the value and safety of niacin for the treatment of mood disorders.

Hoffer, A., A.W. Saul, S. Hickey. *Hospitals and Health: Your Orthomolecular Guide to a Shorter, Safer Hospital Stay*. Laguna Beach, CA: Basic Health Publications, 2011.

This one is essential for anyone expecting (or not expecting) to have a hospital stay, including expectant moms.

Hoffer, A., J. Prousky. *Anxiety: Orthomolecular Diagnosis and Treatment.* Toronto, ON: CCNM Press, 2007.
A natural approach to anxiety written by experts in their field.

Holford, P., S. Lawson. *Optimum Nutrition before, during, and after Pregnancy.* Hachette, UK: Piatkus Books, 2004.
Patrick Holford's work is always worth reading, and this book will interest pregnant women in particular.

Irwin, J.B. *The Natural Way to a Trouble Free Pregnancy: The Toxemia/Thiamine Connection.* Fairfield, CT: Aslan Publishing, 2008.
Written by John Irwin, MD, this book talks in detail about how important and safe thiamin is for a smooth pregnancy.

Jonsson, B.H., A.W. Saul. *The Vitamin Cure for Depression: How to Prevent and Treat Depression Using Nutrition and Vitamin Supplementation.* Laguna Beach, CA: Basic Health Publications, 2012.
This book gives you what you are likely not getting from your doctor: the clear value of vitamins and other nutrients to combat depression.

Klenner, F.R. "Observations on the Dose and Administration of Ascorbic Acid When Employed beyond the Range of a Vitamin in Human Pathology." Article available free of charge at http://www.doctoryourself.com/klennerpaper.html.
Dr. Frederick R. Klenner is a pioneer in the field of orthomolecular medicine. Anyone wanting to know more about high dose vitamin C therapy will want to take the opportunity to read this very important paper.

Levy, T.E. *Curing the Incurable: Vitamin C, Infectious Diseases, and Toxins.* Philadelphia, PA: Xlibris Corporation, 2002.

Levy, T.E. *Primal Panacea.* Henderson NV: MedFox Publishing, 2011.
Both a medical doctor and a lawyer, Thomas Levy knows exactly what he is talking about. Readers will find great comfort in understanding the critical role that optimal vitamin C intake has for the reduction of toxins, the prevention of vaccine side effects, its antiviral and antibiotic properties, and much more, as well as its incredible safety in both adults and children.

Pauling, L. *How to Live Longer and Feel Better.* Corvallis, OR: Oregon State University Press, 2006.
The classic must-read for anyone interested in orthomolecular medicine written by the guy who gave it its name, and how it can do exactly what the title claims.

Prousky, J. *The Vitamin Cure for Chronic Fatigue Syndrome: How to Prevent and Treat Chronic Fatigue Syndrome Using Safe and Effective Natural Therapies.* Laguna, Beach, CA: Basic Health Publications, 2010.

New moms are always exhausted, but, if after those first few crazy months pass on by and sleep still doesn't make you feel rested, you may want to investigate the possibility of chronic fatigue. Written by a naturopath, Johnathan Prousky, this book may be just what you are looking for.

Saul, A.W. *Doctor Yourself: Natural Healing That Works.* 2nd edition. Laguna Beach, CA: Basic Health Publications, 2012.

Saul, A.W. *Fire Your Doctor: How to Be Independently Healthy.* Laguna Beach, CA: Basic Health Publications, 2005.

If you'd like to learn more about your health while actually enjoying reading about it, these books are a great place to start. Both are written by my father, who is always a great inspiration to me.

Saul, A.W., editor. *The Orthomolecular Treatment of Chronic Disease.* Laguna Beach, CA: Basic Health Publications, 2014.

This is a reference book, but it reads as enjoyably as a good novel. It's enormous, it's interesting, and it's packed with articles from over sixty-five experts in nutritional healing.

Saul, A.W., H.S. Case. *Vegetable Juicing for Everyone. How to Get Your Family Healthier and Happier, Faster!* Laguna Beach, CA: Basic Health Publications, 2013.

I wrote this one along with my father. It is not a juicing recipe book. (There are lots of those out there already.) If you want to get motivated and excited about juicing vegetables, while being entertained at the same time with stories about our off-kilter family, it might be just the thing.

References

CHAPTER 1. PREG TREK

1. Carousel Designs. Baby Stackers: Designer Diaper Storage in Dozens of Coordinating Patterns. www.babybedding.com/diaper-stackers?p=all (accessed Sep 15, 2014).

CHAPTER 2. VITAMINS AND PREGNANCY: FACT VERSUS FICTION

1. Hoffer, A., A.W. Saul. *Orthomolecular Medicine for Everyone: Megavitamin Therapeutics for Families and Physicians.* Laguna Beach, CA: Basic Health Publications, 2008.

2. Ibid.

3. Ibid.

4. Finer, L.B., M.R. Zolna. "Unintended Pregnancy in the United States: Incidence and Disparities, 2006." *Contraception* 84(5) (Nov 2011): 478–85. doi: 10.1016/j.contraception.2011.07.013.

5. Centers for Disease Control. CDC Newsroom. "Majority of Americans Not Meeting Recommendations for Fruit and Vegetable Consumption." Press Release, September 29, 2009. www.cdc.gov/media/pressrel/2009/r090929.htm. (accessed Sep 2014). Casagrande, S.S., Y. Wang, C. Anderson, et al. "Have Americans Increased Their Fruit and Vegetable Intake? The Trends between 1988 and 2002." *Am J Prev Med* 32(4) (Apr 2007): 257–63. Available online at: www.fruitsandveggiesmorematters.org/wp-content/uploads/UserFiles/File/pdf/ press/AJPM_32–4_Casagrande_with%20embargo.pdf (accessed Oct 2014).

6. Ibid.

7. U.S. Department of Agriculture. Food and Nutrition Service. "USDA and HHS Announce New Dietary Guidelines to Help Americans Make Healthier Food Choices and Confront Obesity Epidemic." Release No. 0040.11. (Jan 31, 2011): www.fns.usda.gov/pressrelease/2011/004011 (accessed Sep 2014).

8. Wilson, R.D., J.A. Johnson, P. Wyatt, et al. "Pre-Conceptional Vitamin/Folic Acid Supplementation 2007: The Use of Folic Acid in Combination with a Multivitamin Supplement for the Prevention of Neural Tube Defects and Other Congenital Anomalies." *J Obstet Gynaecol Can* 29(12) (Dec 2007): 1003–26.

9. Botto, L.D., J. Mulinare, J.D. Erickson. "Occurrence of Congenital Heart Defects in Relation to Maternal Mulitivitamin Use." *Am J Epidemiol* 151(92) May 1, 2000): 878–84.

10. Saul, A.W. *The Orthomolecular Treatment of Chronic Disease: 65 Experts on Therapeutic and Preventive Nutrition.* Laguna Beach, CA: Basic Health Publications. 2014.

11. Wilson, S.M., B.N. Bivins, K.A. Russell, et al. "Oral Contraceptive Use: Impact on Folate, Vitamin B6, and Vitamin B12 Status." *Nutr Rev* 69(10) (Oct 2011):572–83. doi: 10.1111/j.1753–4887.2011.00419.x. Wynn, V. "Vitamins and Oral Contraceptive Use." *Lancet* 1(7906) (Mar 8, 1975): 561–4. Haas, E.M. "Nutrient Programs: Nutrient Program for Oral Contraceptives." Healthy.net. HealthWorld Online. www.healthy.net/scr/ article.aspx?Id=1260 (accessed Sep 2014). Webb, J.L. "Nutritional Effects of Oral Contraceptive Use: A Review." *J Reprod Med* 25(4) (Oct 1980): 150–6. Palmery, M., A. Saraceno, A. Vaiarelli, et al. "Oral Contraceptives and Changes in Nutritional Requirements." *Eur Rev Med Pharmacol Sci* 17(13) (Jul 2013):1804

12. Mursu, J., K. Robien, L.J. Harnack, et al. "Dietary Supplements and Mortality Rate in Older Women. The Iowa Women's Health Study." *Arch Intern Med* 171(18) (Oct 10, 2011): 1625–33.

13. Mayo Clinic News Network. "Nearly 7 in 10 Americans Take Prescription Drugs, Mayo Clinic, Olmsted Medical Center Find." (Jun 19, 2013) http://newsnetwork.mayoclinic.org/ discussion/nearly-7-in-10-americans-take-prescription-drugs-mayo-clinic-olmsted-medical-center-find/ (accessed Sept 2014).

14. Vlahos, J. "Pill-Popping Pets." *The New York Times Magazine* (July 13, 2008): www.nytimes.com/2008/07/13/magazine/13pets-t.html?pagewanted=all&_r=1&. (accessed Sept 2014).

15. Mayo Clinic News Network. "Nearly 7 in 10 Americans Take Prescription Drugs, Mayo Clinic, Olmsted Medical Center Find." (Jun 19, 2013) http://newsnetwork.mayoclinic .org/discussion/nearly-7-in-10-americans-take-prescription-drugs-mayo-clinic-olmsted-medical-center-find/ (accessed Sept 2014).

16. Ibid.

17. Centers for Disease Control and Prevention (CDC). FastStats. "Therapeutic Drug Use." www.cdc.gov/nchs/fastats/drug-use-therapeutic.htm (accessed Sept 2014). CDC. NCHS. "National Ambulatory Medical Care Survey: 2010 Summary Tables." www.cdc.gov/ nchs/data/ahcd/namcs_summary/2010_namcs_web_tables.pdf (accessed Sept 2014).

18. Dean, C. *Hormone Balance: A Women's Guide to Restoring Health and Vitality.* Avon, MA: Adams Media, 2005.

19. Ibid.

20. Ibid.

21. Ibid.

22. Wu, G., F.W. Bazer, T.A. Cudd, et al. "Maternal Nutrition and Fetal Development." *J Nutr* 134(9) (Sept 2004): 2169–72.

23. Ibid.

24. Ibid.

25. Barker, D.J. "Maternal Nutrition, Fetal Nutrition, and Disease in Later Life." *Nutrition* 13(9) (Sept 1997): 807–13.

26. Ibid.

27. Saul, A.W. "The Doctor Yourself Newsletter." DoctorYourself.com 4(13) (Jun 5, 2004):www.doctoryourself.com/news/v4n13.html (accessed Sept 2014).

28. Challem, J. "Sorting through Conflicting Research." *Nutr Reporter* 18(3) (Mar 2007).

29. Gaby, A.R. "Safe Upper Limits" for Nutritional Supplements: One Giant Step Backward." *J Orthomolecular Med* 18(3–4) (3rd & 4th Quarter 2003): 126–130.

30. Hoffer, A. "Side Effects of Over-the-Counter Drugs." *J Orthomolecular Med* 18(3–4) (3rd & 4th Quarter 2003): 168–172.

31. Orthomolecular Medicine News Service. "Vitamins: It's Dose that Does It." Orthomolecular.org (Feb 2, 2009): http://orthomolecular.org/resources/omns/v05n01.shtml (accessed Oct 2014).

32. Jemal, A., R. Siegel, J. Xu, et al. "Cancer Statistics, 2010." *CA Cancer J Clin* 60(5) (Sep–Oct 2010): 277–300.

33. Ibid.

34. Ibid.

35. Riboli, E., T. Norat. "Epidemiologic Evidence of the Protective Effect of Fruit and Vegetables on Cancer Risk." *Am J Clin Nutr* 78(3 Suppl) (Sep 2003):559S–569S. U.S. Department of Agriculture. Center for Nutrition Policy and Promotion. "Report of the Dietary Guidelines Advisory Committee on the Dietary Guidelines for Americans, 2010. Part D. Section 5: Carbohydrates." Table D4.2. www.cnpp.usda.gov/DietaryGuidelines. (accessed October 2014).

36. Hung, H.C., K.J. Joshipura, R. Jiang, et al. "Fruit and Vegetable Intake and Risk of Major Chronic Disease." *J Natl Cancer Inst* 96(21) (2004):1577–1584.

37. Block, G., B. Patterson, A. Subar. "Fruit, Vegetables, and Cancer Prevention: A Review of the Epidemiological Evidence." *Nutr Cancer* 18(1) (1992):1–29.

38. Kemper, K.J., K.L. Hood. "Does Pharmaceutical Advertising Affect Journal Publication about Dietary Supplements?" *BMC Complement Altern Med* 8(11) (Apr 9, 2008).

39. Centers for Disease Control. CDC Newsroom. "Majority of Americans Not Meeting Recommendations for Fruit and Vegetable Consumption." Press Release. (Sept 29, 2009):www.cdc.gov/media/pressrel/2009/r090929.htm. (accessed Sept 2014). Casagrande, S.S., Y. Wang, C. Anderson, et al. "Have Americans Increased Their Fruit and Vegetable Intake? The Trends between 1988 and 2002." *Am J Prev Med* 32(4) (Apr 2007):257–63.

40. Starfield, B. "Is US Health Really the Best in the World?" *JAMA* 284(4) (Jul 26, 2000):483–5.

41. Associated Press. "Drug Errors Injure More Than 1.5 Million A Year: Report Calls for All Prescriptions to Be Electronic by 2010." (Jul 20, 2006): www.msnbc.msn.com/id/13954142 (accessed Sept 2014). Saul, A.W. "How to Make People Believe Any Anti-Vitamin Scare: It Just Takes Lots of Pharmaceutical Industry Cash." *Orthomolecular Medicine News Service.* (Oct 20, 2011): http://orthomolecular.org/resources/omns/v07n12.shtml (accessed Sept 2014).

42. Challem, J. "Perspectives on Recent Issues." *Nutrition Reporter* 18(8) (Aug 2007).

43. Bronstein, A.C., et al. "2009 Annual Report of the American Association of Poison Control Centers' National Poison Data System (NPDS) (Dec 2010):979–1178.

44. Saul, A.W. "So Where Are the Bodies? Vitamin Supplement Safety Confirmed by

America's Largest Database." *Orthomolecular Medicine News Service* 9(3) (Jan 30, 2013.): http://orthomolecular.org/resources/omns/v09n03.shtml (accessed Oct 2014).

45. Mowry, J.B., D.A. Spyker, L.R. Cantilena, Jr., et al. "2012 Annual Report of the American Association of Poison Control Centers' National Poison Data System (NPDS): 30th Annual Report." *Clin Toxicol (Phila)* 51(10) (Dec 2013):949–1229. doi: 10.3109/15563650.2013.863906. Vitamin data discussed above can be found at the very end of the report on pages 1197–1200, Table 22B.

46. Saul, A.W. "Newsletter v4n20" *The Doctor Yourself Newsletter* 4(20) (Sept 20, 2004): www.DoctorYourself.com/news/v4n20.html. (accessed Oct 2014).

47. Ibid.

CHAPTER 3. VITAMIN C AND PREGNANCY

1. Pauling, L. *Vitamin C and the Common Cold*. San Francisco, CA: W.H. Freeman and Company, 1970.

2. Campbell, R., A.W. Saul. *The Vitamin Cure for Infant and Toddler Health Problems*. Laguna Beach, CA: Basic Health Publications, 2013.

3. Bronstein, A.C., et al. "2009 Annual Report of the American Association of Poison Control Centers' National Poison Data System (NPDS) (Dec 2010):979–1178. Bronstein, A.C., D.A. Spyker, L.R., Cantilena Jr, et al. "2008 Annual Report of the American Association of Poison Control Centers' National Poison Data System (NPDS): 26th Annual Report." *Clin Toxicol* 47 (2009):911–1084. Orthomolecular Medicine News Service. "Zero Deaths from Vitamins, Minerals, Amino Acids or Herbs: Poison Control Statistics Prove Supplements' Safety Yet Again." Orthomolecular.org: (January 5, 2011). http://orthomolecular.org/ resources/omns/v07n01.shtml (accessed Oct 2014).

4. Levine, M., S.C. Rumsey, R. Daruwala, et al. "Criteria and Recommendations for Vitamin C Intake." *JAMA* 281(15) (April 1999):1415–1423.

5. Panel on Dietary Antioxidants and Related Compounds, et al. *Dietary Reference Intakes for Vitamin C, Vitamin E, Selenium, and Carotenoids* (2000) National Academies Press, 2000. www.nap.edu/openbook.php?record_id=9810&page=155 (accessed Oct 2014).

6. Ibid.

7. Ibid.

8. Klenner, F.R. "Observations on the Dose and Administration of Ascorbic Acid When Employed Beyond the Range of a Vitamin in Human Pathology." *J Applied Nutr* 23(3 & 4) (Winter 1971): 61–88.

9. Saul, A.W. *Doctor Yourself: Natural Healing That Works*. 2nd edition. Laguna Beach, CA: Basic Health Publications, 2012.

10. Pauling, L. *How to Live Longer and Feel Better*. Corvallis, OR: Oregon State University Press, 2006.

11. Klenner, F.R. "Observations on the Dose and Administration of Ascorbic Acid When Employed Beyond the Range of a Vitamin in Human Pathology." *J Applied Nutr* 23(3 & 4) (Winter 1971): 61–88.

12. Saul, A.W. *Doctor Yourself: Natural Healing That Works*. 2nd edition. Laguna Beach, CA: Basic Health Publications, 2012.

13. Klenner, F.R. "Observations on the Dose and Administration of Ascorbic Acid When Employed Beyond the Range of a Vitamin in Human Pathology." *J Applied Nutr* 23(3 & 4) (Winter 1971): 61–88.

14. Ibid.

15. Ibid.

16. National Institute of Health. Office of Dietary Supplements. "Vitamin C: Fact Sheet for Health Professionals." http://ods.od.nih.gov/factsheets/VitaminC-HealthProfessional/ (accessed Oct 2014).

17. Ibid.

18. Gaby, A.R. "Safe Upper Limits" for Nutritional Supplements: One Giant Step Backward." *J Orthomolecular Med* 18(3–4) (3rd & 4th Quarter 2003).

19. U.S. National Library of Medicine. National Institutes of Health. Medline Plus. "Miscarriage." www.nlm.nih.gov/medlineplus/ency/article/001488.htm (accessed Oct 2014).

20. Pavlov Jr., A., I.I. Bussel. "Can Vitamin C Induce Abortion?" Science-Based Medicine.org. www.sciencebasedmedicine.org/index.php/can-vitamin-c-induce-abortion/ (accessed Oct 2014).

21. Pauling, L. *How to Live Longer and Feel Better.* Corvallis, OR: Oregon State University Press, 2006.

22. Ibid.

23. DoctorYourself.Com. Doctor Yourself Newsletter. "Junk Science on Vitamin C Megadoses Exposed." 2(3) (Nov 24, 2001):www.doctoryourself.com/news/v2n3.html (accessed Oct 2014).

24. Milton, K. "Nutritional Characteristics of Wild Primate Foods: Do the Diets of Our Closest Living Relatives Have Lessons for Us?" *Nutr* 15(6) (1999): 488–498. Available online at: www.2ndchance.info/wildprimatediets.pdf (accessed Oct 2014).

25. National Center for Health Statistics. "Americans Slightly Taller, Much Heavier Than Four Decades Ago: Mean Body Weight, Height, and Body Mass Index, United States, 1960–2002." Advance Data No. 347. (Oct 27, 2004):www.cdc.gov/nchs/press room/04news/americans.htm (accessed Oct 2014).

26. U.S. Department of Agriculture. Animal and Plant Health Inspection Service. Care Resource Guide, Animal Care, 12.4.2 www.aphis.usda.gov/animal_welfare/down-loads/manuals/dealer/feeding.pdf (accessed Feb, 2010; no longer available on the www). See also: Giroud, A.C. P. Leblond, R. Ratsimamanga. "The Vitamin C Requirement of the Guinea-Pig." *Yale J Biol Med* 9(6) (Jul 1937). Available online at www.ncbi.nlm.nih.gov/pmc/articles/PMC2601737/ (accessed Oct 2014).

27. Lawson S. "The Optimal Intake of Vitamin C." The Linus Pauling Institute. (May 1997):http://lpi.oregonstate.edu/sp-su97/intake.html (accessed Oct 2014).

28. Levy, T.E. *Vitamin C, Infectious Diseases, and Toxins: Curing the Incurable.* Philadelphia, PA: Xlibris Corporation, 2002. Kola, I., R. Vogel, H. Spielmann. "Coadministration of Ascorbic Acid with Cyclophosphamide (CPA) to Pregnant Mice Inhibits the Clastogenic Activity of CPA in Preimplantation Murine Blastocysts." *Mutagenesis* 4(4) (Jul 1989):297–301. Pillans, P.I., S.F. Ponzi, M.I. Parker. "Effects of Ascorbic Acid on the Mouse Embryo and on Cyclophosphamide-Induced Cephalic DNA Strand Breaks In Vivo." *Arch Toxicol* 64(5) (1990):423–5.

29. Ibid.

30. Cass, H., K. Barnes. *8 Weeks to Vibrant Health.* New York, NY: McGraw Hill. 2004.

31. J.F. Shelton, E.M. Geraghty, D.J. Tancredi, et al. "Neurodevelopmental Disorders and Prenatal Residential Proximity to Agricultural Pesticides: The CHARGE Study." *Environ Health Perspect* 122(10) (Oct 2014) doi:10.1289/ehp.1307044 (accessed Oct 2014).

32. Levy, T.E. *Vitamin C, Infectious Diseases, and Toxins: Curing the Incurable.* Philadelphia, PA: Xlibris Corporation, 2002.

33. Steuerwald, U., P. Weihe, P.J. Jørgensen, "Maternal Seafood Diet, Methylmercury Exposure, and Neonatal Neurologic Function." *J Pediatr* 136(5) (May 2000):599–605.

34. U.S. Food and Drug Administration. "What You Need to Know About Mercury in Fish and Shellfish (Brochure)" EPA-823-R-04–005 (March 2004): www.fda.gov/food/resourcesforyou/consumers/ucm110591.htm (accessed Oct 2014).

35. Cass, H., K. Barnes. *8 Weeks to Vibrant Health.* New York, NY: McGraw Hill. 2004.

36. Levy, T.E. *Vitamin C, Infectious Diseases, and Toxins: Curing the Incurable.* Philadelphia, PA: Xlibris Corporation, 2002.

37. Ibid.

38. Hickey, S., A.W. Saul. *Vitamin C: The Real Story: The Remarkable and Controversial Healing Factor* Laguna Beach, CA: Basic Health Publications, 2008.

39. Hickey, S., A.W. Saul. *Vitamin C: The Real Story: The Remarkable and Controversial Healing Factor* Laguna Beach, CA: Basic Health Publications, 2008. Simon, J.A., E.S. Hudes. "Relationship of Ascorbic Acid to Blood Lead Levels." *JAMA* 281(24) (Jun 23–30 1999) 281(24):2289–93.

40. Altmann, P., R.F. Maruna, H. Maruna. "[Lead detoxication effect of a combined calcium phosphate and ascorbic acid therapy in pregnant women with increased lead burden]." [Author's translation; original article in German]. *Wien Med Wochenschr* 131(12) (1981): 311–4.

41. Ibid.

42. West, W.L., E.M. Knight, C.H. Edwards, et al. "Maternal Low-level Lead and Pregnancy Outcomes." *J Nutr* 124(6 Suppl) (Jun 1, 1994):981S–6S.

43. Levy, T.E. *Vitamin C, Infectious Diseases, and Toxins: Curing the Incurable.* Philadelphia, PA: Xlibris Corporation, 2002.

44. Levy, T. *Primal Panacea.* Henderson, NV: MedFox Publishing, 2011.

45. Borane, V.R., S.P. Zambare. "Role of Ascorbic Acid in Lead and Cadmium Induced Changes on the Blood Glucose Level of the Freshwater Fish, Channa orientalis." *J Aquatic Biol* 21(2) (2006): 244–248. Gajawat, S.G. Sancheti, P.K. Goyal. "Vitamin C Against Concomitant Exposure to Heavy Metal and Radiation: A Study on Variations in Hepatic Cellular Counts." *Asian J Exper Sci* 19(2) (2005): 53–58. Shousha, W. "The Curative and Protective Effects of L-Ascorbic Acid & Zinc Sulphate on Thyroid Dysfunction and Lipid Peroxidation in Cadmium-Intoxicated Rats." *Egyptian J Biochem & Molec Biol* 22(1) (2004): 1–16. Vasiljeva, S., N. Berzina, I. Remeza. "Changes in Chicken Immunity Induced by Cadmium, and the Protective Effect of Ascorbic Acid."

Proceed Latvian Acad Sci, Sect B: Natural, Exact and Appl Sci 57(6) (2003): 232–7. Mahajan, A.Y., S.P. Zambare. "Ascorbate Effect on Copper Sulphate and Mercuric Chloride Induced Alterations of Protein Levels in Freshwater Bivalve Corbicula Itriatella." *Asian J Microbiol, Biotech & Environ Sci* 3(1–2) (2001): 95–100. Norwood, J., Jr., A.D. Ledbetter, D.L. Doerfler, G.E. Hatch. "Residual Oil Fly Ash Inhalation in Guinea Pigs: Influence of Ascorbate and Glutathione Depletion." *Toxicol Sci* 61(1) (2001): 144–53. Guillot, I., P. Bernard, W.A. Rambeck. "Influence of Vitamin C on the Retention of Cadmium in Turkeys." Tiergesundheitsdienst Bayern, Germany. Editors: Schubert, Flachowsky, Bitsch. *Vitamine und Zusatzstoffe in der Ernaehrung von Mensch und Tier, Symposium, 5th, Jena* (Sep 28–29, 1995): 233–237.

46. Orthomolecular Medicine News Service. "Vitamin Supplements Help Protect Children from Heavy Metals, Reduce Behavioral Disorders." Orthomolecular.org (Oct 8, 2007): www.orthomolecular.org/resources/omns/v03n07.shtml (accessed Oct 2014).

47. Ibid.

48. Barrett, B., E. Gunter, J. Jenkins, "Ascorbic Acid Concentration in Amniotic Fluid in Late Pregnancy." *Biol Neonate* 60(5) (1991):333–5.

49. Ornoy, A. "Embryonic Oxidative Stress as a Mechanism of Teratogenesis with Special Emphasis on Diabetic Embryopathy." *Reprod Toxicol* 24(1) (Jul 2007):31–41.

50. Hickey, S., A.W. Saul. *Vitamin C: The Real Story: The Remarkable and Controversial Healing Factor* Laguna Beach, CA: Basic Health Publications, 2008. Pauling, L. *How to Live Longer and Feel Better.* Corvallis, OR: Oregon State University Press, 2006.

51. Lide, D.R. CRC *Handbook of Chemistry and Physics* 85th edition. Boca Raton, FL: CRC Press, 2004.

52. Saul, A.W. "Megadoses of C for Little Kids: How to Do It." DoctorYourself.com: www.doctoryourself.com/megakid.html (accessed Oct 2014).

53. Saul, A.W. *Vitamin C: The Real Story: The Remarkable and Controversial Healing Factor* Laguna Beach, CA: Basic Health Publications, 2008. Cathcart, R.F. "Vitamin C, Titrating to Bowel Tolerance, Anascorbemia, and Acute Induced Scurvy." *Med Hypotheses* 7(11) (Nov 1981): 1359–76.

54. Saul, A.W.. *Vitamin C: The Real Story: The Remarkable and Controversial Healing Factor* Laguna Beach, CA: Basic Health Publications, 2008.

55. Dean, C. *The Magnesium Miracle,* Updated edition. New York: Ballantine Books, 2006.

56. Saul, A.W. *Vitamin C: The Real Story: The Remarkable and Controversial Healing Factor* Laguna Beach, CA: Basic Health Publications, 2008. DoctorYourself.Com "Kidney Stones." DoctorYourself.com: www.doctoryourself.com/kidney.html (accessed Oct 2014).

57. Saul, A.W. *Vitamin C: The Real Story: The Remarkable and Controversial Healing Factor* Laguna Beach, CA: Basic Health Publications, 2008. Pauling, L. *How to Live Longer and Feel Better.* Corvallis, OR: Oregon State University Press, 2006.

58. Saul, A.W. "Receding Gums." DoctorYourself.com: www.doctoryourself.com/gums.html (accessed Oct 2014). See also: Riordan, H.D., J.A. Jackson. "Topical Ascorbate Stops Prolonged Bleeding from Tooth Extraction." *J Orthomolecular Med* 6(3–4) (1991): 202. www.doctoryourself.com/news/v3n18.txt or www.orthomolecular.org/library/jom/1991/pdf/1991-v06n03&04-p202.pdf (accessed Oct 2014).

59. Oregon State University. Linus Pauling Institute. Micronutrient Information Center. "The Bioavailability of Different Forms of Vitamin C (Ascorbic Acid)." (Nov 27, 2013): http://lpi.oregonstate.edu/infocenter/vitamins/vitaminC/vitCform.html (accessed Oct 2014).

60. Dean, C. *The Magnesium Miracle,* Updated edition. New York: Ballantine Books, 2006.

61. Saul, A.W. *Vitamin C: The Real Story: The Remarkable and Controversial Healing Factor* Laguna Beach, CA: Basic Health Publications, 2008. DoctorYourself.Com "Kidney Stones." DoctorYourself.com: www.doctoryourself.com/kidney.html (accessed Oct 2014).

62. Oregon State University. Linus Pauling Institute. "The Bioavailability of Different Forms of Vitamin C." http://lpi.oregonstate.edu/infocenter/vitamins/vitaminC/vitCform.html (accessed Oct 2014).

63. Pauling, L. *How to Live Longer and Feel Better.* Corvallis, OR: Oregon State University Press, 2006. Oregon State University. Linus Pauling Institute. "The Bioavailability of Different Forms of Vitamin C." http://lpi.oregonstate.edu/infocenter/vitamins/vitaminC/vitCform.html (accessed Oct 2014).

64. Saul, A.W. "So Exactly What Is a Rose Hip, Anyway?" DoctorYourself.com. 2005: www.doctoryourself.com/bioflavinoids.html (accessed Oct 2014)..

65. Saul, A.W. *Doctor Yourself: Natural Healing That Works.* 2nd edition. Laguna Beach, CA: Basic Health Publications, 2012.

66. Gaby, A.R. "The Myth of Infantile 'Rebound Scurvy'". *Townsend Letter for Doctors and Patients* 203 (Jun 2000): 122.

67. Ibid.

68. Ibid.

69. Ibid.

70. Saul, A.W. *Doctor Yourself: Natural Healing That Works.* 2nd edition. Laguna Beach, CA: Basic Health Publications, 2012.

71. Ibid.

72. Ibid.

73. Ibid.

74. Ibid.

75. CI: Bass, W.T., N. Malati, M.C. Castle, et al. "Evidence for the Safety of Ascorbic Acid Administration to the Premature Infant." *Am J Perinatol* 15(2) (Feb 1998): 133–40.

76. Campbell, R., A.W. Saul. *The Vitamin Cure for Infant and Toddler Health Problems.* Laguna Beach, CA: Basic Health Publications, 2013.

77. Pauling, L. *Vitamin C and the Common Cold.* San Francisco, CA: W. H. Freeman and Company, 1970.

78. Pauling, L. *How to Live Longer and Feel Better.* Corvallis, OR: Oregon State University Press, 2006.

79. Orthomolecular Medicine News Service. "About 'Objections' to Vitamin C Ther-

apy" Orthomolecular.org (Oct 12, 2010): http://orthomolecular.org/resources/omns/v06n24.shtml (accessed Oct 2014).

80. Cathcart, R.F. "Vitamin C, Titrating to Bowel Tolerance," 1981. Available online at: www.doctoryourself.com/titration.html (accessed Oct 2014). See also: Orthomolecular Medicine News Service. "Vitamin C as an Antiviral: It's All About Dose." Orthomolecular.org (Oct 12, 2010): http://orthomolecular.org/resources/omns/v05n09.shtml (accessed Oct 2014). Saul, A.W. "Putting the 'C' in Cure: Quantity and Frequency Are the Keys to Ascorbate Therapy." Orthomolecular.org. (Dec 15, 2009): http://orthomolecular.org/resources/omns/v05n11.shtml (accessed Oct 2014).

81. Saul, A.W. "Hidden in Plain Sight: The Pioneering Work of Frederick Robert Klenner, M.D." *J Orthomolecular Med* 22(12007) (Mar 2007):31–8. Available online at: www.doctoryourself.com/klennerbio.html (accessed Oct 2014). See also: Orthomolecular.org. "Frederic Klenner, M.D., 1907–1984: Hall of Fame, 2005. http://orthomolecular.org/hof/2005/fklenner.html (accessed Oct 2014). Smith, L.H. "Clinical Guide to the Use of Vitamin C: The Clinical Experiences of Frederic R. Klenner, M.D., Abbreviated, Summarized and Annotated." (Nov 20, 2013): www.seanet.com/~alexs/ascorbate/198x/smith-lh-clinical_guide_1988.htm (accessed Oct 2014).

82. Pauling, L. *How to Live Longer and Feel Better.* Corvallis, OR: Oregon State University Press, 2006. Saul, A.W. "How to Live Longer and Feel Better by Linus Pauling: Review." DoctorYourself.com www.doctoryourself.com/livelonger.html (accessed Oct 2014). Saul, A.W. "Linus Pauling, PhD: The Megavitamin, Orthomolecular Medicine and Nutrition-Related Publications: Selection and Abridgement." DoctorYourself.com www.doctoryourself.com/biblio_pauling_ortho.html (accessed Oct 2014). Stone, I. *The Healing Factor: Vitamin C against Disease.* New York: Putnam Pub Group, 1974. Available online at: The Vitamin Foundation. http://vitamincfoundation.org/stone/ (accessed Oct 2014).

83. Orthomolecular Medicine News Service. "No Deaths from Vitamins, Minerals, Amino Acids or Herbs: Poison Control Statistics Prove Supplements' Safety." Orthomolecular.org (Jan 19, 2010): http://orthomolecular.org/resources/omns/v06n04.shtml (accessed Oct 2014).

84. Levine, M., S.C. Rumsey, D. Rushad, et al. "Criteria and Recommendations for Vitamin C Intake." *JAMA* 281(15) (Apr 21, 1999): 1419–23.

85. Brody, S. "High-Dose Ascorbic Acid Increases Intercourse Frequency and Improves Mood: A Randomized Controlled Clinical Trial." *Biol Psychiatry* 52(4) (Aug 15, 2002): 371–4.

86. McCormick, W.J. "Lithogenesis and Hypovitaminosis." *Med World (New York)* 159 (Jul 1946): 410–3.

87. Cheraskin, E., W.M. Ringsdorf, E.L. Sisley. *The Vitamin C Connection: Getting Well and Staying Well with Vitamin C.* New York: Harper and Row, 1983. See also: Ringsdorf, W.M. Jr, E. Cheraskin. "Nutritional Aspects of Urolithiasis." *South Med J* 74(1) (Jan 1981):41–3, 46.

88. Gerster, H. "No Contribution of Ascorbic Acid to Renal Calcium Oxalate Stones." *Ann Nutr Metab* 41(5) (1997):269–82. See also: Hickey, S., H. Roberts. "Vitamin C Does Not Cause Kidney Stones." *Orthomolecular Med News Service* (Jul 5, 2005): http://orthomolecular.org/resources/omns/v01n07.shtml (accessed Oct 2014).

89. Mayland, C.R., M.I. Bennett, K. Allan. "Vitamin C Deficiency in Cancer Patients."

Palliat Med 19(1) (Jan 2005):17–20. See also: Orthomolecular Medicine News Service. "Intravenous Vitamin C Is Selectively Toxic to Cancer Cells." Orthomolecular.org (Sep 22, 2005): http://orthomolecular.org/resources/omns/v01n09.shtml (accessed Oct 2014). Orthomolecular Medicine News Service. "Vitamin C Slows Cancer Down." Orthomolecular.org (Oct 31, 2008): http://orthomolecular.org/resources/omns/v04n19.shtml (accessed Oct 2014).

90. Gokce, N., J.F. Keaney, B. Frei, et al. "Long-Term Ascorbic Acid Administration Reverses Endothelial Vasomotor Dysfunction in Patients with Coronary Heart Disease." *Circulation* 99 (1999): 3234–40. Available online at: http://circ.ahajournals.org/cgi/reprint/99/25/3234 (accessed Oct 2014). See also: Spencer, A., A.W. Saul. "Vitamin C and Cardiovascular Disease: A Personal Viewpoint." *Orthomolecular Med News Service* (Jun 22, 2010): http://orthomolecular.org/resources/omns/v06n20.shtml (accessed Oct 2014). Orthomolecular Medicine News Service. "Vitamin C Saves Lives." Orthomolecular.org (Apr 22, 2005): http://orthomolecular.org/resources/omns/v01n02.shtml (accessed Oct 2014).

91. Duffy, S.J., N. Gokce, M. Holbrook, et al. "Treatment of Hypertension with Ascorbic Acid." *Lancet* 354(9195) (Dec 11, 1999):2048–9.

92. Saul, A.W. "RDA for Vitamin C Is 10% of USDA Standard for Guinea Pigs: Are You Healthier Than a Lab Animal?" *Orthomolecular Med News Service* (Feb 4, 2010): http://orthomolecular.org/resources/omns/v06n08.shtml (accessed Oct 2014).

93. Saul, A.W. "The Pioneering Work of William J. McCormick, M.D." *J Orthomolecular Med* 18(2) (2003): 93–6. Available online at: www.doctoryourself.com/mccormick.html

94. Klenner, F.R. "The Use of Vitamin C as an Antibiotic." *J Applied Nutr* 6 (1953):274–8. Available online at: http://whale.to/v/c/klenner1.html (accessed Oct 2014).

95. Orthomolecular Medicine News Service. "Antibiotics Put 142,000 into Emergency Rooms Each Year: U.S. Centers for Disease Control Waits 60 Years to Study the Problem." Orthomolecular.org (Oct 13, 2008): www.orthomolecular.org/resources/omns/v04n14.shtml (accessed Oct 2014).

96. Cathcart, R.F. "The Third Face of Vitamin C." *J Orthomolecular Med* 7:4 (1993):197–200.

97. Ibid.

98. Shehab, N., P.R. Patel, A. Srinivasan, et al. "Emergency Department Visits for Antibiotic-Associated Adverse Events." *Clin Infect Dis* 47(6) (Sep 15,2008):735–43. doi: AU1086/591126.

99. Cass, H., K. Barnes. *8 Weeks to Vibrant Health*. New York, NY: McGraw Hill, 2004.

100. MacDonald, T.M., P.H.G. Beardon, M.M. McGilchrist, et al. "The Risks of Symptomatic Vaginal Candidiasis after Oral Antibiotic Therapy." *Q J Med* 86(7) (1993):419–24. Onifade, A.K., O.B. Olorunfemi. "Epidemiology of Vulvo-Vaginal Candidiasis in Female Patients in Ondo State Government Hospitals." *J Food Agric Environment* 3(1) (2005):118–9. Kirsch, D.R., R. Kelly, M.B. Kurtz. *The Genetics of Candida*. Boca Raton, FL: CRC Press, 1990.

101. Fidel, P.L., J. Cutright, C. Steele. "Effects of Reproductive Hormones on Experi-

mental Vaginal Candidiasis." *Infect Immun* 68(2) (Feb 2000):651–57. Dean, C. *Hormone Balance: A Women's Guide to Restoring Health and Vitality*. Avon, MA: Adams Media, 2005.

102. Cassone, A., F. De Barnardis, G. Santoni. "Anticandidal Immunity and Vaginitis: Novel Opportunities for Immune Intervention." *Infect Immun* 75(10) (Oct 2007): 4675–86.

103. Centers for Disease Control and Prevention. "Antibiotic/Antimicrobial Resistance." (Aug 6, 2014): www.cdc.gov/drugresistance/index.html (accessed Oct 2014).

104. Harmsen, H.J., A.C. Wildeboer-Veloo, G.C. Raangs, et al. "Analysis of Intestinal Flora Development in Breast-Fed and Formula-Fed Infants by Using Molecular Identification and Detection Methods." *J Pediatr Gastroenterol Nutr* 30(1) (Jan 2000):61–7.

105. Benn, C.S., P. Thorsen, J.S. Jensen, et al. "Maternal Vaginal Microflora during Pregnancy and the Risk of Asthma Hospitalization and Use of Antiasthma Medication in Early Childhood." *J Allergy Clin Immunol* 110(1) (Jul 2002):72–7.

106. Mueller, N.T., R. Whyatt, L. Hoepner, et al. "Prenatal Exposure to Antibiotics, Cesarean Section and Risk of Childhood Obesity." *Int J Obes (Lond)* (Nov 11, 2014): doi: 10.1038/ijo.2014.180. [Epub ahead of print.]

107. Penders, J., C. Thijs, C. Vink, et al. "Factors Influencing the Composition of the Intestinal Microbiota in Early Infancy." *Pediatrics* 118(2) (Aug 2006):511–21.

108. Pauling, L. *How to Live Longer and Feel Better*. Corvallis, OR: Oregon State University Press, 2006. Levy, T.E. *Vitamin C, Infectious Diseases, and Toxins: Curing the Incurable*. Philadelphia, PA: Xlibris Corporation, 2002.

109. Levy, T.E. *Vitamin C, Infectious Diseases, and Toxins: Curing the Incurable*. Philadelphia, PA: Xlibris Corporation, 2002.

110. Cathcart, R.F. "Vitamin C, Titrating to Bowel Tolerance," 1981. Available online at: www.doctoryourself.com/titration.html.

111. Orthomolecular Medicine News Service. "Antibiotics Put 142,000 into Emergency Rooms Each Year: U.S. Centers for Disease Control Waits 60 Years to Study the Problem." www.orthomolecular.org/resources/omns/v04n14.shtml (accessed Oct 2014).

112. Byerley, L.O., A. Kirksey. "Effects of Different Levels of Vitamin C Intake on the Vitamin C Concentration in Human Milk and the Vitamin C Intakes of Breast-Fed Infants." *Am J Clin Nutr* 41(4) (Apr 1985):665–71. Panel on Dietary Antioxidants and Related Compounds, et al. *Dietary Reference Intakes for Vitamin C, Vitamin E, Selenium, and Carotenoids* (2000) National Academies Press, 2000. www.nap.edu/openbook.php?record_id=9810&page=155 (accessed Oct 2014).

113. Byerley, L.O., A. Kirksey. "Effects of Different Levels of Vitamin C Intake on the Vitamin C Concentration in Human Milk," 1985.

114. Hoppu, U., M. Rinne, P. Salo-Väänänen, et al. "Vitamin C in Breast Milk May Reduce the Risk of Atopy in the Infant." *Eur J Clin Nutr* 59(1) (Jan 2005):123–8.

115. Pauling, L. *Vitamin C and the Common Cold*. San Francisco, CA: W. H. Freeman and Company, 1970.

116. Levy, T.E. *Vitamin C, Infectious Diseases, and Toxins: Curing the Incurable*. Philadelphia, PA: Xlibris Corporation, 2002.

117. Levy, T.E. *Vitamin C, Infectious Diseases, and Toxins: Curing the Incurable*.

Philadelphia, PA: Xlibris Corporation, 2002. Werbach, M.R., J. Moss. *Textbook of Nutritional Medicine*. Tarzana, CA: Third Line Press, 1999.

118. Werbach, M.R., J. Moss. *Textbook of Nutritional Medicine*. . Tarzana, CA: Third Line Press, 1999.

119. Saul, A.W. "Notes On Orthomolecular (Megavitamin) Use of Vitamin C." DoctorYourself.com (2004): www.doctoryourself.com/ortho_c.html (accessed Oct 2014).

CHAPTER 4. VITAMIN E AND PREGNANCY

1. Saul, A.W. "Vitamin E: A Cure in Search of Recognition." *J Orthomolecular Med* 18 (3–4) (2003): 205–12.

2. Oregon State University. News & Research Communications. "Excess Vitamin E Intake Not a Health Concern." (Apr 15, 2013): http://oregonstate.edu/ua/ncs/archives/2013/apr/excess-vitamin-e-intake-not-health-concern (accessed Oct 2014).

3. Ibid.

4. Ibid.

5. Saul, A.W. "Vitamin E: A Cure in Search of Recognition." *J Orthomolecular Med* 18 (3–4) (2003): 205–12.

6. Stampfer M.J., C.H. Hennekens, J.E. Manson, et al. "Vitamin E Consumption and the Risk of Coronary Disease in Women." *N Engl J Med* 328(20) (May 20, 1993): 1444–9.

7. Hoffer, A. "The True Cost of Cynicism." Editorial. *J Orthomolecular Med* 7(4) (Nov 19, 1992): 195–6.

8. Smedts, H.P., J.H. de Vries, M. Rakhshandehroo, et al. "High Maternal Vitamin E Intake by Diet or Supplements Is Associated with Congenital Heart Defects in the Offspring." *BJOG* 116(3) (Feb 2009): 416–23.

9. Boskovic, R., L. Cargaun, J. Dulus, et al. "High Doses of Vitamin E and Pregnancy Outcome." *Reprod Toxicol* (July 2004) July;18(5):722.

10. Boskovic R, Gargaun L., Oren D., et al. "Pregnancy Outcome Following High Doses of Vitamin E Supplementation." *Reprod Toxicol* 20(1) (May–Jun 2005): 85–8.

11. Martin, M.M., L.S. Hurley. "Effect of Large Amounts of Vitamin E during Pregnancy and Lactation." *Am J Clin Nutr* 30(10) (Oct 1977): 1629–37.

12. National Institute of Health. Office of Dietary Supplements. "Vitamin E: Fact Sheet for Health Professionals." http://ods.od.nih.gov/factsheets/VitaminE-HealthProfessional/ (accessed Oct 2014).

13. Oregon State University. News & Research Communications. "Excess Vitamin E Intake Not a Health Concern." (Apr 15, 2013): http://oregonstate.edu/ua/ncs/archives/2013/apr/excess-vitamin-e-intake-not-health-concern (accessed Oct 2014).

14. Ibid.

15. Ibid.

16. Ibid.

17. Institute of Medicine. Food and Nutrition Board. *Dietary Reference Intakes: Vitamin C, Vitamin E, Selenium, and Carotenoids*. Washington, DC: National Academies Press, 2000.

18. Ibid.

19. Saul, A.W. "Vitamin E: A Cure in Search of Recognition." *J Orthomolecular Med* 18 (3–4) (2003): 205–212.

20. Gao, X., P.E. Wilde, A.H. Lichtenstein, et al. "The Maximal Amount of Dietary Alpha-Tocopherol Intake in U.S. Adults (NHANES 2001–2002)." *J Nutr* 136(4) (2006):1021–1026. Interagency Board for Nutrition Monitoring and Related Research. *Third Report on Nutrition Monitoring in the United States*. Washington, DC: U.S. Government Printing Office, 1995.

21. Maras, J.E., O.I. Bermudez, N. Qiao, et al. "Intake of Alpha-Tocopherol Is Limited among US Adults." *J Am Diet Assoc* 104(4) (Apr 2004): 567–75.

22. Saul, A.W. "Can Vitamin Supplements Take the Place of a Bad Diet? *J Orthomolecular Med* 18(3–4) (2003): 213–16.

23. Bicknell, F., F. Prescott. *The Vitamins in Medicine*. 3rd ed. Milwaukee, WI: Lee Foundation for Nutritional Research, 1976. Saul, A.W. *Doctor Yourself: Natural Healing That Works*. 2nd edition. Laguna Beach, CA: Basic Health Publications, 2012.

24. Challem, J. "Natural vs. Synthetic Vitamin E." *Nutrition Science News* (November 2001).

25. Cass, H., K. Barnes. *8 Weeks to Vibrant Health*. New York, NY: McGraw Hill. 2004.

26. Barbas, C., E. Herrera. "Lipid Composition and Vitamin E Content in Human Colostrum and Mature Milk." *J Physiol Biochem* 54(3) (Sep 1998): 167–73. Martin, M.M., L.S. Hurley. "Effect of Large Amounts of Vitamin E during Pregnancy and Lactation." *Am J Clin Nutr* 30(10) (Oct 1977): 1629–37.

27. Barbas, C., E. Herrera. "Lipid Composition and Vitamin E Content in Human Colostrum and Mature Milk." *J Physiol Biochem* 54(3) (Sep 1998): 167–73.

28. Bayer Aspirin. "I Am ProHeart." www.iamproheart.com (accessed Oct 2014).

29. Federal Trade Commission. Bureau of Consumer Protection Business Center. "Dietary Supplements: An Advertising Guide for Industry." (Apr 2001): www.business.ftc.gov/documents/bus09-dietary-supplements-advertising-guide-industry (accessed Oct 2014).

30. Williams, H.T.G., D. Fenna, R.A. Macbeth. "Alpha Tocopherol in the Treatment of Intermittent Claudication." *Surg Gynecol Obstet* 132(4) (Apr 1971): 662–6.

31. Pacini, A.J. "Why We Need Vitamin E." *Health Culture Mag* (January 1936).

32. British Medical Journal, i, 1940: 890. cited in: Bicknell, F., F. Prescott. *The Vitamins in Medicine*. Milwaukee, WI: Lee Foundation for Nutritional Research, 1953: 632.

33. Roche Vitamins. "Vitamin E in Human Nutrition." www.roche-vitamins.com/home/what/what-hnh/what-hnh-vitamins/what-hnh-vitamin-e (URL no longer available).

34. Horwitt, M.K. "Vitamin E: A Reexamination." *Am J Clin Nutr* 29(5) (1976): 569–78.

35. Horwitt, M. "Interviews with Nutritional Experts: 'Vitamin E and the RDA.'" HealthWorld Online. www.healthy.net/Health/Interview/Vitamin_E_and_the_RDA/178 (accessed Oct 2014).

36. United States Postal Service. P.O.D. Docket No. 1/187. March 15, 1961. www.usps.gov/judicial/1961deci/1-187.htm (accessed Oct 2014).

37. Shute, E. *The Heart and Vitamin E*. London, Canada: Shute Foundation for Medical Research, 1963. Shute, W.E. *Dr. Wilfred E. Shute's Complete Updated Vitamin E Book*. New Canaan, CT: Keats, 1975. Shute, W.E., H.J. Taub. *Vitamin E for Ailing & Healthy Hearts*. New York: Jove, 1983. Shute, W.E., K.S. Berry, B.S. Carnahan. *Health Preserver: Defining the Versatility of Vitamin E*. Emmaus, PA: Rodale Press, 1977. Shute, W.E. *The Vitamin E Book*. New Canaan, CT: Keats Publishing, 1978. Shute, W.E. *Your Child and Vitamin E*. New Canaan, CT: Keats Publishing, 1979

38. Shute, W.E. *Your Child and Vitamin E*. New Canaan, CT: Keats Publishing, 1979

39. Ochsner, E.W.A. "Thromboembolism." Letter. *N Engl J Med* 271(4) (July 23, 1964): 211.

40. Shute, E.V., A.B. Vogelsang, F.R. Skelton, et al. "The Influence of Vitamin E on Vascular Disease." *Surg Gyn Obst* 86 (1948): 1–8.

41. United States Postal Service. P.O.D. Docket No. 1/187. March 15, 1961. www.usps.gov/judicial/1961deci/1–187.htm (accessed Oct 2014).

42. Bursell, S.E., A.C. Clermont, L.P. Aiello, et al. "High-Dose Vitamin E Supplementation Normalizes Retinal Blood Flow and Creatinine Clearance in Patients with Type 1 Diabetes." *Diabetes Care* 22(8) (Aug 1999): 1245–51.

43. Koo, J.R., Z. Ni, F. Oviesi, et al. "Antioxidant Therapy Potentiates Antihypertensive Action of Insulin in Diabetic Rats." *Clin Exp Hypertens* 24(5) (Jul 2002): 333–44.

44. GISSI-Prevenzione Investigators. "Dietary Supplementation with n-3 Polyunsaturated Fatty Acids and Vitamin E after Myocardial Infarction: Results of the GISSI-Prevenzione Trial." *Lancet* 354(9177) (Aug 1999): 447–55.

45. Hoffer, A. Personal Communication, June 2003.

46. Rosenbloom, M. "Vitamin Toxicity." Medscape. (Jun 3, 2013): http://emedicine .medscape.com/article/819426-overview. (accessed Oct 2014).

47. ABC News. "Vita-Mania: RDA for C, E Raised; Limits Set." The Associated Press, Washington, April 11, 2000: http://abcnews.go.com/sections/living/DailyNews/vitamin000411.html (URL no longer available).

48. Rosenberg, H. *The Book of Vitamin Therapy*. New York: Berkley Windhover Books, 1975.

49. Ogunmekan, A.O., P.A. Hwang. "A Randomized, Double-Blind, Placebo-Controlled, Clinical Trial of D-Alpha-Tocopheryl Acetate (Vitamin E), as Add-On therapy, for Epilepsy in Children." *Epilepsia* 30(1) (Jan–Feb 1989): 84–9.

50. Hittner, H.M., L.B. Godio, A.J. Rudolph, et al. "Retrolental Fibroplasia: Efficacy of Vitamin E in a Double-Blind Clinical Study of Preterm Infants." *N Engl J Med;* 305(23) (Dec 3 1981) 1365–71.

51. Williams, S.R. *Nutrition and Diet Therapy*. 7th edition. St. Louis: Mosby, 1993. (p 186). 6th edition, 1989. p 225.

CHAPTER 5. VITAMIN A AND PREGNANCY

1. Werbach, M.R., J. Moss. *Textbook of Nutritional Medicine*. Tarzana, CA: Third Line Press, 1999.

2. BabyCenter Medical Advisory Board. "Vitamin A in Your Pregnancy Diet." Baby-

Center: www.babycenter.com/0_vitamin-a-in-your-pregnancy-diet_675.bc (accessed Oct 2014).

3. Saul, A.W. *Fire Your Doctor: How to Be Independently Healthy.* Laguna Beach, CA: Basic Health Publications, 2005.

4. BabyCenter Medical Advisory Board. "Vitamin A in Your Pregnancy Diet." Baby-Center. www.babycenter.com/0_vitamin-a-in-your-pregnancy-diet_675.bc (accessed Oct 2014).

5. Ibid.

6. Georgetown University Medical Center. "Vitamin A Pushes Breast Cancer to Form Blood Vessel Cells." ScienceDaily, (July 17, 2008): www.sciencedaily.com/releases/2008/07/080715204719.htm (accessed Oct 2014). Tanvetyanon, T., G. Bepler. "Beta-carotene in Multivitamins and the Possible Risk of Lung Cancer among Smokers versus Former Smokers: A Meta-Analysis and Evaluation of National Brands." *Cancer* 113(1) (Jul 1, 2008): 150–7.

7. Orthomolecular Medicine News Service. "Vitamin A: Cancer Cure or Cancer Cause?" (Aug 20, 2008): http://orthomolecular.org/resources/omns/v04n09.shtml (accessed Oct 2014). Orthomolecular Medicine News Service. "Which Kills Smokers: 'Camels' or Carrots? Are Smokers Getting Lung Cancer from Beta-Carotene?" (Nov 18, 2008): http://orthomolecular.org/resources/omns/v04n23.shtml (accessed Oct 2014).

8. Rothman, K.J., L.L. Moore, M.R. Singer, et al. "Teratogenicity of High Vitamin A Intake." *N Engl J Med* 333 (Nov 23, 1995): 1369–73.

9. Werler, M.M., E.J. Lammer, A.A. Mitchell. "Teratogenicity of High Vitamin A Intake." Comment. *N Engl J Med* 334(18) (May 2, 1996):1195–6; author reply 1197.

10. Werbach, M.R., J. Moss. *Textbook of Nutritional Medicine,* 1999. Mills, J.L., J.L. Simpson, G.C. Cunningham, et al. "Vitamin A and Birth Defects." *Am J Obstet Gynecol* 177(1) (Jul 1997): 31–6.

11. Werbach, M.R., J. Moss. *Textbook of Nutritional Medicine.* Tarzana, CA: Third Line Press, 1999. Miller, R.K., A.G. Hendrickx, J.L. Mills, et al. "Periconceptional Vitamin A Use: How Much Is Teratogenic?" *Reprod Toxicol* 12(1) (Jan-Feb 1998): 75–88. Mills, J.L., J.L. Simpson, G.C. Cunningham, et al. "Vitamin A and Birth Defects." *Am J Obstet Gynecol* 177(1) (Jul 1997): 31–36.

12. World Health Organization. The Micronutrient Initiative. "Safe Vitamin A Dosage during Pregnancy and Lactation. Recommendations and Report of a Consultation." World Health Organization. WHO/Nut/98.4 (1998): http://whqlibdoc.who.int/hq/1998/WHO_NUT_98.4_eng.pdf (accessed Oct 2014).

13. Saul, A.W. *Doctor Yourself: Natural Healing That Works.* Laguna Beach, CA: Basic Health Publications, 2003. West, K.P., Jr. "Extent of Vitamin a Deficiency among Preschool Children and Women of Reproductive Age." *J Nutr* 132(9 Suppl) (Sep 2002): 2857S–2866S.

14. Hustead, V.A., G.R. Gutcher, S.A. Anderson, et al. "Relationship of Vitamin A (Retinol) Status to Lung Disease in the Preterm Infant." *J Pediatr* 105(4) (Oct 1984): 610–5. Radhika, M.S., P. Bhaskaram, N. Balakrishna, et al. "Effects of Vitamin A Deficiency during Pregnancy on Maternal and Child Health." *BJOG* 109(6) (Jun 2002): 689–93.

15. Sommer A. "Vitamin A Deficiency and Clinical Disease: An Historical Overview." *J Nutr* 138(10): 1835–9.

16. West, K.P. Jr., J. Katz, S.K. Khatry, et al. "Double Blind, Cluster Randomised Trial of Low Dose Supplementation with Vitamin A or Beta-Carotene on Mortality Related to Pregnancy in Nepal." *BMJ* 318(7183) (Feb 27, 1999): 570–5.

17. V. Azaïs-Braesco, G. Pascal. "Vitamin A in Pregnancy: Requirements and Safety Limits." *Am J Clin Nutr* 71(5) (May 2000): 1325s–1333s.

18. World Health Organization. Nutrition. "Micronutrient Deficiencies: Vitamin A Deficiency." www.who.int/nutrition/topics/vad/en/ (accessed Oct 2014).

19. Challem, J. "Teratogenicity of High Vitamin A Intake. Comment on" *N Engl J Med* 334(18) (May 1996): 1196–7. Block, G. "The Data Support a Role for Antioxidants in Reducing Cancer Risk." *Nutr Rev* 50(7) (July 2007): 207–13.

20. Strobel, M., J. Tinz, H.K. Biesalski. "The Importance of Beta-Carotene as a Source of Vitamin A with Special Regard to Pregnant and Breastfeeding Women." *Eur J Nutr* 46(Suppl 1) (Jul 2007): I1–20

21. Ibid.

22. V. Azaïs-Braesco, G. Pascal. "Vitamin A in Pregnancy: Requirements and Safety Limits." *Am J Clin Nutr* 71(5) (May 2000): 1325s–1333s.

23. U.S. Department of Agriculture. Agricultural Research Service. "Community Nutrition Mapping Project. CNMap." (3/10/2010): http://ars.usda.gov/Services/docs.htm ?docid=15656 (accessed Oct 2014).

24. World Health Organization. The Micronutrient Initiative. "Safe Vitamin A Dosage during Pregnancy and Lactation. Recommendations and Report of a Consultation." World Health Organization. WHO/Nut/98.4 (1998): http://whqlibdoc.who.int/hq/ 1998/WHO_NUT_98.4_eng.pdf (accessed Oct 2014).

25. The Teratology Society. "Teratology Society Position Paper: Recommendations for Vitamin A Use during Pregnancy." *Teratology* 35 (1987): 269–75. Available online at: www.teratology.org/pubs/vitamina.asp (accessed Oct 2014).

26. National Institute of Health. Office of Dietary Supplements. "Vitamin A: Fact Sheet for Health Professionals." (Jun 5, 2013): http://ods.od.nih.gov/factsheets/VitaminA-HealthProfessional/ (accessed Oct 2014).

27. Rothman, K.J., L.L. Moore, M.R. Singer, et al. "Teratogenicity of High Vitamin A Intake." *N Engl J Med* 333 (Nov 23, 1995): 1369–73.

28. National Institute of Health. Office of Dietary Supplements. "Vitamin A: Fact Sheet for Health Professionals." (Jun 5, 2013): http://ods.od.nih.gov/factsheets/VitaminA-HealthProfessional/ (accessed Oct 2014).

29. Miller, R.K., A.G. Hendrickx, J.L. Mills, et al. "Periconceptional Vitamin A Use: How Much Is Teratogenic?" *Reprod Toxicol* 12(1) (Jan–Feb 1998): 75–88. National Institute of Health. Office of Dietary Supplements. "Vitamin A: Fact Sheet for Health Professionals." (Jun 5, 2013): http://ods.od.nih.gov/factsheets/VitaminA-HealthProfessional/ (accessed Oct 2014). Grune, T., G. Lietz, A. Palou, et al. "Beta-Carotene Is an Important Vitamin A Source for Humans." *J Nutr* 140(12) (Dec 2010): 2268S–85S.

30. Super Nutrition's Fact vs. Fiction. "The Truth about Vitamin A (Retinol) & Beta-Carotene." 6d (Mar 2009): www.supernutritionusa.com/images/pdfs/VitaminALongVersion.pdf (accessed Oct 2014).

31. Ibid.

32. Tanvetyanon, T., G. Bepler. "Beta-carotene in Multivitamins and the Possible Risk of Lung Cancer among Smokers versus Former Smokers: A Meta-Analysis and Evaluation of National Brands." *Cancer* 113(1) (Jul 1, 2008): 150–7.

33. Ibid.

34. Orthomolecular Medicine News Service. "Which Kills Smokers: 'Camels' or Carrots? Are Smokers Getting Lung Cancer from Beta-Carotene?" (Nov 18, 2008): http://orthomolecular.org/resources/omns/v04n23.shtml (accessed Oct 2014).

35. Patrick, L. "Beta-Carotene: The Controversy Continues." *Altern Med Rev* 5(6) (Dec 2000): 530–45.

36. American Association of Poison Control Centers (AAPCC). "Annual Reports." www.aapcc.org/annual-reports/ (accessed Oct 2014).

37. Orthomolecular Medicine News Service. "Which Kills Smokers: 'Camels' or Carrots? Are Smokers Getting Lung Cancer from Beta-Carotene?" (Nov 18, 2008): http://orthomolecular.org/resources/omns/v04n23.shtml (accessed Oct 2014).

38. McLarty, J.W., D.B. Holiday, W.M. Girard, et al. "Beta-Carotene, Vitamin A, and Lung Cancer Chemoprevention: Results of an Intermediate Endpoint Study." *Am J Clin Nutr* 62(6 Suppl) (Dec 1995): 1431S–1438S.

39. Orthomolecular Medicine News Service. "Which Kills Smokers: 'Camels' or Carrots? Are Smokers Getting Lung Cancer from Beta-Carotene?" (Nov 18, 2008): http://orthomolecular.org/resources/omns/v04n23.shtml (accessed Oct 2014).

40. Oliveira-Menegozzo, J.M., D.P. Bergamaschi, P. Middleton, et al. "Vitamin A Supplementation for Postpartum Women." *Cochrane Database Syst Rev* CD005944 (Oct 8, 2010): doi: 10.1002/14651858.

41. Butte, N.F., M.G. Lopez-Alarcon, C. Garza. "Nutrient Adequacy of Exclusive Breastfeeding for the Term Infant during the First Six Months of Life." World Health Organization. Department of Nutrition for Health and Development. (2002): http://whqlibdoc.who.int/publications/9241562110.pdf (accessed Oct 2014).

42. National Institute of Health. Office of Dietary Supplements. "Vitamin A: Fact Sheet for Health Professionals." (Jun 5, 2013): http://ods.od.nih.gov/factsheets/VitaminA-HealthProfessional/ (accessed Oct 2014).

43. Orthomolecular Medicine News Service. "Vitamin A: Cancer Cure or Cancer Cause?" (Aug 20, 2008): http://orthomolecular.org/resources/omns/v04n09.shtml (accessed Oct 2014).

44. Semba, R.D. "Vitamin A, Immunity, and Infection." *Clin Infect Dis* 19(3) (Sep 1994): 489–99.

CHAPTER 6. VITAMIN D AND PREGNANCY

1. Hollis, B.W. "Circulating 25-Hydroxyvitamin D Levels Indicative of Vitamin D Sufficiency: Implications for Establishing a New Effective Dietary Intake Recommendation for Vitamin D" *J. Nutr* 135(2) (Feb 2005): 317–22

2. Yu, C.K., L. Sykes, M. Sethi, et al. "Vitamin D Deficiency and Supplementation during Pregnancy." *Clin Endocrinol (Oxf)* 70(5) (May 2009): 685–90. doi: 10.1111/j.1365–2265.2008.03403.x.

3. Office of Dietary Supplements. National Institutes of Health. "Vitamin D: Fact Sheet for Health Professionals." (Jun 24, 2011): http://ods.od.nih.gov/factsheets/VitaminD-HealthProfessional/ (accessed Oct 2014).

4. Hollis, B.W. "Circulating 25-Hydroxyvitamin D Levels Indicative of Vitamin D Sufficiency: Implications for Establishing a New Effective Dietary Intake Recommendation for Vitamin D" *J. Nutr* 135(2) (Feb 2005): 317–22.

5. Ibid.

6. Hollis, B.W. "Circulating 25-Hydroxyvitamin D Levels Indicative of Vitamin D Sufficiency: Implications for Establishing a New Effective Dietary Intake Recommendation for Vitamin D" *J. Nutr* 135(2) (Feb 2005): 317–22. Datta, S., M. Alfaham, D.P. Davies, et al. "Vitamin D Deficiency in Pregnant Women from a Non-European Ethnic Minority Population—An International Study." *BJOG* 109(8) (2002): 905–8.

7. Lee, J.M., J.R. Smith, B.L. Philipp,et al. "Vitamin D Deficiency in a Healthy Group of Mothers and Newborn Infants." *Clin Pediatr (Phila)* 46(1) (Jan 2007): 42–4. Bodnar, L.M., H.N. Simhan, R.W. Powers, et al. "High Prevalence of Vitamin D Insufficiency in Black and White Pregnant Women Residing in the Northern United States and Their Neonates." *J Nutr;*137(2) (Feb 2007): 447–52.

8. Bodnar, L.M., H.N. Simhan, R.W. Powers, et al. "High Prevalence of Vitamin D Insufficiency in Black and White Pregnant Women Residing in the Northern United States and Their Neonates." *J Nutr;*137(2) (Feb 2007): 447–52.

9. Johnson, D.D., C.L. Wagner, T.C. Hulsey, et al. "Vitamin D Deficiency and Insufficiency Is Common during Pregnancy." *Am J Perinatol* 28(1) (Jan 2011): 7–12. doi: 10.1055/s-0030-1262505.

10. Dawodu, A., C.L. Wagner. "Mother-Child Vitamin D Deficiency: An International Perspective." *Arch Dis Child* 92(9) (Sep 2007): 737–40. van der Meer, I.M., N.S. Karamali, A.J. Boeke, et al. "High Prevalence of Vitamin D Deficiency in Pregnant Non-Western Women in The Hague, Netherlands." *Am J Clin Nutr* 84(2) (Aug 2006): 350–9. Bassir, M., S. Laborie, A. Lapillonne, et al. "Vitamin D Deficiency in Iranian Mothers and Their Neonates: A Pilot Study." *Acta Paediatr* 90(5) (May 2001): 577–9. Markestad, T., A. Elzouki, M. Legnain, et al. "Serum Concentrations of Vitamin D Metabolites in Maternal and Umbilical Cord Blood of Libyan and Norwegian Women." *Hum Nutr Clin Nutr* 38(1) (Jan 1984): 55–62. Sachan, A., R. Gupta, V. Das, et al. "High Prevalence of Vitamin D Deficiency among Pregnant Women and Their Newborns in Northern India." *Am J Clin Nutr* 81(5) (May 2005): 1060–4.

11. M.L. Mulligan, S.K. Felton, A.E. Riek, et al. "Implications of Vitamin D Deficiency in Pregnancy and Lactation." *Am J Obstet Gynecol* 202(5) (May 2010): 429.e1–9.

12. Lau, S.L., J.E. Gunton, N.P. Athayde, et al. "Serum 25-Hydroxyvitamin D and Glycated Haemoglobin Levels in Women with Gestational Diabetes Mellitus." *Med J Aust* 194(7) (Apr 4, 2011): 334–7. Hollis, B.W. "Vitamin D Requirement during Pregnancy and Lactation." *J Bone Miner Res* 22(Suppl 2) (Dec 2007): V39–44.

13. Holick, M.F. "Medical Progress: Vitamin D Deficiency." *NEJM* 357(3) (Jul 19, 2007): 266–81.

14. Aghajafari, F., T. Nagulesapillai, P.E. Ronskley, et al. "Association between Maternal Serum 25-Hydroxyvitamin D Level and Pregnancy and Neonatal Outcomes: Systematic Review and Meta-Analysis of Observational Studies." *BMJ* 346 (Mar 26, 2013): doi 10.1136/bmj.f1169.

15. Challem, J. "Vitamin D Benefits Pregnant Women and Their Fetuses." *The Nutrition Reporter* 24(7) (July 2013).

16. Saul, A.W. "Vitamin D: Deficiency, Diversity and Dosage."*J Orthomolecular Med* 18(3/4) (Sep 2003): 194–204.

17. R.P. Heaney. "Vitamin D* Action. FAQ's (Frequently Asked Questions) Vitamin D." Grassroots Health. (8/2/2011): www.grassrootshealth.net/media/download/daction_faq _trifold.pdf (accessed Oct 2014).

18. Holick, M.F. "Medical Progress: Vitamin D Deficiency." *NEJM* 357(3) (Jul 19, 2007): 266–81.

19. Office of Dietary Supplements. National Institutes of Health. "Vitamin D: Fact Sheet for Health Professionals." (Jun 24, 2011): http://ods.od.nih.gov/factsheets/VitaminD-HealthProfessional/ (accessed Oct 2014).

20. Ibid.

21. Aghajafari, F., T. Nagulesapillai, P.E. Ronskley, et al. "Association between Maternal Serum 25-Hydroxyvitamin D Level and Pregnancy and Neonatal Outcomes: Systematic Review and Meta-Analysis of Observational Studies." *BMJ* 346 (Mar 26, 2013): doi 10.1136/bmj.f1169.

22. Garbedian, K., M. Boggild, J. Moody, et al. "Effect of Vitamin D Status on Clinical Pregnancy Rates Following In Vitro Fertilization." *CMAJ Open* 1(2) (Jun 28, 2013): E77–E82.

23. Cassidy-Bushrow, A.E., R.M. Peters, D.A. Johnson, et al. "Vitamin D Nutritional Status and Antenatal Depressive Symptoms in African American Women." *J Womens Health (Larchmt)* 21(11) (Nov 20112): 1189–95. doi: 10.1089/jwh.2012.3528. Brandenbarg, J., T.G. Vrijkotte, G. Goedhart, et al. "Maternal Early-Pregnancy Vitamin D Status Is Associated with Maternal Depressive Symptoms in the Amsterdam Born Children and Their Development Cohort." *Psychosom Med* 74(7) (Sep 2012):751–7. doi: 10.1097/PSY.0b013e3182639fdb.

24. CCHR International. The Mental Health Watchdog. "Drug Studies on Antidepressants Causing Birth Defects." (Jan 12, 2012): www.cchrint.org/psychiatric-drugs/antidepressantsbirthdefects/drug-studies-on-antidepressants-causing-birth-defects/ (accessed Oct 2014).

25. Mercola, J. "Five Ways to Help Beat Depression without Antidepressants." Mercola.com. (Mar 9, 2010): http://articles.mercola.com/sites/articles/archive/2010/03/09/antidepressants-are-no-better-than-placebo.aspx (accessed Oct 2014).

26. Mercola, J. "This Vital Vitamin Reduces Diabetes, High Blood Pressure, and Preeclampsia in Pregnancy by 30 Percent." Mercola.com. (Jul 22, 2010): http://carlwattsartist.com/Mercola-This-Vital-Vitamin-Reduces-Diabetes-High-Blood-Pressure.htm l (accessed Oct 2014).

27. Camargo, C.A. Jr, S.L. Rifas-Shiman, A.A. Litonjua, et al. "Maternal Intake of Vitamin D during Pregnancy and Risk of Recurrent Wheeze in Children at 3 Y of Age." *Am J Clin Nutr* 85(3) (Mar 2007): 788–95.

28. Grant, W.B. "Vitamin D Requirements during Pregnancy and Lactation." Sunlight, Nutrition and Health Research Center (SUNARC). www.sunarc.org/Vitamin%20D% 20pregnancy.htm (accessed Oct 2014).

29. Ibid

30. Drake, V.J. "Micronutrient Needs during Pregnancy and Lactation." Linus Pauling Institute. Micronutrient Information Center. (Jul 2011): http://lpi.oregonstate.edu/infocenter/lifestages/pregnancyandlactation/ (accessed Oct 2014).

31. Linus Pauling Institute. Micronutrient Information Center. Oregon State University. "Vitamin K." http://lpi.oregonstate.edu/infocenter/vitamins/vitaminK/ (accessed November 2014).

32. Ibid.

33. Mercola, J.M. "The Potential Dark Side of the Routine Newborn Vitamin K Shot." (Mar 27, 2010): http://articles.mercola.com/sites/articles/archive/2010/03/27/high-risks-to-your-baby-from-vitamin-k-shot-they-dont-warn-you-about.aspx (accessed October 2014).

34. Saul, A.W. "Vitamin D: Deficiency, Diversity and Dosage." *J Orthomolecular Med* 18(3/4) (Sep 2003): 194–204.

35. Hollis, B.W. "Circulating 25-Hydroxyvitamin D Levels Indicative of Vitamin D Sufficiency: Implications for Establishing a New Effective Dietary Intake Recommendation for Vitamin D" *J. Nutr* 135(2) (Feb 2005): 317–22. Datta, S., M. Alfaham, D.P. Davies, et al. "Vitamin D Deficiency in Pregnant Women from a Non-European Ethnic Minority Population—An International Study." *BJOG* 109(8) (2002): 905–8.

36. Hollis, B.W., D. Johnson, T.C. Hulsey, et al. "Vitamin D Supplementation during Pregnancy: Double-Blind, Randomized Clinical Trial of Safety and Effectiveness." *J Bone Miner Res* 26(10) (Oct 2011): 2341–57.

37. Ibid.

38. Hollis, B.W., C.L. Wagner. "Vitamin D and Pregnancy: Skeletal Effects, Nonskeletal Effects, and Birth Outcomes." *Calcif Tissue Int* 92(2) (Feb 2013):128–39.

39. Ibid.

40. Ibid.

41. Office of Dietary Supplements. National Institutes of Health. "Vitamin D: Fact Sheet for Health Professionals." (Jun 24, 2011): http://ods.od.nih.gov/factsheets/VitaminD-HealthProfessional/ (accessed Oct 2014).

42. Hollis, B.W. "Circulating 25-Hydroxyvitamin D Levels Indicative of Vitamin D Sufficiency: Implications for Establishing a New Effective Dietary Intake Recommendation for Vitamin D" *J. Nutr* 135(2) (Feb 2005): 317–22. Datta, S., M. Alfaham, D.P. Davies, et al. "Vitamin D Deficiency in Pregnant Women from a Non-European Ethnic Minority Population—An International Study." *BJOG* 109(8) (2002): 905–8.

43. Hollis, B.W., C.L. Wagner. "Vitamin D Requirements during Lactation: High-Dose Maternal Supplementation as Therapy to Prevent Hypovitaminosis D for Both the Mother and the Nursing Infant." *Am J Clin Nutr* 80(6 Suppl) (Dec 2004): 1752S–8S.B. W. Hollis. "Circulating 25-Hydroxyvitamin D Levels Indicative of Vitamin D Sufficiency: Implications for Establishing a New Effective Dietary Intake Recommendation for Vitamin D" *J. Nutr* 135(2) (Feb 2005): 317–22.

44. Basile, L.A., S.N. Taylor, C.L. Wagner, et al. "The Effect of High-Dose Vitamin D Supplementation on Serum Vitamin D Levels and Milk Calcium Concentration in Lactating Women and Their Infants." *Breastfeed Med* 1(1) (Spring 2006): 27–35.

45. Wagner, C.L., T.C. Hulsey, D. Fanning, et al. "High-Dose Vitamin D3 Supplementation in a Cohort of Breastfeeding Mothers and Their infants: A 6-Month Follow-Up Pilot Study." *Breastfeed Med* 1(2) (Summer 2006): 59–70.

46. Vitamin D Council. "Vitamin D during Pregnancy and Breastfeeding." (Jan 30, 2013): https://www.vitamindcouncil.org/further-topics/vitamin-d-during-pregnancy-and-breastfeeding/(accessed Oct 2014).

47. Rosenbloom, M. "Vitamin Toxicity." VCU Department of Nurse Anesthesia. (Oct 14, 2014): www.emedicine.com/emerg/topic638.htm (accessed Oct 2014).

48. The Merck Manual of Diagnosis and Therapy. 3rd ed. Section 1. Chapter 3. "Vitamin Deficiency, Dependency, and Toxicity. Vitamin D Toxicity." www.merck.com/pubs/mmanual/section1/chapter3/3e.htm

49. Ibid.

50. Williams, S.R. *Nutrition and Diet Therapy.* 6th edition. St. Louis, MO: Mosby, 1989.

51. Bicknell, F.F. Prescott. *The Vitamins in Medicine.* 3rd edition. Milwaukee, WI: Lee Foundation, 1953:544, 578–591.

52. Marya, R.K., S. Rathee, V. Lata, et al. "Effects of Vitamin D Supplementation in Pregnancy." *Gynecol Obstet Invest* 12(3) (1981):155–61.

53. Commonwealth of Massachusetts. "Tarpey v. Crescent Ridge Dairy, Inc., 47 Mass. App. Ct. 380. (1999): http://masscases.com/cases/app/47/47massappct380.html. (accessed Oct 2014).

54. Doherty, Wallace, Pillsbury, and Murphy, P.C. Attorneys at Law: www.dwpm.com/content/main/litigation00_news.php3 (accessed Jun 2003) (No longer available on the www).

55. Martini, F.H. "Metabolism and Energetics. Diet and Nutrition: Vitamins. Hypervitaminosis." In *Anatomy and Physiology* Chapter 25. NY: Prentice Hall, 2000. Available online   at: http://media.pearsoncmg.com/ph/esm/esm_martini_fundanaphy_5/bb/obj/25/CH25/html/ch25_8_4.html

56. Saul, A.W. "Vitamin D: Deficiency, Diversity and Dosage." *J Orthomolecular Med* 18(3/4) (Sep 2003): 194–204.

57. Hollis, B.W., C.L. Wagner. "Assessment of Dietary Vitamin D Requirements during Pregnancy and Lactation." *Am J Clin Nutr* 79(5) (May 2004): 717–26.

58. Yu, C.K., L. Sykes, M. Sethi, et al. "Vitamin D Deficiency and Supplementation during Pregnancy." *Clin Endocrinol (Oxf)* 70(5) (May 2009): 685–90. doi: 10.1111/j.1365–2265.2008.03403.x.

59. Vitamin D Council. "Vitamin D during Pregnancy and Breastfeeding." (Jan 30, 2013): https://www.vitamindcouncil.org/further-topics/vitamin-d-during-pregnancy-and-breastfeeding/ (accessed Oct 2014).

60. The American Congress of Obstetricians and Gynecologists (ACOG). "Vitamin D: Screening and Supplementation during Pregnancy." 495 (July 2011). www.acog.org/Resources-And-Publications/Committee-Opinions/Committee-on-Obstetric-Practice/Vitamin-D-Screening-and-Supplementation-During-Pregnancy (accessed Oct 2014).

61. Holick, M.F. "Calcium and Vitamin D. Diagnostics and Therapeutics." *Clin Lab Med* 20(3) (Sep 2000): 569–90.

62. "Vitamin D* Action. FAQ's (Frequently Asked Questions) Vitamin D." Grassroots Health. www.grassrootshealth.net/index.php/daction#hqone (accessed Oct 2014).

63. Wolpowitz, D., B.A. Gilchrest. "The Vitamin D Questions: How Much Do You Need and How Should You Get It?" *J Am Acad Derm* 54(2) (Feb 2006): 301–17.

64. Grant, W.B. "Why Is the Public Misinformed About UV and Vitamin D?" Sunlight, Nutrition and Health Research Center (SUNARC). www.sunarc.org/public%20misinformed.htm (accessed Oct 2014).

65. Key, S.W., M. Marble. "Studies Link Sun Exposure to Protection Against Cancer." *Cancer Weekly Plus* (Nov 17, 1997): 5–6. Studzinski, G.P., D.C. Moore. "Sunlight: Can It Prevent As Well As Cause Cancer?" *Cancer Res* 55(18) (Sep 1995):4014–22.

66. Mercola, J. "Sun Can Actually Help Protect You Against Skin Cancer." (Jun 16, 2011): http://articles.mercola.com/sites/articles/archive/2011/06/16/sun-can-protect-you-against-skin-cancer.aspx. (accessed Nov 2014).

CHAPTER 7. THE B VITAMINS AND PREGNANCY

1. American Association of Poison Control Centers (AAPCC). "Annual Reports." www.aapcc.org/annual-reports/ (accessed Oct 2014).

2. BabyCenter Medical Advisory Board. "Thiamine in Your Pregnancy Diet." BabyCenter. www.babycenter.com/0_thiamine-in-your-pregnancy-diet_668.bc (accessed Oct 2014).

3. National Institutes of Health. Medline Plus. U.S. National Library of Medicine. "Thiamin." www.nlm.nih.gov/medlineplus/ency/article/002401.htm (accessed Oct 2014).

4. Harrell, R.F. "Mental Response to Added Thiamine." *J Nutr* 31 (Mar 1946): 283.

5. Harrell, R.F, E. Woodyard, A.I. Gates. *The Effect of Mothers' Diets on the Intelligence of Offspring: A Study of Vitamin Supplementation of the Diets of Pregnant and Lactating Women on the Intelligence of Their Children.* NY: Bureau of Publications, Teachers College, Columbia University, 1955. Bryan, A.H. "The Effect of Mothers' Diets on the Intelligence of Offspring. A Study of the Influence of Vitamin Supplementation of the Diets of Pregnant and Lactating Women on the Intelligence of Their Children. (Review)" *Am J Public Health Nations Health* 46(9) (Sep 1956): 1162–64.

6. Saul, A.W. "The Pioneering Work of Ruth Flinn Harrell: Champion of Children." *J Orthomolecular Med.* 19(4) (Mar 2004): 21–6.

7. Irwin, J.B. *The Natural Way to a Trouble Free Pregnancy: The Toxemia/Thiamine Connection.* Aslan Publishing, 2008.

8. Ibid.

9. Linus Pauling Institute. Micronutrient Information Center. Oregon State University. "Thiamin." http://lpi.oregonstate.edu/infocenter/vitamins/thiamin/ (accessed Oct 2014).

10. Ibid.

11. Linus Pauling Institute. Micronutrient Information Center. Oregon State University. "Thiamin." http://lpi.oregonstate.edu/infocenter/vitamins/thiamin/ (accessed Oct 2014).

12. National Institutes of Health. Medline Plus. U.S. National Library of Medicine. "Thiamin." www.nlm.nih.gov/medlineplus/ency/article/002401.htm (accessed Oct 2014).

13. Irwin, J.B. *The Natural Way to a Trouble Free Pregnancy: The Toxemia/Thiamine Connection.* Aslan Publishing, 2008.

14. Saul, A.W. *The Vitamin Cure for Alcoholism.* Laguna Beach, CA: Basic Health Publications, 2009.

15. Breedon, C. "Thinking About Prenatal Nutrition and Fetal Alcohol Syndrome (FAS)" West Virginia WIC. Office of Nutrition Services. Nutritionist Training Handouts. http://ons.wvdhhr.org/HealthNutrition/NutritionistTraining/tabid/2000/Default.aspx (accessed Oct 2014).

16. Linus Pauling Institute. Micronutrient Information Center. Oregon State University. "Riboflavin." http://lpi.oregonstate.edu/infocenter/vitamins/riboflavin/ (accessed Oct 2014).

17. Gaby, A.R. "'Safe Upper Levels' for Nutritional Supplements: One Giant Step Backward." *J Orthomolecular Med* 18(3–4) (2003):126–30.

18. U.S. National Library of Medicine. National Institutes of Health. "Riboflavin (Vitamin B2)" www.nlm.nih.gov/medlineplus/druginfo/natural/957.html (accessed Oct 2014).

19. Schoenen, J., J. Jacquy, M. Lenaerts. "Effectiveness of High-Dose Riboflavin in Migraine Prophylaxis. A Randomized Controlled Trial." *Neurology* 50(2) (Feb 1998): 466–70. Boehnke, C., U. Reuter, U. Flach, et al. "High-Dose Riboflavin Treatment Is Efficacious in Migraine Prophylaxis: An Open Study in a Tertiary Care Centre." *Eur J Neurol* 11(7) (Jul 2004): 475–7. Gaby, A.R. "'Safe Upper Levels' for Nutritional Supplements: One Giant Step Backward." *J Orthomolecular Med* 18(3–4) (2003):126–30.

20. Linus Pauling Institute. Micronutrient Information Center. Oregon State University. "Riboflavin." http://lpi.oregonstate.edu/infocenter/vitamins/riboflavin/ (accessed Oct 2014). Wacker, J., J. Frühauf, M. Schulz, et al. "Riboflavin Deficiency and Preeclampsia." *Obstet Gynecol* 96(1) (Jul 2000): 38–44.

21. Singer, N. "Botox Shots Approved for Migraine." The New York Times. (Oct 15, 2010): www.nytimes.com/2010/10/16/health/16drug.html?_r=0 (accessed Oct 2014).

22. United Kingdom Tertology Information Service. "Exposure to Botulinum Toxin or Botox in Pregnancy." Version 2. August 2012. (No longer available on the www).

23. Morgan, J.C., S.S. Iyer, E.T. Moser, et al. "Botulinum Toxin A during Pregnancy: A Survey of Treating Physicians." *J Neurol Neurosurg Psychiatry* 77(1) (Jan 2006): 117–9.

24. Morgan, J.C., S.S. Iyer, E.T. Moser, et al. "Botulinum Toxin A during Pregnancy: A Survey of Treating Physicians." *J Neurol Neurosurg Psychiatry* 77(1) (Jan 2006): 117–9.

25. Allergan. "Results with Botox." www.botoxchronicmigraine.com/botox-chronic-migraine-patients/?cid=sem_CMB_goo_s_7935 (accessed Oct 20143).

26. Cady, R., C. Schreiber. "Botulinum Toxin Type A as Migraine Preventive Treatment in Patients Previously Failing Oral Prophylactic Treatment Due to Compliance Issues." *Headache* 48(6) (Jun 2008): 900–13. Aurora, S.K., M. Gawel, J.L. Brandes, et al. "Botulinum Toxin Type A Prophylactic Treatment of Episodic Migraine: A Randomized, Double-Blind, Placebo-Controlled Exploratory Study." *Headache* 47(4) (Apr 2007): 486–99.

27. Allergan. "Results with Botox." www.botoxchronicmigraine.com/botox-chronic-migraine-patients/?cid=sem_CMB_goo_s_7935 (accessed Oct 20143).

28. Singer, N. "Botox Shots Approved for Migraine." The New York Times. (Oct 15, 2010): www.nytimes.com/2010/10/16/health/16drug.html?_r=0 (accessed Oct 2014).

29. Langham, R.Y. "Vitamins for Dystonia." (Sep 1, 2011): www.livestrong.com/article/531321-vitamins-for-dystonia/ (accessed Oct 2014).

30. Hoffer, A. *Vitamin B-3 and Schizophrenia: Discovery, Recovery, Controversy.* Kingston, Ontario, Canada: Quarry Press, 1998.

31. Hoffer., A. "Vitamin B-3: Niacin and Its Amide." DoctorYourself.com. www.doctoryourself.com/hoffer_niacin.html (accessed Oct 2014).

32. Hoffer, A. "Chronic Schizophrenia Patients Treated Ten Years or More." *J Orthomolecular Med* 9(1) 1994: 7–37.

33. Ibid.

34. Louik, C., A.E. Lin, M.M. Werler, et al. "First-Trimester Use of Selective Serotonin-Reuptake Inhibitors and the Risk of Birth Defects." *N Engl J Med* 356(26) (Jun 28, 2007): 2675–83.

35. ACOG Committee on Ethics. The American Congress of Obstetricians and Gynecologists. "ACOG Committee Opinion #321: Maternal Decision Making, Ethics, and the Law." *Obstet Gynecol* 106(5 Pt 1) (Nov 2005): 1127–37. Available online at: www.acog.org/resources_and_publications/committee_opinions/committee_on_ethics/maternal_decision_making_ethics_and_the_law (accessed November 2013).

36. Savage, D.G. "Supreme Court Rules Generic-Drug Makers Can't Be Sued over Defects." *Portland Press Herald* (Jun 24, 2013): www.pressherald.com/2013/06/24/supreme-court-rules-generic-drug-makers-cant-be-sued-over-defects/ (accessed Oct 2014).

37. Mercola, J. "The Latest in Atrocious Supreme Court Decisions—Only 2 Justices Stand Up for Your Rights. . . ." (Mar 22, 2011): http://articles.mercola.com/sites/articles/archive/2011/03/22/betrayal-of-consumers-by-us-supreme-court-gives-total-liability-shield-to-big-pharma.aspx (accessed Oct 2014).

38. Savage, D.G. "Supreme Court Rules Generic-Drug Makers Can't Be Sued over Defects." *Portland Press Herald* (Jun 24, 2013): www.pressherald.com/2013/06/24/supreme-court-rules-generic-drug-makers-cant-be-sued-over-defects/ (accessed Oct 2014).

39. Ibid.

40. Mercola, J. "The Latest in Atrocious Supreme Court Decisions—Only 2 Justices Stand Up for Your Rights. . . ." (Mar 22, 2011): http://articles.mercola.com/sites/articles/archive/2011/03/22/betrayal-of-consumers-by-us-supreme-court-gives-total-liability-shield-to-big-pharma.aspx (accessed Oct 2014).

41. CCHR International. The Mental Health Watchdog. "Drug Studies on Antidepressants Causing Birth Defects." (Jan 12, 2012): www.cchrint.org/psychiatric-drugs/antidepressantsbirthdefects/drug-studies-on-antidepressants-causing-birth-defects/ (accessed Oct 2014).

42. Alwan, S., J. Reefhuis, S.A. Rasmussen, et al. "Use of Selective Serotonin-Reuptake Inhibitors in Pregnancy and the Risk of Birth Defects." *N Engl J Med* 356 (Jun 28, 2007): 2684–92.

43. Ibid.

44. Louik, C., A.E. Lin, M.M. Werler, et al. "First-Trimester Use of Selective Serotonin-Reuptake Inhibitors and the Risk of Birth Defects." *N Engl J Med* 356(26) (Jun 28, 2007): 2675–83.

45. Ibid.

46. Ibid.

47. Ibid.

48. Ibid.

49. Reller, M.D., M.J. Strickland, T. Riehle-Colarusso, et al. "Prevalence of Congenital Heart Defects in Metropolitan Atlanta, 1998–2005." *J Pediatr* 153(6) (Dec 2008): 807–13. doi: 10.1016/j.jpeds.2008.05.059.

50. CCHR International. The Mental Health Watchdog. "Drug Studies on Antidepressants Causing Birth Defects." (Jan 12, 2012): www.cchrint.org/psychiatric-drugs/antidepressantsbirthdefects/drug-studies-on-antidepressants-causing-birth-defects/ (accessed Oct 2014).

51. Pedersen, L.H., T.B. Henriksen, M. Vestergaard, et al. "Selective Serotonin Reuptake Inhibitors in Pregnancy and Congenital Malformations: Population Based Cohort Study." *BMJ* 339 (Sep 23, 2009): b3569. doi: 10.1136/bmj.b3569.

52. Kieler, H., M. Artama., A. Engeland, et al. "Selective Serotonin Reuptake Inhibitors during Pregnancy and Risk of Persistent Pulmonary Hypertension in the Newborn: Population Based Cohort Study from the Five Nordic Countries," *BMJ* 344 (Jan 12, 2012): d8012.

53. CCHR International. The Mental Health Watchdog. "Drug Studies on Antidepressants Causing Birth Defects." (Jan 12, 2012): www.cchrint.org/psychiatric-drugs/antidepressantsbirthdefects/drug-studies-on-antidepressants-causing-birth-defects/ (accessed Oct 2014).

54. Harrington, R.A., L. Li-Ching, R.M. Crum, et al. "Prenatal SSRI Use and Offspring with Autism Spectrum Disorder or Developmental Delay." *Pediatrics* (pub online Apr 14, 2014): doi: 10.1542/peds.2013–3406).

55. Clements, C.C., V.M. Castro, S.R. Blumenthal, et al. "Prenatal Antidepressant Exposure Is Associated with Risk for Attention-Deficit Hyperactivity Disorder but Not Autism Spectrum Disorder in a Large Health System." *Mol Psychiatry* (pub online Aug 26, 2014): doi: 10.1038/mp.2014.90.

56. Zhong, W., H. Maradit-Kremers, J.L. St. Sauver, et al. "Age and Sex Patterns of Drug Prescribing in a Defined American Population" *Mayo Clinic Proceedings* 88(7) (Jun 2013): 697–707.

57. Fournier, J.C., R.J. DeRubeis, S.D. Hollon, et al. "Antidepressant Drug Effects and Depression SeverityA Patient-Level Meta-analysis." *JAMA* 303(1) (Jan 6, 2010): 47–53. Kirsch, I., B.J. Deacon, T.B. Huedo-Medina, et al. "Initial Severity and Antidepressant Benefits: A Meta-Analysis of Data Submitted to the Food and Drug Administration." *PLoS Med* 5(2) (Feb 2008): e45. doi: 10.1371/journal.pmed.0050045

58. Jonsson, B.H., A.W. Saul. *The Vitamin Cure for Depression.* Laguna Beach, CA: Basic Health Publications, 2012.

59. Hoffer, A., A.W. Saul, H.D. Foster. *Niacin: The Real Story.* Laguna Beach, CA: Basic Health Publications, 2012.

60. Hoffer, A., J. Prousky. *Naturopathic Nutrition: A Guide to Nutrient-Rich Food and Nutritional Supplements for Optimum Health.* Toronto, ON: CCNM Press, 2006.

61. Ibid.

62. Jonsson, B.H., A.W. Saul. *The Vitamin Cure for Depression.* Laguna Beach, CA: Basic Health Publications, 2012.

63. Hoffer., A. "Vitamin B-3: Niacin and Its Amide." DoctorYourself.com. www.doctoryourself.com/hoffer_niacin.html (accessed Oct 2014).

64. Orthomolecular Medicine News Service. "Mental Health Treatment that Works." *Orthomolecular Med News Service* (Oct 7, 2005): http://orthomolecular.org/resources/omns/v01n11.shtml (accessed Oct 2014).

65. Hoffer, A., A.W. Saul, H.D. Foster. *Niacin: The Real Story.* Laguna Beach, CA: Basic Health Publications, 2012.

66. Ibid.

67. Ibid.

68. Ibid.

69. Saul, A.W., J.N. Vaman, "No Deaths from Vitamins—None at All in 27 Years." *Orthomolecular Med News Service* (Jun 14, 2011): http://orthomolecular.org/resources/omns/v07n05.shtml (accessed Oct 2014).

70. Starfield, B. "Is US Health Really the Best in the World?" *JAMA* 284(4) (Jul 26, 2000):483–85.

71. Jonsson, B.H., A.W. Saul. *The Vitamin Cure for Depression.* Laguna Beach, CA: Basic Health Publications, 2012.

72. Hoffer, A., A.W. Saul, H.D. Foster. *Niacin: The Real Story.* Laguna Beach, CA: Basic Health Publications, 2012.

73. Ibid.

74. Hoffer, A. "Negative and Positive Side Effects of Vitamin B3." *J Orthomolecular Med* 18(3–4) 2003: 146–160. Available online at: http://orthomolecular.org/library/jom/2003/pdf/2003-v18n0304-p144.pdf (accessed Oct 2014).

75. Hoffer, A., A.W. Saul, H.D. Foster. *Niacin: The Real Story.* Laguna Beach, CA: Basic Health Publications, 2012.

76. Hoffer, A. "Facts and Factoids: An Information Sheet for Patients." www.doctoryourself.com/hoffer_factoids.html (accessed Oct 2014).

77. Jonsson, B.H., A.W. Saul. *The Vitamin Cure for Depression.* Laguna Beach, CA: Basic Health Publications, 2012.

78. Hoffer, A., A.W. Saul, H.D. Foster. *Niacin: The Real Story.* Laguna Beach, CA: Basic Health Publications, 2012.

79. Ibid.

80. Hoffer, A. "Negative and Positive Side Effects of Vitamin B3." *J Orthomolecular Med* 18(3–4) 2003: 146–160. Available online at: http://orthomolecular.org/library/jom/2003/pdf/2003-v18n0304-p144.pdf (accessed Oct 2014).

81. Drugs.com. "Niacin Pregnancy and Breastfeeding Warnings." www.drugs.com/pregnancy/niacin.html (accessed Oct 2014).

82. Linus Pauling Institute. Micronutrient Information Center. Oregon State University. "Niacin." http://lpi.oregonstate.edu/infocenter/vitamins/niacin/ (accessed Oct 2014).

83. Hoffer, A., A.W. Saul, H.D. Foster. *Niacin: The Real Story*. Laguna Beach, CA: Basic Health Publications, 2012.

84. Drugs.com. "Niacin." www.drugs.com/niacin.html (accessed Oct 2014).

85. Starfield, B. "Is US Health Really the Best in the World?" *JAMA* 284(4) (Jul 26, 2000):483–485.

86. Saul, A.W., J.N. Vaman, "No Deaths from Vitamins—None at All in 27 Years." *Orthomolecular Med News Service* (Jun 14, 2011): http://orthomolecular.org/resources/omns/v07n05.shtml (accessed Oct 2014).

87. Werbach, M.R., J. Moss. *Textbook of Nutritional Medicine*. Tarzana, CA: Third Line Press, 1999.

88. Expert Group on Vitamins and Minerals. "Safe Upper Levels for Vitamins and Minerals." London, UK: Food Standards Agency. (May 2003): http://http://cot.food.gov.uk/sites/default/files/cot/vitmin2003.pdf (accessed Oct 2014).

89. Moghissi, K.S. "Risks and Benefits of Nutritional Supplements during Pregnancy." *Obstet Gynecol* 58(5 Suppl) (Nov 1981): 68s–78s.

90. Toxnet. Toxicology Data Network. "Nicotinic Acid." http://toxnet.nlm.nih.gov/cgi-bin/sis/search/a?dbs+hsdb:@term+@DOCNO+3134 (accessed Oct 2014).

91. Cosmetic Ingredient Review Expert Panel. "Final Report of the Safety Assessment of Niacinamide and Niacin." *Int J Toxicol* 24(Suppl 5) (2005): 1–31.

92. Personal e-mail correspondence with Todd Penberthy.

93. Hoffer, A., A.W. Saul. *Orthomolecular Medicine for Everyone: Megavitamin Therapeutics for Families and Physicians*. Laguna Beach, CA: Basic Health Publications, 2008.

94. Hoffer., A. "Vitamin B-3: Niacin and Its Amide." DoctorYourself.com. www.doctoryourself.com/hoffer_niacin.html (accessed Oct 2014).

95. Hoffer, A., A.W. Saul, H.D. Foster. *Niacin: The Real Story*. Laguna Beach, CA: Basic Health Publications, 2012.

96. Ibid.

97. Hoffer., A. "Vitamin B-3: Niacin and Its Amide." DoctorYourself.com. www.doctoryourself.com/hoffer_niacin.html (accessed Oct 2014).

98. Hoffer, A., A.W. Saul, H.D. Foster. *Niacin: The Real Story*. Laguna Beach, CA: Basic Health Publications, 2012.

99. Penberthy, W.T. "Laropiprant Is the Bad One; Niacin Is/Was/Will Always Be the Good One." *Orthomolecular Med News Service* (Jul 25, 2014): http://orthomolecular.org/resources/omns/v10n12.shtml (accessed Oct 2014).

100. Ibid.

101. Carlson, L.A. "Nicotinic Acid: the Broad-Spectrum Lipid Drug. A 50th Anniversary Review." *J Intern Med* 258(2) (Aug 2005): 94–114.

102. Penberthy, W.T. "Laropiprant Is the Bad One; Niacin Is/Was/Will Always Be the

Good   One."   *Orthomolecular   Med   News   Service*   (Jul   25,   2014):
http://orthomolecular.org/resources/omns/v10n12.shtml (accessed Oct 2014).

103. Guyton, J.R., H.E. Bays. "Safety Considerations with Niacin Therapy." *Am J Cardiol* 99(6A) (Mar 19, 2007) 22C–31C. Penberthy, W.T. "Laropiprant Is the Bad One; Niacin Is/Was/Will Always Be the Good One." *Orthomolecular Med News Service* (Jul 25, 2014): http://orthomolecular.org/resources/omns/v10n12.shtml (accessed Oct 2014).

104. Penberthy, W.T. "Laropiprant Is the Bad One; Niacin Is/Was/Will Always Be the Good   One."   *Orthomolecular   Med   News   Service*   July   25,   2014.
http://orthomolecular.org/resources/omns/v10n12.shtml (accessed Oct 2014).

105. Saul, A.W. "How to Determine a Saturation Level of Niacin." DoctorYourself.com (2013): www.doctoryourself.com/niacin.html (accessed Oct 2014).

106. Passwater, R.A. *Supernutrition*. New York, NY: Pocket Books, 1976.

107. Hoffer., A. "Vitamin B-3: Niacin and Its Amide." DoctorYourself.com. www.doctoryourself.com/hoffer_niacin.html (accessed Oct 2014).

108. Hoffer, A., A.W. Saul, H.D. Foster. *Niacin: The Real Story*. Laguna Beach, CA: Basic Health Publications, 2012.

109. Ibid.

110. Ibid.

111. Linus Pauling Institute. Micronutrient Information Center. Oregon State University. "Pantothenic Acid." http://lpi.oregonstate.edu/infocenter/vitamins/pa/ (accessed Oct 2014).

112. National Institutes of Health. Medline Plus. U.S. National Library of Medicine. "Pantothenic Acid (Vitamin B5)." www.nlm.nih.gov/medlineplus/druginfo/natural/853.html (accessed Oct 2014).

113. Linus Pauling Institute. Micronutrient Information Center. Oregon State University. "Pantothenic Acid." http://lpi.oregonstate.edu/infocenter/vitamins/pa/ (accessed Oct 2014).

114. Vutyavanich, T., S. Wongtra-ngan, R. Ruangsri. "Pyridoxine for Nausea and Vomiting of Pregnancy: A Randomized, Double-Blind, Placebo-Controlled Trial." *Am J Obstet Gynecol* 173(3 Pt 1) (Sept 1995): 881–4. Sahakian, V., D. Rouse, S. Sipes, et al. "Vitamin B6 Is Effective Therapy for Nausea and Vomiting of Pregnancy: A Randomized, Double-Blind Placebo-Controlled Study." *Obstet Gynecol* 78(1) (Jul 1991): 33–36.

115. Sahakian, V., D. Rouse, S. Sipes, et al. "Vitamin B6 Is Effective Therapy for Nausea and Vomiting of Pregnancy: A Randomized, Double-Blind Placebo-Controlled Study." *Obstet Gynecol* 78(1) (Jul 1991): 33–36.

116. Office of Dietary Supplements. National Institutes of Health. "Vitamin B6: Fact Sheet for Consumers." http://ods.od.nih.gov/factsheets/VitaminB6-QuickFacts/ (accessed Oct 2014).

117. Linus Pauling Institute. Micronutrient Information Center. Oregon State University. "Vitamin B6." http://lpi.oregonstate.edu/infocenter/vitamins/vitaminB6/ (accessed Oct 2014).

118. Davis, S.D., T. Nelson, T.H. Shepard. "Teratogenicity of Vitamin B6 Deficiency: Omphalocele, Skeletal and Neural Defects, and Splenic Hypoplasia." *Science* 169(3952) (Sep 25, 1970): 1329–30.

119. Morris, M.S., M.F. Picciano, P.F. Jacques. "Plasma Pyridoxal 5'-Phosphate in the US Population: The National Health and Nutrition Examination Survey, 2003–2004." *Am J Clin Nutr* 87(5) (May 2008): 1446–54.

120. Office of Dietary Supplements. National Institutes of Health. "Vitamin B6: Fact Sheet for Health Professionals." http://ods.od.nih.gov/factsheets/VitaminB6-HealthProfessional/ (accessed Oct 2014).

121. Morris, M.S., M.F. Picciano, P.F. Jacques. "Plasma Pyridoxal 5'-Phosphate in the US Population: The National Health and Nutrition Examination Survey, 2003–2004." *Am J Clin Nutr* 87(5) (May 2008): 1446–54.

122. Cohen, M., A. Bendich. "Safety of Pyridoxine—A Review of Human and Animal Studies." *Toxicol Lett* 32(2–3) (Dec 1986): 129–39. Gaby, A.R. "'Safe Upper Levels' for Nutritional Supplements: One Giant Step Backward." *J Orthomolecular Med* 18(3–4) (2003):126–30. Saul, A.W. *Fire Your Doctor: How to Be Independently Healthy*. Laguna Beach, CA: Basic Health Publications, 2005. Pauling, L. *How to Live Longer and Feel Better*. Corvallis, OR: Oregon State University Press, 2006. Office of Dietary Supplements. National Institutes of Health. "Vitamin B6: Fact Sheet for Health Professionals." http://ods.od.nih.gov/factsheets/VitaminB6-HealthProfessional/ (accessed Oct 2014). Bender, D.A. "Non-Nutritional Uses of Vitamin B6." *Br J Nutr* 81(1) (Jan 1999):7–20.

123. Gaby, A.R. "'Safe Upper Levels' for Nutritional Supplements: One Giant Step Backward." *J Orthomolecular Med* 18(3–4) (2003):126–30.

124. Linus Pauling Institute. Micronutrient Information Center. Oregon State University. "Vitamin B6." http://lpi.oregonstate.edu/infocenter/vitamins/vitaminB6/ (accessed September 2014).

125. Pauling, L. *How to Live Longer and Feel Better*. Corvallis, OR: Oregon State University Press, 2006.

126. Ibid.

127. Office of Dietary Supplements. National Institutes of Health. "Vitamin B6: Fact Sheet for Health Professionals." http://ods.od.nih.gov/factsheets/VitaminB6-HealthProfessional/ (accessed Oct 2014).

128. Shrim, A., R. Boskovic, C. Maltepe, et al. "Pregnancy Outcome Following Use of Large Doses of Vitamin B6 in the First Trimester." *J Obstet Gynaecol* 26(8) (Nov 2006): 749–51.

129. A.N. Chaudary, A. Porter-Blake, P. Holford. "Indices of Pyridoxine Levels on Symptoms Associated with Toxicity: A Retrospective Study." *J Orthomolecular Med* 18(2) (2003): 65–76.

130. Institute of Medicine. Food and Nutrition Board. "Dietary Reference Intakes: Thiamin, Riboflavin, Niacin, Vitamin B6, Folate, Vitamin B12, Pantothenic Acid, Biotin, and Choline." Washington, DC: National Academy Press; 1998.

131. Office of Dietary Supplements. National Institutes of Health. "Vitamin B6: Fact Sheet for Health Professionals" http://ods.od.nih.gov/factsheets/VitaminB6-HealthProfessional/ (accessed Oct 2014).

132. Davis, S.D., T. Nelson, T.H. Shepard. "Teratogenicity of Vitamin B6 Deficiency: Omphalocele, Skeletal and Neural Defects, and Splenic Hypoplasia." *Science* 169(3952) (Sep 25, 1970): 1329–30.

133. Linus Pauling Institute. Micronutrient Information Center. Oregon State University. "Vitamin B6." http://lpi.oregonstate.edu/infocenter/vitamins/vitaminB6/ (accessed Oct 2014).

134. BabyCenter Medical Advisory Board. "Folic Acid: Why You Need It before and during Pregnancy." BabyCenter. (March 2013): www.babycenter.com/0_folic-acid-why-you-need-it-before-and-during-pregnancy_476.bc (accessed Oct 2014).

135. March of Dimes. "Folic Acid." www.marchofdimes.com/pregnancy/take-folic-acid-before-youre-pregnant.aspx (accessed Oct 2014).

136. Ibid.

137. Scholl, T.O., W.G. Johnson. "Folic Acid: Influence on the Outcome of Pregnancy." *Am J Clin Nutr* 71(5 Suppl): (May 2000): 1295S–303S.

138. Shaw, G.M., et al. "Risks of Orofacial Clefts in Children Born to Women Using Multivitamins Containing Folic Acid Periconceptionally." *Lancet* 346(8972) (Aug 12, 1995): 393–6.

139. Czeizel, A.E., L. Tímár, A. Sárközi. "Dose-Dependent Effect of Folic Acid on the Prevention of Orofacial Clefts." *Pediatrics* 104(6) (Dec 1, 1999): e66.

140. Shaw, G.M., C.D. O'Malley, C.R. Wasserman, et al. (1995). "Maternal Periconceptional Use of Multivitamins and Reduced Risk for Conotruncal Heart Defects and Limb Deficiencies among Offspring." *Am J Med Genet* 59(4) (Dec 4, 1995): 536–545. Botto, L.D., J. Mulinare, J.D. Erickson. "Occurrence of Congenital Heart Defects in Relation to Maternal Mulitivitamin Use." *Am J Epidemiol* 151(92) May 1, 2000): 878–84.

141. Wen, S.W., X.K. Chen, M. Rodger, et al. "Folic Acid Supplementation in Early Second Trimester and the Risk of Preeclampsia." *Am J Obstet Gynecol;*198(1) (Jan 2008): 45.e1–7.

142. Office of Dietary Supplements. National Institutes of Health. "Folate." http://ods.od.nih.gov/factsheets/Folate-HealthProfessional/ (accessed Oct 2014).

143. The American College of Obstetricians and Gynecologists. Frequently Asked Questions. "Nutrition during Pregnancy." www.acog.org/~/media/For%20Patients/faq001 .pdf?dmc=1&ts=20131208T1531017232 (accessed Oct 2014).

144. Office of Dietary Supplements. National Institutes of Health. "Folate." http://ods.od.nih.gov/factsheets/Folate-HealthProfessional/ (accessed Oct 2014). Bailey, R.L., K.W. Dodd, J.J. Gahche, et al. "Total Folate and Folic Acid Intake from Foods and Dietary Supplements in the United States: 2003–2006." *Am J Clin Nutr* 91(1) (Jan 2010): 231–7.

145. Office of Dietary Supplements. National Institutes of Health. "Folate." http://ods.od.nih.gov/factsheets/Folate-HealthProfessional/ (accessed Oct 2014).

146. Seremak-Mrozikiewicz, A. "[Metafolin—Alternative for Folate Deficiency Supplementation in Pregnant Women]." [Article in Polish] *Ginekol Pol* 84(7) (Jul 2013): 641–6. Bailey, L.B., J.F. Gregory, 3rd. "Polymorphisms of Methylenetetrahydrofolate Reductase and Other Enzymes: Metabolic Significance, Risks and Impact on Folate Requirement." *J Nutr* 129(5) (May 1999): 919–22. Kauwell, G.P., C.E. Wilsky, J.J. Cerda, et al. "Methylenetetrahydrofolate Reductase Mutation (677C—>T) Negatively Influences Plasma Homocysteine Response to Marginal Folate Intake in Elderly Women." *Metabolism* 49(11) (Nov 2000): 1440–3.

147. Butterworth, C.E. Jr., T. Tamura. "Folic Acid Safety and Toxicity: A Brief Review." *Am J Clin Nutr* 50(2) (Aug 1989): 353–8.

148. Office of Dietary Supplements. National Institutes of Health. "Vitamin B12: Fact Sheet for Health Professionals." http://ods.od.nih.gov/factsheets/VitaminB12-HealthProfessional/#en5 (accessed Oct 2014).

149. Ibid.

150. Wilson, R.D., J.A. Johnson, P. Wyatt, et al. "Pre-Conceptional Vitamin/Folic Acid Supplementation 2007: The Use of Folic Acid in Combination with a Multivitamin Supplement for the Prevention of Neural Tube Defects and Other Congenital Anomalies." *J Obstet Gynaecol Can* 29(12) (Dec 2007): 1003–26.

151. Linus Pauling Institute. Micronutrient Information Center. Oregon State University. "Folic Acid." http://lpi.oregonstate.edu/infocenter/vitamins/fa/ (accessed Oct 2014).

152. Tamura, T., R.L. Goldenberg, L.E. Freeberg, et al. "Maternal Serum Folate and Zinc Concentrations and Their Relationships to Pregnancy Outcome." *Am J Clin Nutr* 56(2) (Aug 1992): 365–70.

153. Hathcock, J.N. "Vitamins and Minerals: Efficacy and Safety." *Am J Clin Nutr* 66(2) (Aug 1997): 427–37.

154. Ebbing. M., K.H. Bønaa, O. Nygård., et al. "Cancer Incidence and Mortality after Treatment with Folic Acid and Vitamin B12." *JAMA* 302(19) (Nov 18, 2009): 2119–26. Cole, B.F., J.A. Baron, R.S. Sandler, et al. "Folic Acid for the Prevention of Colorectal Adenomas: A Randomized Clinical Trial." *JAMA* 297(21) (Jun 6, 2007): 2351–9.

155. Saul, A.W. "Folic Acid Does Not Cause Cancer. So Who Made the Mistake?" *Orthomolecular Med News Service* (May 6, 2010): http://orthomolecular.org/resources/omns/v06n17.shtml (accessed Oct 2014).

156. Ibid.

157. Ibid.

158. Ibid.

159. Fox News. Associated Press. "High Doses of Folic Acid May Increase Colon Cancer Risk." (Jun 5, 2007): www.foxnews.com/story/2007/06/05/high-doses-folic-acid-may-increase-colon-cancer-risk/ (accessed Oct 2014).

160. Vollset, S.E., R. Clarke, S. Lewington, et al. "Effects of Folic Acid Supplementation on Overall and Site-Specific Cancer Incidence during the Randomised Trials: Meta-Analyses of Data on 50,000 Individuals." *Lancet* 381(9871) (Mar 23, 2013): 1029–36.

161. Fox News. Reuters. "High Doses of Folic Acid Don't Raise Cancer Risk, Study Finds." (Jan 28, 2013): www.foxnews.com/health/2013/01/28/high-doses-folic-acid-dont-raise-cancer-risk-study-finds/ (accessed Oct 2014).

162. Ibid.

163. Kaufman, W. "What Took the FDA So Long to Come Out in Favor of Folic Acid?" www.doctoryourself.com/kaufman4.html (accessed Oct 2014).

164. Office of Dietary Supplements. National Institutes of Health. "Vitamin B12: Fact Sheet for Health Professionals." http://ods.od.nih.gov/factsheets/VitaminB12-HealthProfessional/#en5 (accessed Oct 2014).

165. U.S. Department of Health and Human Services. National Institutes of Health.

National Heart Lung and Blood Institute. "What Is Pernicious Anemia?" www.nhlbi
.nih.gov/health/health-topics/topics/prnanmia/ (accessed Oct 2014).

166. Office of Dietary Supplements. National Institutes of Health. "Vitamin B12: Fact
Sheet for Health Professionals." http://ods.od.nih.gov/factsheets/VitaminB12-HealthPro-
fessional/#en5 (accessed Oct 2014). Johnson, M.A. "If High Folic Acid Aggravates Vitamin B12 Deficiency What Should Be Done About It?" *Nutr Rev* 65(10) (Oct 2007):
451–8.

167. Linus Pauling Institute. Micronutrient Information Center. Oregon State University. "Vitamin B12." http://lpi.oregonstate.edu/infocenter/vitamins/vitaminB12/ (accessed
Oct 2014).

168. Ibid.

169. American Pregnancy Association. "Mercury Levels in Fish." (Jan 2014):
http://americanpregnancy.org/pregnancy-health/mercury-levels-in-fish/ (accessed Oct
2014).

170. Institute of Medicine. Food and Nutrition Board. "Dietary Reference Intakes: Thiamin, Riboflavin, Niacin, Vitamin B6, Folate, Vitamin B12, Pantothenic Acid, Biotin,
and Choline." Washington, DC: National Academy Press; 1998.

171. Ibid.

172. Vidal-Alaball, J., C.C. Butler, R. Cannings-John, et al. "Oral Vitamin B12 versus
Intramuscular Vitamin B12 for Vitamin B12 Deficiency." *Cochrane Database Syst Rev*
3 (Jul 20, 2005): CD004655. Butler, C.C., J. Vidal-Alaball, R. Cannings-John, et al.
"Oral vitamin B12 versus Intramuscular Vitamin B12 for Vitamin B12 Deficiency: A
Systematic Review of Randomized Controlled Trials." *Fam Pract* 23(3) (Jun 2006):
279–85.

173. Institute of Medicine. Food and Nutrition Board. "Dietary Reference Intakes: Thiamin, Riboflavin, Niacin, Vitamin B6, Folate, Vitamin B12, Pantothenic Acid, Biotin,
and Choline." Washington, DC: National Academy Press; 1998. von Schenck, U., C.
Bender-Gotze, B. Koletzko. "Persistence of Neurological Damage Induced by Dietary
Vitamin B12 Deficiency in Infancy." *Arch Dis Childhood* 77 (Aug 1997): 137–9. Kaiser,
L., L.H. Allen. "Position of the American Dietetic Association: Nutrition and Lifestyle
for a Healthy Pregnancy Outcome." *J Am Diet Assoc* 102(10) (Oct 2002): 1479–90.

174. Mock, D.M. "Biotin." In: Shils, M.E., M. Shike, A.C. Ross, et al., eds. *Modern
Nutrition in Health and Disease*. 10th ed. Baltimore, MD: Lippincott Williams &
Wilkins; 2006:498–506.

175. Mock, D.M., J.G. Quirk, N.I. Mock. "Marginal Biotin Deficiency during Normal
Pregnancy." *Am J Clin Nutr* 75(2) (Feb 2002): 295–9. Zempleni, J., D.M. Mock. "Marginal Biotin Deficiency Is Teratogenic." *Proc Soc Exp Biol Med* 223(1) (Jan 2000):
14–21.

176. Linus Pauling Institute. Micronutrient Information Center. Oregon State University. "Biotin." http://lpi.oregonstate.edu/infocenter/vitamins/biotin/ (accessed Oct 2014).

177. Mock, D.M. "Biotin Status: Which Are Valid Indicators and How Do We Know?"
J Nutr 129(2S Suppl) (Feb 1999): 498S–503S.

178. Linus Pauling Institute. Micronutrient Information Center. Oregon State University. "Biotin." http://lpi.oregonstate.edu/infocenter/vitamins/biotin/ (accessed Oct 2014).

179. American Association of Poison Control Centers (AAPCC). "Annual Reports." www.aapcc.org/annual-reports/ (accessed Oct 2014). Linus Pauling Institute. Micronutrient Information Center. Oregon State University. "Biotin." http://lpi.oregonstate.edu/infocenter/vitamins/biotin/ (accessed Oct 2014).

180. Linus Pauling Institute. Micronutrient Information Center. Oregon State University. "Biotin." http://lpi.oregonstate.edu/infocenter/vitamins/biotin/ (accessed Oct 2014).

181. Watanabe, T. "Morphological and Biochemical Effects of Excessive Amounts of Biotin on Embryonic Development in Mice." *Experientia* 52(2) (Feb 15, 1996): 149–54.

182. Ibid.

183. Challem, J. *The Food Mood Solution.* Hoboken, NJ: John Wiley & Sons, 2007.

184. Zeisel, S.H. "Choline: Needed for Normal Development of Memory." *J Am Coll Nutr* 19(5 Suppl) (Oct 2000):528S–531S.

185. Saul, A.W. *Doctor Yourself.* Laguna Beach, CA: Basic Health Publications, 2012.

186. Ziesel, S.H. "Choline, Homocysteine, and Pregnancy." *Am J Clin Nutr* 82(4) (Oct 2005): 719–20.

187. Zeisel, S.H., K.A. da Costa. "Choline: An Essential Nutrient for Public Health." *Nutr Rev* 67(11) (Nov 2009): 615–23.

188. Ibid.

189. Shaw, G.M. S.L. Carmichael, W. Yang, et al. "Periconceptional Dietary Intake of Choline and Betaine and Neural Tube Defects in Offspring." *Am J Epidemol* 160(2) (Feb 2004): 102–9.

190. Ibid.

191. Zeisel, S.H., K.A. da Costa. "Choline: An Essential Nutrient for Public Health." *Nutr Rev* 67(11) (Nov 2009): 615–23.

192. Chan, J., L. Deng, L.G. Mikael, et al. "Low Dietary Choline and Low Dietary Riboflavin during Pregnancy Influence Reproductive Outcomes and Heart Development in Mice." *Am J Clin Nutr* 91(4) (Jan 2010): 1035–43.

193. Moon J, M. Chen, S.U. Gandhy, et al. "Perinatal Choline Supplementation Improves Cognitive Functioning and Emotion Regulation in the Ts65Dn Mouse Model of Down Syndrome." *Behav Neurosci* 124(3) (Jun 2010): 346–361.

194. Ibid.

195. Saul, A.W. *Doctor Yourself.* Laguna Beach, CA: Basic Health Publications, 2012.

196. Case, H.S. *The Vitamin Cure for Women's Health Problems.* Laguna Beach, CA: Basic Health Publications, 2012. Balch, J.F., P.A. Balch. *Prescriptions for Natural Healing.* New York, NY: Avery Publishing Group, 1990.

197. Saul, A.W. *Doctor Yourself.* Laguna Beach, CA: Basic Health Publications, 2012.

CHAPTER 8. MINERALS AND MORE

1. Cass, H., K. Barnes. *8 Weeks to Vibrant Health.* New York, NY: McGraw Hill. 2004.

2. Hoffer, A., A.W. Saul. *Orthomolecular Medicine for Everyone: Megavitamin Therapeutics for Families and Physicians.* Laguna Beach, CA: Basic Health Publications, 2008.

3. Cass, H., K. Barnes. *8 Weeks to Vibrant Health.* New York, NY: McGraw Hill. 2004.

4. National Institutes of Health. Medline Plus. U.S. National Library of Medicine. "Boron." www.nlm.nih.gov/medlineplus/druginfo/natural/894.html (accessed Oct 2014).

5. BabyCenter Medical Advisory Board. "Calcium in Your Pregnancy Diet." BabyCenter. www.babycenter.com/0_calcium-in-your-pregnancy-diet_665.bc (accessed Oct 2014).

6. National Institutes of Health. Office of Dietary Supplements. "Calcium: Fact Sheet for Health Professionals." (Nov 21, 2013): http://ods.od.nih.gov/factsheets/Calcium-HealthProfessional/ (accessed Oct 2014).

7. NIH Osteoporosis and Related Bone Diseases National Resource Center. "Pregnancy, Breastfeeding, and Bone Health." (Jan 2012): www.niams.nih.gov/Health_Info/Bone/Bone_Health/Pregnancy/default.asp (accessed Oct 2014).

8. Hacker, A.N., E.B. Fung, J.C. King. "Role of Calcium during Pregnancy: Maternal and Fetal Needs." *Nutr Rev* 70(7) (Jul 2012):397–409.

9. NIH Osteoporosis and Related Bone Diseases National Resource Center. "Pregnancy, Breastfeeding, and Bone Health." (Jan 2012): www.niams.nih.gov/Health_Info/Bone/Bone_Health/Pregnancy/default.asp (accessed Oct 2014).

10. Prevention Health Books. *Prevention's Best Vitamin Cures: The Ultimate Compendium of Vitamin and Mineral Cures with More Than 500 Remedies for Whatever Ails You!* New York: Rodale; St. Martin's Paperbacks, 2000.

11. Hammar, M., G. Berg, F. Solheim, et al. "Calcium and Magnesium Status in Pregnant Women. A Comparison between Treatment with Calcium and Vitamin C in Pregnant Women with Leg Cramps." *Int J Vitam Nutr Res* 57(2) (1987): 179–83.

12. National Institutes of Health. Office of Dietary Supplements. "Calcium: Fact Sheet for Health Professionals." (Nov 21, 2013): http://ods.od.nih.gov/factsheets/Calcium-HealthProfessional/ (accessed Oct 2014).

13. Dean, C. *The Magnesium Miracle*, Updated edition. New York: Ballantine Books, 2006.

14. Ibid.

15. Thys-Jacobs, S., P. Starkey, D. Bernstein, et al. "Calcium Carbonate and the Premenstrual Syndrome: Effects on Premenstrual and Menstrual Symptoms. Premenstrual Syndrome Study Group." *Am J Obstet Gynecol* 179:2 (1998): 444–52.

16. Dean, C. *The Magnesium Miracle*, Updated edition. New York: Ballantine Books, 2006.

17. Linus Pauling Institute. Micronutrient Information Center. Oregon State University. "Chromium." http://lpi.oregonstate.edu/infocenter/minerals/chromium/ (accessed Oct 2014).

18. Ibid.

19. Hoffer, A., A.W. Saul. *Orthomolecular Medicine for Everyone: Megavitamin Therapeutics for Families and Physicians.* Laguna Beach, CA: Basic Health Publications, 2008.

20. McLeod, M.N. *Lifting Depression: The Chromium Connection.* Laguna Beach, CA: Basic Health Publications, 2005.

21. Docherty, J.P., D.A. Sack, M. Roffman, et al. "A Double-Blind, Placebo-Controlled, Exploratory Trial of Chromium Picolinate in Atypical Depression: Effect on Carbohydrate Craving." *J Psychiatr Pract* 11(5) (Sep 2005):302–314.

22. Challem, J. *The Food Mood Solution.* Hoboken, NJ: John Wiley & Sons, 2007. McLeod, M.N. *Lifting Depression: The Chromium Connection.* Laguna Beach, CA: Basic Health Publications, 2005.

23. Office of Dietary Supplements. National Institutes of Health. "Chromium: Fact Sheet for Health Professionals." http://ods.od.nih.gov/factsheets/Chromium-HealthProfessional/ (accessed September 2013).

24. Saul, A.W. *Doctor Yourself: Natural Healing That Works.* Laguna Beach, CA: Basic Health Publications, 2003. Anderson, R., A. Kozlovsky. "Chromium Intake, Absorption, and Excretion of Subjects Consuming Self-Selected Diets," *Am J Clin Nutr* 41(6) (Jun 1985):1177–1183. Saul, A. *Fire Your Doctor: How to Be Independently Healthy.* Laguna Beach, CA: Basic Health Publications, 2005.

25. National Academy of Sciences. Institute of Medicine. Office of Dietary Supplements. "Dietary Reference Intakes for Vitamin A, Vitamin K, Arsenic, Boron, Chromium, Copper, Iodine, Iron, Manganese, Molybdenum, Nickel, Silicon, Vanadium, and Zinc." Washington, DC: National Academy Press, 2001. Available online at: www.nap.edu/openbook.php?record_id=10026&page=209 (accessed Oct 2014).

26. Office of Dietary Supplements. National Institutes of Health. "Chromium: Fact Sheet for Health Professionals."http://ods.od.nih.gov/factsheets/Chromium-HealthProfessional/ (accessed September 2013).

27. Linus Pauling Institute. Micronutrient Information Center. Oregon State University. "Chromium." http://lpi.oregonstate.edu/infocenter/minerals/chromium/ (accessed Oct 2014).

28. National Academy of Sciences. Institute of Medicine. Office of Dietary Supplements. "Dietary Reference Intakes for Vitamin A, Vitamin K, Arsenic, Boron, Chromium, Copper, Iodine, Iron, Manganese, Molybdenum, Nickel, Silicon, Vanadium, and Zinc." Washington, DC: National Academy Press, 2001. Available online at: www.nap.edu/openbook.php?record_id=10026&page=216 (accessed Oct 2014).

29. McLeod, M.N. *Lifting Depression: The Chromium Connection.* Laguna Beach, CA: Basic Health Publications, 2005.

30. Linus Pauling Institute. Micronutrient Information Center. "Micronutrient Needs during Pregnancy and Lactation."http://lpi.oregonstate.edu/infocenter/lifestages/pregnancyandlactation/

31. Hoffer, A., A.W. Saul. *Orthomolecular Medicine for Everyone: Megavitamin Therapeutics for Families and Physicians.* Laguna Beach, CA: Basic Health Publications, 2008.

32. Pfeiffer, C., R. Mailloux. "Excess Copper as a Factor in Human Diseases." *J Orthomolecular Med* 2(3) 1987: 171–82.)

33. Ibid.

34. Ibid.

35. National Institutes of Health. Office of Dietary Supplements. "Iodine: Fact Sheet

for Health Professionals." http://ods.od.nih.gov/factsheets/Iodine-HealthProfessional/ (accessed Oct 2014).

36. Ibid.

37. Ibid.

38. Flechas, J.D. "Iodine Insufficiency FAQ." http://iodineresearch.com/orthoflechas .html (Oct 2014).

39. Gaby, Alan R. *Nutritional Medicine,* Concord, NH: Fritz Perlberg Publishing, 2011.

40. National Institutes of Health. Office of Dietary Supplements. "Iodine: Fact Sheet for Health Professionals." http://ods.od.nih.gov/factsheets/Iodine-HealthProfessional/ (accessed Oct 2014).

41. Patrick, L. "Iodine: Deficiency and Therapeutic Considerations." *Altern Med Rev* 13(2) (Jun 2008): 116–27.

42. American Academy of Pediatrics. "Pregnant and Breastfeeding Women May Be Deficient in Iodine; AAP Recommends Supplements." (May 26, 2014):. www.aap.org/en-us/about-the-aap/aap-press-room/Pages/Pregnant-and-Brestfeeding-Women-May-Be-.asp x#sthash.z2OmctKF.dpuf (accessed Oct 2014).

43. National Institutes of Health. Office of Dietary Supplements. "Iodine: Fact Sheet for Health Professionals." http://ods.od.nih.gov/factsheets/Iodine-HealthProfessional/ (accessed Oct 2014).

44. Ibid.

45. Flechas, J.D. "Iodine Insufficiency FAQ." http://iodineresearch.com/orthoflechas .html (Oct 2014).

46. Obican, S.G., G.D. Jahnke, O.P. Soldin, et al. "Teratology Public Affairs Committee Position Paper: Iodine Deficiency in Pregnancy." *Birth Defects Research A Clin Mol Teratol* 94(9) (Sep 2012): 677–82.

47. National Institutes of Health. Office of Dietary Supplements. "Iodine: Fact Sheet for Health Professionals." http://ods.od.nih.gov/factsheets/Iodine-HealthProfessional/ (accessed Oct 2014).

48. Public Health Comm. of the American Thyroid Association, D.V. Becker, L.E. Braverman, et al. "Iodine Supplementation for Pregnancy and Lactation—United States and Canada: Recommendations of the American Thyroid Association." *Thyroid* 16(10) (Oct 2006): 949–51. doi:10.1089/thy.2006.16.949.

49. Obican, S.G., G.D. Jahnke, O.P. Soldin, et al. "Teratology Public Affairs Committee Position Paper: Iodine Deficiency in Pregnancy." *Birth Defects Research A Clin Mol Teratol* 94(9) (Sep 2012): 677–82.

50. National Institutes of Health. Office of Dietary Supplements. "Iodine: Fact Sheet for Health Professionals." http://ods.od.nih.gov/factsheets/Iodine-HealthProfessional/ (accessed Oct 2014).

51. Obican, S.G., G.D. Jahnke, O.P. Soldin, et al. "Teratology Public Affairs Committee Position Paper: Iodine Deficiency in Pregnancy." *Birth Defects Research A Clin Mol Teratol* 94(9) (Sep 2012): 677–82.

52. Abraham, G.E. "The Bioavailability of Iodine Applied to the Skin." www.optimox.com/pics/Iodine/updates/UNIOD-02/UNIOD_02.htm (accessed Oct 2014).

53. Linus Pauling Institute. Micronutrient Information Center. Oregon State University. "Iron." http://lpi.oregonstate.edu/infocenter/minerals/iron/ (accessed Oct 2014).

54. Ibid.

55. Campbell, R., A.W. Saul. *The Vitamin Cure for Children's Health Problems.* Laguna Beach, CA: Basic Health Publications, 2011.

56. Centers for Disease Control and Prevention. "Toddler Deaths Resulting from Ingestion of Iron Supplements—Los Angeles, 1992–1993." *MMWR Weekly.* 42(06) (Feb 19, 1993): 111–3. Available online at: www.cdc.gov/mmwr/preview/mmwrhtml/00019593.htm (accessed Oct 2014).

57. Ibid.

58. Tenenbein, M. "Unit-Dose Packaging of Iron Supplements and Reduction of Iron Poisoning in Young Children." *Arch Pediatr Adolesc Med* 159(6) (Jun 2005): 557–60.

59. Food and Drug Administration, HHS. "Iron-Containing Supplements and Drugs; Label Warning Statements and Unit-Dose Packaging Requirements; Removal of Regulations for Unit-Dose Packaging Requirements for Dietary Supplements and Drugs. Final Rule; Removal of Regulatory Provisions in Response to Court Order." *Fed Regist* 68(201) (Oct 17, 2003):59714–5.

60. Centers for Disease Control and Prevention. Child Injury Infographic. "Injury: the #1 Killer of Children in the U.S." Vital Signs. (Apr 16, 2012): www.cdc.gov/vitalsigns/ChildInjury/infographic.html?s_cid=bb-vitalsigns-123 (accessed Oct 2014).

61. American Association of Poison Control Centers (AAPCC). "Annual Reports." www.aapcc.org/annual-reports/ (accessed Oct 2014).

62. Ibid.

63. Ibid.

64. Ibid.

65. Centers for Disease Control and Prevention. Child Injury Infographic. "Injury: the #1 Killer of Children in the U.S." Vital Signs. (Apr 16, 2012): www.cdc.gov/vitalsigns/ChildInjury/infographic.html?s_cid=bb-vitalsigns-123 (accessed Oct 2014).

66. Werbach, M.R., J. Moss. *Textbook of Nutritional Medicine.* Tarzana, CA: Third Line Press, 1999.

67. Werbach, M.R., J. Moss. *Textbook of Nutritional Medicine.* Tarzana, CA: Third Line Press, 1999. McCombs, J. "Treatment of Preeclampsia and Eclampsia." *Clin Pharm* 11(3) (Mar 1992): 236–45. Sibai, B.M. "Magnesium Sulfate Is the Ideal Anticonvulsant in Preeclampsia-Eclampsia." *Am J Obstet Gynecol* 162(5) (May 1990):1141–5. Omu A.E., Al-Harmi, J., Vedi, H.L., "Magnesium Sulphate Therapy in Women with Pre-Eclampsia and Eclampsia in Kuwait." *Med Princ Pract* 17(3) (2008):227–32. doi: 10.1159/000117797. Thapa, K., R. Jha. "Magnesium Sulphate: A Life Saving Drug." *JNMA J Nepal Med Assoc* 47(171) (Jul–Sep 2008):104–8.

68. Schendel, D.E., C.J. Berg, M. Yeargin-Allsopp. "Prenatal Magnesium Sulfate Exposure and the Risk for Cerebral Palsy or Mental Retardation among Very Low-Birth-Weight Children Aged 3 to 5 Years." *JAMA* 276(22) (1996):1805–10. Rouse, D.J., D.G.

Hirtz, E. Thom, et al. "A Randomized, Controlled Trial of Magnesium Sulfate for the Prevention of Cerebral Palsy." *N Engl J Med* 359(9) (Aug 28, 2008):895–905. doi: 10.1056/NEJMoa0801187. Costantine, M.M., S.J. Weiner. "Effects of Antenatal Exposure to Magnesium Sulfate on Neuroprotection and Mortality in Preterm Infants: A Meta-Analysis." *Obstet Gynecol* 114(2 Pt 1) (Aug 2009): 354–64. doi: 10.1097/AOG.0b013e3181ae98c2.

69. Dahle, L.O., G. Berg, M. Hammar. "The Effect of Oral Magnesium Substitution on Pregnancy-Induced Leg Cramps." *Am J Obstet Gynecol* 173(1) (Ki; 1995): 175–80.

70. Bardicef, M., O. Bardicef, Y. Sorokin. "Extracellular and Intracellular Magnesium Depletion in Pregnancy and Gestational Diabetes." *Am J Obstet Gynecol* 172(3) (Mar 1995): 1009–13. Wibell, L., M. Gebre-Medhin, G. Lindmark. "Magnesium and Zinc in Diabetic Pregnancy." *Acta Paediatr Scand Suppl* 320 (1985): 100–6.

71. Dean, C. *The Magnesium Miracle,* Updated edition. New York: Ballantine Books, 2006. Seelig, M.S. "Consequences of Magnesium Deficiency on the Enhancement of Stress Reactions; Preventive and Therapeutic Implications (A Review)." *J Am Coll Nutr* 13(5) (Oct 1994): 429–46.

72. Dean, C. *The Magnesium Miracle.* Updated edition. New York: Ballantine Books, 2006.

73. Ibid.

74. National Institutes of Health. Office of Dietary Supplements. "Magnesium: Fact Sheet for Health Professionals." http://ods.od.nih.gov/factsheets/magnesium. (accessed Oct 2014).

75. Dean, C. *The Magnesium Miracle,* Updated edition. New York: Ballantine Books, 2006.

76. Hammar, M., G. Berg, F. Solheim, et al. "Calcium and Magnesium Status in Pregnant Women. A Comparison between Treatment with Calcium and Vitamin C in Pregnant Women with Leg Cramps." *Int J Vitam Nutr Res* 57(2) (1987): 179–83.

77. Ibid.

78. Werbach, M.R., J. Moss. *Textbook of Nutritional Medicine.* Tarzana, CA: Third Line Press, 1999. Weaver, K. "Pregnancy-Induced Hypertension and Low Birth Weight in Magnesium-Deficient Ewes." *Magnesium* 5(3–4) (1986): 191–200. Takaya, J., F. Yamato, K. Kaneko. "Possible Relationship between Low Birth Weight and Magnesium Status: from the Standpoint of "Fetal Origin" Hypothesis." *Magnes Res* 19(1) (Mar 2006): 63–9.

79. Werbach, M.R., J. Moss. *Textbook of Nutritional Medicine.* Tarzana, CA: Third Line Press, 1999. Jovanovic-Peterson, L., C.M. Peterson. "Vitamin and Mineral Deficiencies Which May Predispose to Glucose Intolerance of Pregnancy." *J Am Coll Nutr* 15(1) (Feb 1996): 14–20.

80. Dean, C. *The Magnesium Miracle,* Updated edition. New York: Ballantine Books, 2006.

81. Holford, P., S. Lawson. *Optimum Nutrition before during and after Pregnancy: Everything You Need to Achieve Optimum Well-Being.* UK: Hachette, 2004.

82. Dean, C. *The Magnesium Miracle,* Updated edition. New York: Ballantine Books, 2006.

83. National Institutes of Health. Office of Dietary Supplements. "Magnesium: Fact Sheet for Health Professionals." http://ods.od.nih.gov/factsheets/Magnesium-HealthProfessional/ (accessed Oct 2014).

84. Dean, C. *The Magnesium Miracle,* Updated edition. New York: Ballantine Books, 2006.

85. Ibid.

86. Ibid.

87. Ibid.

88. Handwerker, S.M., B.T. Altura, B. Royo. "Ionized Serum Magnesium Levels in Umbilical Cord Blood of Normal Pregnant Women at Delivery: Relationship to Calcium, Demographics, and Birthweight." *Am J Perinatol* 10(5) (Sep 1993): 392–7.

89. Tuormaa, T.E. "The Adverse Effects of Manganese Deficiency on Reproduction and Health: A Literature Review Deficiency." *J Orthomolecular Med* 11(2nd Q) (1996): http://orthomolecular.org/library/jom/1996/articles/1996-v11n02-p069.shtml (accessed Oct 2014).

90. Linus Pauling Institute. Micronutrient Information Center. Oregon State University. "Manganese." http://lpi.oregonstate.edu/infocenter/minerals/manganese/ (accessed Oct 2014).

91. Hoffer, A., A.W. Saul. *Orthomolecular Medicine for Everyone: Megavitamin Therapeutics for Families and Physicians.* Laguna Beach, CA: Basic Health Publications, 2008.

92. Pfeiffer, C.C., S. LaMola. "Zinc and Manganese in the Schizophrenias." *J Orthomolecular Psych* 12(3) (1983): 215–34.

93. Linus Pauling Institute. Micronutrient Information Center. Oregon State University. "Manganese." http://lpi.oregonstate.edu/infocenter/minerals/manganese/ (accessed Oct 2014).

94. Hoffer, A., A.W. Saul. *Orthomolecular Medicine for Everyone: Megavitamin Therapeutics for Families and Physicians.* Laguna Beach, CA: Basic Health Publications, 2008.

95. Linus Pauling Institute. Micronutrient Information Center. "Micronutrient Needs during Pregnancy and Lactation." http://lpi.oregonstate.edu/infocenter/lifestages/pregnancyandlactation/ (accessed Oct 2014).

96. Hoffer, A., A.W. Saul. *Orthomolecular Medicine for Everyone: Megavitamin Therapeutics for Families and Physicians.* Laguna Beach, CA: Basic Health Publications, 2008.

97. Tuormaa, T.E. "The Adverse Effects of Manganese Deficiency on Reproduction and Health: A Literature Review Deficiency." *J Orthomolecular Med* 11(2nd Q) (1996): http://orthomolecular.org/library/jom/1996/articles/1996-v11n02-p069.shtml (accessed Oct 2014).

98. Keen, C.L., J.L. Ensunsa, M.H. Watson, et al. "Nutritional Aspects of Manganese from Experimental Studies." *Neurotoxicology* 20(2–3) (Apr–Jun 1999): 213–23.

99. Linus Pauling Institute. Micronutrient Information Center. Oregon State University. "Manganese." http://lpi.oregonstate.edu/infocenter/minerals/manganese/ (accessed Oct 2014).

100. Ibid.

101. Holford, P., S. Lawson. *Optimum Nutrition before during and after Pregnancy: Everything You Need to Achieve Optimum Well-Being.* UK: Hachette, 2004. National Institutes of Health. Office of Dietary Supplements. "Selenium: Fact Sheet for Consumers." http://ods.od.nih.gov/factsheets/Selenium-Consumer/ (accessed Oct 2014).

102. Orthomolecular Medicine News Service. "Vitamin Supplements Help Protect Children from Heavy Metals, Reduce Behavioral Disorders." (Oct 8, 2007): www.orthomolecular.org/resources/omns/v03n07.shtml (accessed Oct 2014).

103. Ibid.

104. Negro, R., G. Greco, T. Mangieri, et al. "The Influence of Selenium Supplementation on Postpartum Thyroid Status in Pregnant Women with Thyroid Peroxidase Autoantibodies." *J Clin Endocrinol Metab* 92(4) (Apr 2007): 1263–8.

105. National Institutes of Health. Office of Dietary Supplements. "Selenium: Dietary Supplement Fact Sheet." http://ods.od.nih.gov/factsheets/Selenium-HealthProfessional/ (Oct 2104).

106. Holford, P., S. Lawson. *Optimum Nutrition before during and after Pregnancy: Everything You Need to Achieve Optimum Well-Being.* UK: Hachette, 2004.

107. Linus Pauling Institute. Micronutrient Information Center. Oregon State University. "Zinc." http://lpi.oregonstate.edu/infocenter/minerals/zinc/ (accessed Oct 2014).

108. Tuormaa, T.E. "Adverse Effects of Zinc Deficiency: A Review from the Literature (to 1995)." *J Orthomolecular Med* 10(3–4) (1995): 149–164. Available online at: http://orthomolecular.org/library/jom/1995/pdf/1995-v10n0304-p149.pdf (accessed Oct 2014).

109. Linus Pauling Institute. Micronutrient Information Center. Oregon State University. "Zinc." http://lpi.oregonstate.edu/infocenter/minerals/zinc/ (accessed Oct 2014).

110. Brighthope, I.E. *The Vitamin Cure for Diabetes.* Laguna Beach, CA: Basic Health Publications Inc., 2012.

111. Linus Pauling Institute. Micronutrient Information Center. Oregon State University. "Zinc." http://lpi.oregonstate.edu/infocenter/minerals/zinc/ (accessed Oct 2014).

112. American Pregnancy Association. "Mercury Levels in Fish." (Jan 2014): http://americanpregnancy.org/pregnancyhealth/fishmercury.htm (accessed Oct 2014).

113. National Institutes of Health. U.S Department of Health and Human Services. "Zinc: Fact Sheet for Health Professionals." http://ods.od.nih.gov/factsheets/Zinc-HealthProfessional/ (accessed August 2014).

114. Stocker, R. "Possible Health Benefits of Coenzyme Q10." Linus Pauling Institute. 2002. http://lpi.oregonstate.edu/f-w02/coenzymeq10.html

115. Linus Pauling Institute. Oregon State University. Micronutrient Information Center. Coenzyme Q10. http://lpi.oregonstate.edu/infocenter/othernuts/coq10/index.html (accessed December 2013).

116. Ibid.

117. MayoClinic. www.mayoclinic.com/health/coenzyme-q10/NS_patient-coenzymeq10

118. Teran, E., M. Racines-Orbe, S. Vivero, et al. "Preeclampsia Is Associated with a

Decrease in Plasma Coenzyme Q10 Levels." *Free Radic Biol Med* 35(11) (Dec 1, 2003): 1453–6.

119. Teran, E., I. Hernandez, B. Nieto, et al. "Coenzyme Q10 Supplementation during Pregnancy Reduces the Risk of Pre-eclampsia." *Int J Gynaecol Obstet* 105(1) (Apr 2009): 43–5.

120. Sa ndor, P.S., L. Di Clemente, G. Coppola, et al. "Efficacy of Coenzyme Q10 in Migraine Prophylaxis: A Randomized Controlled Trial." *Neurology* 64(4) (Feb 22, 2005): 713–15.

121. Cass, H., K. Barnes. *8 Weeks to Vibrant Health*. New York, NY: McGraw Hill. 2004.

122. Greenberg, J.A., S.J. Bell, W. Van Ausdal. "Omega-3 Fatty Acid Supplementation during Pregnancy." *Rev Obstet Gynecol* 1(4) (Fall 2008): 162–9.

123. American Pregnancy Association. "Omega-3 Fish Oil and Pregnancy." http://americanpregnancy.org/pregnancyhealth/omega3fishoil.html (accessed Oct 2014).

124. Su, K.P., S.Y. Huang, T.H. Chiu, et al. "Omega-3 Fatty Acids for Major Depressive Disorder during Pregnancy: Results from a Randomized, Double-Blind, Placebo-Controlled Trial." *J Clin Psychiatry* 69(4) (Apr 2008):644–51.

125. Holford, P., S. Lawson. *Optimum Nutrition before during and after Pregnancy: Everything You Need to Achieve Optimum Well-Being*. UK: Hachette, 2004.

126. American Pregnancy Association. "Omega-3 Fish Oil and Pregnancy." http://americanpregnancy.org/pregnancyhealth/omega3fishoil.html (accessed Oct 2014).

127. Ibid.

128. Ibid.

129. Greenberg, J.A., S.J. Bell, W. Van Ausdal. "Omega-3 Fatty Acid Supplementation during Pregnancy." *Rev Obstet Gynecol* 1(4) (Fall 2008): 162–9. Melanson, S.F., E.L. Lewandrowski, J.G. Flood, et al. "Measurement of Organochlorines in Commercial Over-the-Counter Fish Oil Preparations: Implications for Dietary and Therapeutic Recommendations for Omega-3 Fatty Acids and a Review of the Literature." *Arch Pathol Lab Med* 129(1) (Jan 2005): 74–7.

130. American Pregnancy Association. "Omega-3 Fish Oil and Pregnancy." http://americanpregnancy.org/pregnancyhealth/omega3fishoil.html (accessed Oct 2014).

131. Ibid.

132. Ibid.

133. Mercola, J. "No-Nonsense Guide to a Naturally Healthy Pregnancy and Baby." Mercola.com. (Nov 7, 2009): http://articles.mercola.com/sites/articles/archive/2009/11/07/No-Nonsense-Guide-to-a-Naturally-Healthy-Pregnancy-and-Baby.aspx (accessed Oct 2014).

134. Mercola, J. "Why Therapeutic Benefits of Coffee Do NOT Apply to Pregnant Women." (Feb 3, 2014): http://articles.mercola.com/sites/articles/archive/2014/02/03/coffee-in-pregnancy.aspx?e_cid=20140203Z1_DNL_art_1&utm_source=dnl&utm_medium=email&utm_content=art1&utm_campaign=20140203Z1&et_cid=DM 38952&et_rid=416942030 (accessed Oct 2014).

135. Greenberg, J.A., S.J Bell, W. Van Ausdal. "Omega-3 Fatty Acid Supplementation during Pregnancy." *Rev Obstet Gynecol* 1(4) (Fall 2008): 162–9.

136. American Pregnancy Association. "Omega-3 Fish Oil and Pregnancy." http://americanpregnancy.org/pregnancyhealth/omega3fishoil.html (accessed Oct 2014).

137. Denomme, J., K.D. Stark, B.J. Holub. "Directly Quantitated Dietary (n-3) Fatty Acid Intakes of Pregnant Canadian Women Are Lower Than Current Dietary Recommendations." *J Nutr* 135(2) (Feb 2005): 206–11.

138. American Pregnancy Association. "Omega-3 Fish Oil and Pregnancy." http://americanpregnancy.org/pregnancyhealth/omega3fishoil.html (accessed Oct 2014).

CHAPTER 9. PREGNANCY ISSUES

1. Bánhidy, F., N. Acs, E.H. Puhó. "Iron Deficiency Anemia: Pregnancy Outcomes with or without Iron Supplementation." *Nutrition* 27(1) (Jan 2011): 65–72. doi: 10.1016/j.nut.2009.12.005.

2. Holford, P., S. Lawson. *Optimum Nutrition before during and after Pregnancy: Everything You Need to Achieve Optimum Well-Being.* UK: Hachette, 2004.

3. Livengood, C.H., D.E. Soper, K. Sheehan, et al. "Comparison of Once-Daily and Twice-Daily Dosing of 0.75% Metronidazole Gel in the Treatment of Bacterial Vaginosis." *Sex Transm Dis* 26(3) (Mar 1999): 137–42. Schmitt, C., J.D. Sobel, C. Meriwether. "Bacterial Vaginosis: Treatment with Clindamycin Cream versus Oral Metronidazole." *Obstet Gynecol* 79(6) (Jun 1992): 1020–3.

4. Sobel, J.D., D. Ferris, J. Schwebke, et al. "Suppressive Antibacterial Therapy with 0.75% Metronidazole Vaginal Gel to Prevent Recurrent Bacterial Vaginosis." *Am J Obstet Gynecol* 194(5) (2006): 1283–9.

5. MacDonald, T.M., P.H.G. Beardon, M.M. McGilchrist, et al. "The Risks of Symptomatic Vaginal Candidiasis after Oral Antibiotic Therapy." *Q J Med* 86(7) (1993): 419–24. Onifade, A.K. O.B. Olorunfemi. "Epidemiology of Vulvo-Vaginal Candidiasis in Female Patients in Ondo State Government Hospitals." *J Food Agric Environment* 3(1) (2005):118–9. Kirsch, D.R., R. Kelly, M.B. Kurtz. *The Genetics of Candida.* Boca Raton, FL: CRC Press, 1990.

6. McLean, N.W., I.J. Rosenstein. "Characterisation and Selection of a *Lactobacillus* Species to Re-colonise the Vagina of Women with Recurrent Bacterial Vaginosis." *J Med Microbiol* 49(6) (2000): 543–52.

7. Bradshaw, C.S., A.N. Morton, J. Hocking, et al. "High Recurrence Rates of Bacterial Vaginosis over the Course of 12 Months after Oral Metronidazole Therapy and Factors Associated with Recurrence." *J Infect Dis* 193(11) (Jun 1, 2006): 1478–86. Baylson, F.A., P. Nyirjesy, M.V. Weitz. "Treatment of Recurrent Bacterial Vaginosis with Tinidazole." *Obstet Gynecol* 104(5 Pt 1) (Nov 2004): 931–2. Hay, P. "Recurrent Bacterial Vaginosis." *Curr Infect Dis Rep* 2(6) (Dec 2000): 506–12.

8. Neri, A., G. Sabah, Z. Samra. "Bacterial Vaginosis in Pregnancy Treated with Yoghurt." *Acta Obstet Gynecol Scand* 72(1) (Jan 1993): 17–9.

9. Hoh, J.K., H.J. Cho, S.R. Chung, et al. "The Effect of Vitamin-C Vaginal Tablets (Vagi-C(R)) in Patients with Each Vaginitis in Pregnancy and in Normal Pregnant Women." *Korean J Perinatol* 17(1) (Mar 2006): 62–7.

10. Bodnar, L.M., M.A. Krohn, H.N. Simhan. "Maternal Vitamin D Deficiency Is Associated with Bacterial Vaginosis in the First Trimester of Pregnancy." *J Nutr* 139(6) (Jun 2009):1157–61.

11. Verstraelen, H., J. Delanghe, K. Roelens, et al. "Subclinical Iron Deficiency Is a Strong Predictor of Bacterial Vaginosis in Early Pregnancy." *BMC Infect Dis* 5(Jul 6, 2005): 55.

12. Johnson, D.D., C.L. Wagner, T.C. Hulsey, et al. "Vitamin D Deficiency and Insufficiency Is Common during Pregnancy." *Am J Perinatol* 28(1) (Jan 2011): 7–12. doi: 10.1055/s-0030-1262505.

13. Lee, J.M., J.R. Smith, B.L. Philipp,et al. "Vitamin D Deficiency in a Healthy Group of Mothers and Newborn Infants." *Clin Pediatr (Phila)* 46(1) (Jan 2007): 42–4. 50. Bodnar, L.M., H.N. Simhan, R.W. Powers, et al. "High Prevalence of Vitamin D Insufficiency in Black and White Pregnant Women Residing in the Northern United States and Their Neonates." *J Nutr* 137(2) (Feb 2007): 447–52.

14. Bodnar, L.M., H.N. Simhan, R.W. Powers, et al. "High Prevalence of Vitamin D Insufficiency in Black and White Pregnant Women Residing in the Northern United States and Their Neonates." *J Nutr* 137(2) (Feb 2007): 447–52.

15. Culhane, J.F., V. Rauh, K.F. McCollum, et al. "Maternal Stress Is Associated with Bacterial Vaginosis in Human Pregnancy." *Matern Child Health J* 5(2) (Jun 2001):127–34.

16. Balch, J.F., P.A. Balch. *Prescriptions for Natural Healing*. New York, NY: Avery Publishing Group, 1990.

17. Werbach, M.R., J. Moss. *Textbook of Nutritional Medicine*. Tarzana, CA: Third Line Press, 1999.

18. Centers for Disease Control and Prevention. "Pregnant? Get a Flu Shot!" (Nov. 4, 2013): www.cdc.gov/Features/PregnancyAndFlu/ (accessed Oct 2014).

19. Centers for Disease Control and Prevention. Seasonal Influenza (Flu). "Thimerosal and 2013–2014 Seasonal Flu Vaccines. Questions and Answers." (Sep 9, 2014): www.cdc.gov/flu/protect/vaccine/thimerosal.htm (accessed Oct 2014).

20. Mercola, J. "Why Giving the Flu Vaccine during Pregnancy Doesn't Make Any Sense." Mercola.com (July 11, 2006): http://articles.mercola.com/sites/articles/archive/2006/07/11/why-giving-the-flu-vaccine-during-pregnancy-doesnt-make-any-sense.aspx (accessed Oct 2014).

21. Downing, D. "Flu Vaccine: No Good Evidence." *Orthomolecular Med News Service* (Jan 14, 2012): http://orthomolecular.org/resources/omns/v08n02.shtml (accessed Oct 2014).

22. Mercola, J. "Flu Vaccine Exposed." Mercola.com (Sep 26, 2009): http://articles.mercola.com/sites/articles/archive/2009/09/26/flu-vaccine-exposed.aspx (accessed Oct 2014).

23. Ibid.

24. Mercola, J. "Why Giving the Flu Vaccine during Pregnancy Doesn't Make Any Sense." Mercola.com (July 11, 2006): http://articles.mercola.com/sites/articles/archive/2006/07/11/why-giving-the-flu-vaccine-during-pregnancy-doesnt-make-any-sense.aspx (accessed Oct 2014).

25. Ibid.

26. Centers for Disease Control and Prevention. "Pregnant? Get a Flu Shot!" (Nov. 4, 2013): www.cdc.gov/Features/PregnancyAndFlu/ (accessed Oct 2014).

27. Mercola, J. "Why Giving the Flu Vaccine during Pregnancy Doesn't Make Any Sense." Mercola.com (July 11, 2006): http://articles.mercola.com/sites/articles/archive/2006/07/11/why-giving-the-flu-vaccine-during-pregnancy-doesnt-make-any-sense.aspx (accessed Oct 2014).

28. Centers for Disease Control and Prevention. "Pregnant? Get a Flu Shot!" (Nov. 4, 2013): www.cdc.gov/Features/PregnancyAndFlu/ (accessed Oct 2014).

29. Mercola, J. "Flu Vaccine Exposed." Mercola.com (Sep 26, 2009): http://articles.mercola.com/sites/articles/archive/2009/09/26/flu-vaccine-exposed.aspx (accessed Oct 2014).

30. Drugs.com "Oseltamivir Pregnancy and Breastfeeding Warnings." www.drugs.com/pregnancy/oseltamivir.html (accessed Oct 2014).

31. Downing, D. "Flu Vaccine: No Good Evidence." *Orthomolecular Med News Service* (Jan 14, 2012): http://orthomolecular.org/resources/omns/v08n02.shtml (accessed Oct 2014).

32. Burch, J., M. Corbett, C. Stock, et al. "Prescription of Anti-Influenza Drugs for Healthy Adults: A Systematic Review and Meta-Analysis." *Lancet Infect Dis* 9(9) (Sep 2009): 537–45.

33. Ibid.

34. National Institutes of Health. Office of Dietary Supplements. "Magnesium: Fact Sheet for Health Professionals." http://ods.od.nih.gov/factsheets/magnesium. (accessed Oct 2014).

35. Hammar, M., G. Berg, F. Solheim, et al. "Calcium and Magnesium Status in Pregnant Women. A Comparison between Treatment with Calcium and Vitamin C in Pregnant Women with Leg Cramps." *Int J Vitam Nutr Res* 57(2) (1987): 179–83.

36. Ibid.

37. Werbach, M.R., J. Moss. *Textbook of Nutritional Medicine.* Tarzana, CA: Third Line Press, 1999.

38. Ibid.

39. Holford, P., S. Lawson. *Optimum Nutrition before during and after Pregnancy: Everything You Need to Achieve Optimum Well-Being.* UK: Hachette, 2004.

40. Saul, A.W. "Vitamin E: A Cure in Search of Recognition." *J Orthomolecular Med* 18 (3–4) (2003): 205–12.

41. RxList. "Coumadin." www.rxlist.com/coumadin-drug/warnings-precautions.htm (accessed Oct 2014).

42. Ibid.

43. Saul, A.W. "Vitamin E: A Cure in Search of Recognition." *J Orthomolecular Med* 18 (3–4) (2003): 205–12.

44. Beckles, G.L.A., P.E. Thompson-Reid. *Diabetes and Women's Health across the Life Stages: A Public Health Perspective.* Atlanta: National Center for Chronic Disease

Prevention and Health Promotion (U.S.), Division of Diabetes Translation, Centers for Disease Control and Prevention (U.S.), 2001. Available online at: http://stacks.cdc .gov/view/cdc/6426 (accessed Nov 2014).

45. Bell, R., S.V. Glinianaia, P.W. Tennant, et al. "Peri-Conception Hyperglycaemia and Nephropathy Are Associated with Risk of Congenital Anomaly in Women with Pre-Existing Diabetes: A Population-Based Cohort Study." *Diabetologia* (Feb 8,2012): doi: http://dx.doi.org/10.1007/s00125-012-2455-y.

46. Stevens, M.S. "Vitamin Deficiencies in People with Diabetes: The Supplements You Need." *Diabetes Health* (Apr 28, 2012) http://diabeteshealth.com/read/2012/04/28/ 7513/vitamin-deficiencies-in-people-with-diabetes-the-supplements-you-need/ (accessed Oct 2014).

47. Ibid.

48. Viana, M., E. Herrera, B. Bonet. "Teratogenic Effects of Diabetes Mellitus in the Rat. Prevention by Vitamin E." *Diabetologia* 39(9) (Sep 1996): 1041–6.

49. Cederberg, J., C.M. Simán, U.J. Eriksson. "Combined Treatment with Vitamin E and Vitamin C Decreases Oxidative Stress and Improves Fetal Outcome in Experimental Diabetic Pregnancy." *Pediatr Res* 49(6) (Jun 2001):755–62.

50. Ibid.

51. Cederberg, J., U.J. Eriksson. "Antioxidative Treatment of Pregnant Diabetic Rats Diminishes Embryonic Dysmorphogenesis." *Birth Defects Res A Clin Mol Teratol* 73(7) (Jul 2005): 498–505.

52. U.S. Department of Health and Human Services. National Institutes of Health. "NIDDK and ORWH Team Up for Mother's Day and National Women's Health Week to Raise Awareness of Gestational Diabetes and Steps to Reduce Risks for Women and Their Children." *NIH News* (May 6, 2010): www.nih.gov/news/health/may2010/niddk-06.htm (accessed Oct 2014).

53. Zhang, C., M.A. Williams, I.O. Frederick, et al. "Vitamin C and the Risk of Gestational Diabetes Mellitus: A Case-Control Study." *J Reprod Med* 49(4) (Apr 2004): 257–66.

54. Guven, M.A., M. Kilinc, C. Batukan, et al. "Elevated Second Trimester Serum Homocysteine Levels in Women with Gestational Diabetes Mellitus." *Arch Gynecol Obstet* 274(6) (Oct 2006): 333–7. Seghieri, G., M.C. Breschi, R. Anichini, et al. "Serum Homocysteine Levels Are Increased in Women with Gestational Diabetes Mellitus." *Metabolism* 52(6) (Jun 2003): 720–3.

55. Idzior-Walu s B., K. Cyganek, K. Sztefko, et al. "Total Plasma Homocysteine Correlates in Women with Gestational Diabetes." *Arch Gynecol Obstet* 278(4) (Oct 2008): 309–13. doi: 10.1007/s00404-008-0571-1.

56. Krishnaveni, G.V., J.C. Hill, S.R. Veena, et al. "Low Plasma Vitamin B12 in Pregnancy Is Associated with Gestational 'Diabesity' and Later Diabetes." *Diabetologia* 52(11) (Nov 2009): 2350–8. doi: 10.1007/s00125-009-1499-0.

57. Holford, P., S. Lawson. *Optimum Nutrition before during and after Pregnancy: Everything You Need to Achieve Optimum Well-Being*. UK: Hachette, 2004.

58. Brighthope, I.E. *The Vitamin Cure for Diabetes*. Laguna Beach, CA: Basic Health Publications Inc., 2012.

59. Bo, S., A. Lezo, G. Menato, et al. "Gestational Hyperglycemia, Zinc, Selenium, and Antioxidant Vitamins." *Nutrition* 21(2) (Feb 2005): 186–91.

60. Parlea, L., I.L. Bromberg, D.S. Feig, et al. "Association between Serum 25-hydrox-yvitamin D in Early Pregnancy and Risk of Gestational Diabetes Mellitus." *Diabet Med* 29(7) (Jul 2012): e25–32. doi: 10.1111/j.1464–5491.2011.03550.x. Soheilykhah, S., M. Mojibian, M. Rashidi, et al. "Maternal Vitamin D Status in Gestational Diabetes Mellitus." *Nutr Clin Pract* 25(5) (Oct 2010): 524–7. doi: 10.1177/0884533610379851. Burris, H., S.L. Rifas-Shiman, K. Kleinman, et al. "Vitamin D Deficiency in Pregnancy and Gestational Diabetes Mellitus." *Am J Obstet Gynecol* 207(3) (Sep 2012): 182.e1–8. doi: 10.1016/j.ajog.2012.05.022.

61. Ley, S.H., A.J. Hanley, M. Sermer, et al. "Lower Dietary Vitamin E Intake during the Second Trimester Is Associated with Insulin Resistance and Hyperglycemia Later in Pregnancy." *Eur J Clin Nutr* 67(11) (Nov 2013): 1154–6.

62. Bo, S., A. Lezo, G. Menato, et al. "Gestational Hyperglycemia, Zinc, Selenium, and Antioxidant Vitamins." *Nutrition* 21(2) (Feb 2005): 186–91.

63. Santanam, N., N. Kavtaradze, C. Dominguez, et al. "Antioxidant Supplementation Reduces Total Chemokines and Inflammatory Cytokines in Women with Endometriosis." *Fertil Steril* 80(Supp 3) (Sep 2003):32–3.

64. Ibid.

65. Ibid.

66. Balch, J.F., P.A. Balch. *Prescriptions for Natural Healing.* New York, NY: Avery Publishing Group, 1990.

67. U.S. National Library of Medicine. National Institutes of Health. Medline Plus. "Endometritis." www.nlm.nih.gov/medlineplus/ency/article/001484.htm (accessed Oct 2014).

68. Ibid.

69. Ness, R.B., D.E. Soper, R.L. Holley, et al. "Douching and Endometritis: Results from the PID Evaluation and Clinical Health (PEACH) Study." *Sex Transm Dis* 28(4) (Apr 2001): 240–5.

70. U.S. National Library of Medicine. National Institutes of Health. Medline Plus. "Endometritis." www.nlm.nih.gov/medlineplus/ency/article/001484.htm (accessed Oct 2014).

71. Zeisel, S.H. "Choline: Needed for Normal Development of Memory." *J Am Coll Nutr* 19(5 Suppl) (Oct 2000): 528S–531S.

72. Walcher, T., M.M. Haenle, M. Kron, et al. "Vitamin C Supplement Use May Protect against Gallstones: An Observational Study on a Randomly Selected Population." *BMC Gastroenterol* 9 (Oct 2009): 74. doi: 10.1186/1471–230X-9–74. Simon, J.A., E.S. Hudes. "Serum Ascorbic Acid and Gallbladder Disease Prevalence among US Adults: The Third National Health and Nutrition Examination Survey (NHANES III)." *Arch Intern Med* 160(7) (Apr 2000): 931–6.

73. Simon, J.A. "Ascorbic Acid and Cholesterol Gallstones." *Med Hypotheses* 40(2) (Feb 1993): 81–4.

74. Maclure, K.M., K.C. Hayes, G.A. Colditz, et al. "Dietary Predictors of Symptom-Associated Gallstones in Middle-Aged Women." *Am J Clin Nutr* 52(5) (Nov 1990):

916–22. Pixley, F., D. Wilson, K. McPherson, et al. "Effect of Vegetarianism on Development of Gall Stones in Women." *Br Med J (Clin Res Ed)* 291(6487) (July 1985): 11–2.

75. Werbach, M.R., J. Moss. *Textbook of Nutritional Medicine.* Tarzana, CA: Third Line Press, 1999.

76. Davis, A. *Let's Get Well.* New York, NY: Harcourt Brace Jovanovich, Inc. 1965.

77. American Pregnancy Association. "Group B Strep Infection: GBS" (2014):http://americanpregnancy.org/pregnancy-complications/group-b-strep-infection/ (accessed Nov 2014).

78. Ibid.

79. Biasucci, G., B. Benenati, L. Morelli, et al. "Cesarean Delivery May Affect the Early Biodiversity of Intestinal Bacteria." *J Nutr* 138(9) (Sep 2008):1796S–1800S.

80. Neu, J., J. Rushing. "Cesarean versus Vaginal Delivery: Long-Term Infant Outcomes and the Hygiene Hypothesis." *Clin Perinatol* 38(2) (Jun 2011):321–31. Biasucci, G., B. Benenati, L. Morelli, et al. "Cesarean Delivery May Affect the Early Biodiversity of Intestinal Bacteria." *J Nutr* 138(9) (Sep 2008):1796S–1800S.

81. Bezirtzoglou, E., E. Stavropoulou. "Immunology and Probiotic Impact of the Newborn and Young Children Intestinal Microflora." *Anaerobe* 17(6) (Dec 2011):369–74. Cabrera-Rubio, R., M.C. Collado, K. Laitinen, et al. "The Human Milk Microbiome Changes over Lactation and Is Shaped by Maternal Weight and Mode of Delivery." *Am J Clin Nutr* 96(3) (Sep 2012):544–51.

82. Levy, T. *Primal Panacea.* Henderson, NV: MedFox Publishing, 2011.

83. Griffith, R.S., A.L. Norins, C. Kagan. "A Multicentered Study of Lysine Therapy in Herpes Simplex Infection." *Dermatologica* 156(5) (1978):257–67.

84. McCune, M.A., H.O. Perry, S.A. Muller, et al. "Treatment of Recurrent Herpes Simplex Infections with L-lysine Monohydrochloride." *Cutis* 34(4) (Ocr 1984):366–73.

85. Milman, N., J. Scheibel, O. Jessen. "Lysine Prophylaxis in Recurrent Herpes Simplex Labialis: A Double-Blind, Controlled Crossover Study." *Acta Derm Venereol* 60(1) (1980):85–7.

86. Griffith, R.S., D.E. Walsh, K.H. Myrmel, et al. "Success of L-lysine Therapy in Frequently Recurrent Herpes Simplex Infection. Treatment and Prophylaxis." *Dermatologica* 175(4) (1987):183–90.

87. Thein, D.J., W.C. Hurt. "Lysine as a Prophylactic Agent in the Treatment of Recurrent Herpes Simplex Labialis." *Oral Surg Oral Med Oral Pathol* 58(6) (Dec 1984):659–66.

88. Prevention Health Books. *Prevention's Best Vitamin Cures: The Ultimate Compendium of Vitamin and Mineral Cures with More Than 500 Remedies for Whatever Ails You!.* New York: Rodale; St. Martin's Paperbacks, 2000.

89. National Agricultural Library. US Department of Agriculture. "Potassium." www.nal.usda.gov/fnic/DRI/DRI_Water/186–268.pdf (accessed October 2013).

90. Franz, K.B. "Magnesium Intake during Pregnancy." *Magnesium.* 6(1) (1987): 18–27.

91. Prevention Health Books. *Prevention's Best Vitamin Cures: The Ultimate Compendium of Vitamin and Mineral Cures with More Than 500 Remedies for Whatever Ails You!* New York: Rodale; St. Martin's Paperbacks, 2000.

92. Ibid.

93. Levy, T. *Primal Panacea*. Henderson, NV: MedFox Publishing, 2011.

94. Vasdev, S., V. Gill, S. Parai, et al. "Dietary Vitamin E Supplementation Lowers Blood Pressure in Spontaneously Hypertensive Rats." *Mol Cell Biochem* 238(1–2) (Sep 2002): 111–7. Vaziri, N.D., Z. Ni, F. Oveisi, et al. "Enhanced Nitric Oxide Inactivation and Protein Nitration by Reactive Oxygen Species in Renal Insufficiency." *Hypertension* 39(1) (Jan 2002): 135–41. Galley, H.F., J. Thornton, P.D. Howdle, et al. "Combination Oral Antioxidant Supplementation Reduces Blood Pressure." *Clin Sci (Lond)* 92(4) (Apr 1997): 361–5.

95. Saul, A.W. "Vitamin E: A Cure in Search of Recognition." *J Orthomolecular Med* 18 (3–4) (2003): 205–12.

96. Vimaleswaran, K.S., A. Cavadino, D.J. Berry, et al. "Association of Vitamin D Status with Arterial Blood Pressure and Hypertension Risk: A Mendelian Randomisation Study." *Lancet Diabetes Endocrinol* 2(9) (Sep 2014): 719–29.)

97. Andrade, A.Z., J.K. Rodrigues, L.A. Dib, et al. "[Serum Markers of Oxidative Stress in Infertile Women with Endometriosis]." *Rev Bras Ginecol Obstet* 32(6) (Jun 2010):279–285. Sekhon, L.H., S. Gupta, Y. Kim, et al. "Female Infertility and Antioxidants." *Curr Women's Health Rev* 6(2) (2010):84–95. Vural, P., C. Akgül, A. Yildirim, et al. "Antioxidant Defence in Recurrent Abortion." *Clin Chim Acta* 295(1–2) (May 2000):169–177. Nelen, W.L., H.J. Blom, E.A. Steegers, et al. "Hyperhomocysteinemia and Recurrent Early Pregnancy Loss: A Meta-Analysis." *Fertil Steril* 74(6) (Dec 2000):1196–1199.

98. Westphal, L.M., M.L. Polan, A.S. Trant, et al. "A Nutritional Supplement for Improving Fertility in Women: A Pilot Study." *J Reprod Med* 49(4) (Apr 2004):289–293.

99. Chavarro J.E., J.W. Rich-Edwards, B. Rosner, et al. "Use of Multivitamins, Intake of B Vitamins, and Risk of Ovulatory Infertility." *Fertil Steril* 89(3) (Mar 2008):668–676.

100. Czeizel, A.E. "Periconceptional Folic Acid Containing Multivitamin Supplementation." *Eur J Obstet Gynecol Reprod Biol* 78(2) (Jun 1998):151–161.

101. Henmi, H., T. Endo, Y. Kitajima, et al. "Effects of Ascorbic Acid Supplementation on Serum Progesterone Levels in Patients with a Luteal Phase Defect." *Fertil Steril* 80(2) (Aug 2003):459–461.

102. Al-Azemi, M.K., A.E. Omu, T. Fatinikun, et al. "Factors Contributing to Gender Differences in Serum Retinol and ?-Ttocopherol in Infertile Couples." *Reprod Biomed Online* 19(4) (Oct 2009):583–590.

103. Howard, J.M., S. Davies, A. Hunnisett. "Red Cell Magnesium and Glutathione Peroxidase in Infertile Women—Effects of Oral Supplementation with Magnesium and Selenium." *Magnes Res* 7(1) (1994):49–57.

104. Balch, J.F., P.A. Balch. *Prescriptions for Natural Healing*. New York, NY: Avery Publishing Group, 1990.

105. Lanzafame, F.M., S. La Vignera, E. Vicari, et al. "Oxidative Stress and Medical Antioxidant Treatment in Male Infertility." *Reprod Biomed Online* (Nov 2009); 19(5):638–59.

106. Ross C, A. Morriss, M. Khairy, et al. "A Systematic Review of the Effect of Oral

Antioxidants on Male Infertility." *Reprod Biomed Online* 2010 Jun;20(6):711–23. doi: 10.1016/j.rbmo.2010.03.008. Epub Mar 10, 2010.

107. Werbach, M.R., J. Moss. *Textbook of Nutritional Medicine.* Tarzana, CA: Third Line Press, 1999. Al-Azemi M.K., A.E. Omu, T. Fatinikun, et al. "Factors Contributing to Gender Differences in Serum Retinol and Alpha-Tocopherol in Infertile Couples." *Reprod Biomed Online* (Oct 2009);19(4):583–90.

108. Pottenger, Jr, F.M. *Pottenger's Cats: A Study in Nutrition.* 2nd edition. Price Pottenger Nutrition; 2nd edition: 1995

109. Dean, C. *The Magnesium Miracle,* Updated edition. New York: Ballantine Books, 2006.

110. Hickey, S. *The Vitamin Cure for Migraines.* Laguna Beach, CA: Basic Health Publications, Inc. 2010.

111. *The Doctor Yourself Newsletter* 1(19) (July 25, 2001): www.doctoryourself.com/news/v1n19.html (accessed Nov 2014)

112. Evers, S., J. Afra, A. Frese, et al. "EFNS Guideline on the Drug Treatment of Migraine—Revised Report of an EFNS Task Force." *Eur J Neurol* 16(9) (Sep 2009): 968–81.

113. Werbach, M.R., J. Moss. *Textbook of Nutritional Medicine.* Tarzana, CA: Third Line Press, 1999. Levy, T.E. *Vitamin C, Infectious Diseases, and Toxins: Curing the Incurable [Kindle Edition].* Xlibris (August 31, 2011)

114. Hickey, S. *The Vitamin Cure for Migraines.* Laguna Beach, CA: Basic Health Publications, Inc. 2010.

115. Schoenen, J., J. Jacquy, M. Lenaerts. "Effectiveness of High-Dose Riboflavin in Migraine Prophylaxis. A Randomized Controlled Trial." *Neurology* 50(2) (Feb 1998): 466–70. Boehnke, C., U. Reuter, U. Flach, et al. "High-Dose Riboflavin Treatment Is Efficacious in Migraine Prophylaxis: An Open Study in a Tertiary Care Centre." *Eur J Neurol* 11(7) (Jul 2004): 475–7.

116. Sa ndor, P.S., L. Di Clemente, G. Coppola, et al. "Efficacy of Coenzyme Q10 in Migraine Prophylaxis: A Randomized Controlled Trial." *Neurology* 64(4) (Feb 22, 2005): 713–15.

117. Sengpiel, V., E. Elind, J. Bacelis, et al. "Maternal Caffeine Intake during Pregnancy Is Associated with Birth Weight but Not with Gestational Length: Results from a Large Prospective Observational Cohort Study." *BMC Med* 11 (Feb 2013): 42. Wendler, C.C., M. Busovsky-McNeal, S. Ghatpande, et al. "Embryonic Caffeine Exposure Induces Adverse Effects in Adulthood." *FASEB J* 23(4) (Apr 2009): 1272–8. doi: 10.1096/fj.08-124941.

118. Sekhon, L.H., S. Gupta, Y. Kim, et al. "Female Infertility and Antioxidants." *Curr Women's Health Rev* 6(2) (2010):84–95. Bedwal, R.S., and A. Bahuguna. "Zinc, Copper and Selenium in Reproduction." *Experientia* 50(7) (Jul 15, 1994):626–640.

119. Vural, P., C. Akgül, A. Yildirim, et al. "Antioxidant Defence in Recurrent Abortion." *Clin Chim Acta* 295(1–2) (May 2000):169–177.

120. Sekhon, L.H., S. Gupta, Y. Kim, et al. "Female Infertility and Antioxidants." *Curr Women's Health Rev* 6(2) (2010):84–95.

121. Nelen, W.L., H.J. Blom, E.A. Steegers, et al. "Hyperhomocysteinemia and Recurrent Early Pregnancy Loss: A Meta-Analysis." *Fertil Steril* 74(6) (Dec 2000):1196–1199.

122. Reznikoff-Etiévant M.F., J. Zittoun, C. Vaylet, et al. "Low Vitamin B(12) Level as a Risk Factor for Very Early Recurrent Abortion." *Eur J Obstet Gynecol Reprod Biol* 104(2) (Sep 10, 2002):156–159. Ronnenberg, A.G., M.B. Goldman, D. Chen, et al. "Preconception Folate and Vitamin B(6) Status and Clinical Spontaneous Abortion in Chinese Women." *Obstet Gynecol* (Jul 2002) 100(1):107–113.

123. Vutyavanich, T., S. Wongtra-ngan, R. Ruangsri. "Pyridoxine for Nausea and Vomiting of Pregnancy: A Randomized, Double-blind, Placebo-controlled Trial." *Am J Obstet Gynecol* 173(3 Pt 1) (Sept 1995): 881–884.

124. Sahakian, V., D. Rouse, S. Sipes, et al. "Vitamin B6 Is Effective Therapy for Nausea and Vomiting of Pregnancy: A Randomized, Double-blind Placebo-controlled Study." *Obstet Gynecol* 78(1) (Jul 1991): 33–36.

125. Ibid.

126. National Institutes of Health. Office of Dietary Supplements. "Vitamin B6: Fact Sheet for Health Professionals." http://ods.od.nih.gov/factsheets/VitaminB6-HealthProfessional/ (accessed Nov 2014).

127. Holford, P., S. Lawson. *Optimum Nutrition before during and after Pregnancy: Everything You Need to Achieve Optimum Well-Being.* UK: Hachette, 2004.

128. Diclegis Home Page. (Sep 2014): https://www.diclegis.com/en/ (accessed Nov 2014).

129. Ibid.

130. Diclegis [package insert]. Bryn Mawr, PA: Duchesnay USA, 2013.

131. Diclegis Home Page. (Sep 2014): https://www.diclegis.com/en/ (accessed Nov 2014).

132. Ibid.

133. Drugs.com. "Zofran." www.drugs.com/zofran.html (accessed Nov 2014).

134. Ibid.

135. Franks, M.E., G.R. Macpherson, W.D. Figg. "Thalidomide." *Lancet* 363(9423) (May 29, 2004): 1802–11.

136. Houlton, S. "Drug Maker Apologises for Thalidomide Tragedy." *Royal Soc Chem* (Sept 4, 2012): www.rsc.org/chemistryworld/2012/09/thalidomide-manufacturer-grunenthal-apology (accessed Nov 2014).

137. U.S. National Library of Medicine. A.D.A.M. Medical Encyclopedia. "Preeclampsia. Toxemia; Pregnancy-Induced Hypertension (PIH)." (Aug 23, 2012): www.ncbi.nlm.nih.gov/pubmedhealth/PMH0001900/ (accessed Nov 2014).

138. U.S. National Library of Medicine. National Institutes of Health. "Preeclampsia." www.nlm.nih.gov/medlineplus/ency/article/000898.htm

139. Brantsaeter, A.L., M. Haugen, S.O. Samuelsen, et al. "A Dietary Pattern Characterized by High Intake of Vegetables, Fruits, and Vegetable Oils Is Associated with Reduced Risk of Preeclampsia in Nulliparous Pregnant Norwegian Women." *J Nutr* 139(6) (Jun 2009): 1162–8.

140. Mayo Clinic Staff. "Preeclampsia." www.mayoclinic.com/health/preeclampsia/DS00583/DSECTION=risk-factors (accessed Nov 2014).

141. Standley, C.A., J.E. Whitty, B.A. Mason, et al. "Serum Ionized Magnesium Levels in Normal and Preeclamptic Gestation." *Obstet Gynecol* 89(1) (Jan 1997): 24–7. Sukonpan, K., V. Phupong. "Serum Calcium and Serum Magnesium in Normal and Preeclamptic Pregnancy." *Arch Gynecol Obstet* 273(1) (Nov 2005): 12–6.

142. Tara, F., G. Maamouri, M.P. Rayman, et al. "Selenium and Hyoertension Selenium Supplementation and the Incidence of Preeclampsia in Pregnant Iranian Women: A Randomized, Double-blind, Placebo-controlled Pilot Trial." *Taiwan J Obstet Gynecol* 49(2) (Jun 2010):181–187.

143. Bodnar, L.M., J.M. Catov, H.N. Simhan, et al. "Maternal Vitamin D Deficiency Increases the Risk of Preeclampsia." *J Clin Endocrinol Metab* 92(9) (Sep 2007): 3517–22. Baker, A.M., S. Haeri, C.A. Camargo, et al. "A Nested Case-Control Study of Midgestation Vitamin D Deficiency and Risk of Severe Preeclampsia." *J Clin Endocrinol Metab* 95(11) (Nov 2010): 5105–9.

144. Haugen, M., A.L. Brantsaeter, L. Trogstad, et al. "Vitamin D Supplementation and Reduced Risk of Preeclampsia in Nulliparous Women." *Epidemiology* 20(5) (Sept 2009): 720–6.

145. Lee, J.M., J.R. Smith, B.L. Philipp,et al. "Vitamin D Deficiency in a Healthy Group of Mothers and Newborn Infants." *Clin Pediatr (Phila)* 46(1) (Jan 2007): 42–4.

146. Hollis, B.W., D. Johnson, T.C. Hulsey, et al. "Vitamin D Supplementation during Pregnancy: Double-Blind, Randomized Clinical Trial of Safety and Effectiveness." *J Bone Miner Res* 26(10) (Oct 2011): 2341–57. Hollis, B.W., C.L. Wagner. "Vitamin D and Pregnancy: Skeletal Effects, Nonskeletal Effects, and Birth Outcomes." *Calcif Tissue Int* 92(2) (Feb 2013):128–39.

147. Office of Dietary Supplements. National Institute of Health. "Dietary Supplement Fact Sheet: Vitamin D." http://ods.od.nih.gov/factsheets/VitaminD-HealthProfessional/ (accessed October 2013).

148. Hollis, B.W. "Circulating 25-Hydroxyvitamin D Levels Indicative of Vitamin D Sufficiency: Implications for Establishing a New Effective Dietary Intake Recommendation for Vitamin D." *J. Nutr* 135(2) (Feb 1, 2005): 317–22.

149. Rajkovic, A., P.M. Catalano, M.R. Malinow. "Elevated Homocyst(e)ine Levels with Preeclampsia." *Obstet Gynecol* 90(2) (Aug 1997): 168–171. Sorensen, T.K., M.R. Malinow, M.A. Williams, et al. "Elevated Second-Trimester Serum Homocyst(e)ine Levels and Subsequent Risk of Preeclampsia." *Gynecol Obstet Invest* 48(2) (1999): 98–103.

150. den Heijer, M., I.A. Brouwer, G.M. Bos, et al. "Vitamin Supplementation Reduces Blood Homocysteine Levels: A Controlled Trial in Patients with Venous Thrombosis and Healthy Volunteers." *Arterioscler Thromb Vasc Biol* 18(3) (Mar 1998):356–61. Brouwer, I.A., M. van Dusseldorp, C.M.G. Thomas, et al. "Low-Dose Folic Acid Supplementation Decreases Plasma Homocysteine Concentrations: A Randomised Trial." *Indian Heart J* 52(Suppl 7) (Nov–Dec 2000): S53–8. Vermeulen, E.G., C.D. Stehouwer, J.W. Twisk, et al. "Effect of Homocysteine-Lowering Treatment with Folic Acid Plus Vitamin B6 on Progression of Subclinical Atherosclerosis: A Randomised, Placebo-Controlled Trial." *Lancet* 355(9203) (Feb 12, 2000): 517–22. Guo, H., J.D. Lee, H. Uzui, et al. "Effects of Folic Acid and Magnesium on the Production of Homocysteine-Induced

Extracellular Matrix Metalloproteinase-2 in Cultured Rat Vascular Smooth Muscle Cells." *Circ J* 70(1) (Jan 2006):141–6.

151. den Heijer, M., I.A. Brouwer, G.M. Bos, et al. "Vitamin Supplementation Reduces Blood Homocysteine Levels: A Controlled Trial in Patients with Venous Thrombosis and Healthy Volunteers." *Arterioscler Thromb Vasc Biol* 18(3) (Mar 1998): 356–61.

152. Linus Pauling Institute. Micronutrient Information Center. Oregon State University. "Riboflavin." http://lpi.oregonstate.edu/infocenter/vitamins/riboflavin/ (accessed Nov 2014). Wacker, J., J. Frühauf, M. Schulz, et al. "Riboflavin Deficiency and Preeclampsia." *Obstet Gynecol* 96(1) (Jul 2000): 38–44.

153. Irwin, J.B. *The Natural Way to a Trouble Free Pregnancy: The Toxemia/Thiamine Connection.* Aslan Publishing, 2008.

154. Teran, E., I. Hernandez, B. Nieto, et al. "Coenzyme Q10 Supplementation during Pregnancy Reduces the Risk of Pre-eclampsia." *Int J Gynaecol Obstet* 105(1) (Apr 2009): 43–5.

155. Brantsaeter, A.L., R. Myhre, M. Haugen, et al. "Intake of Probiotic Food and Risk of Preeclampsia in Primiparous Women: The Norwegian Mother and Child Cohort Study." *Am J Epidemiol* 174(7) (Oct 2011): 807–15.

156. Ibid.

157. Roberts J.M., L. Myatt, C.Y. Spong, et al. "Vitamins C and E to Prevent Complications of Pregnancy-Associated Hypertension." *N Engl J Med* 362(14) (Apr 2010): 1282–91.

158. Chappell, L.C., P.T. Seed, A,L. Briley, et al. "Effect of Antioxidants on the Occurrence of Pre-eclampsia in Women at Increased Risk: A Randomised Trial." *Lancet* 354(9181) (Sept 1999): 810–6.

159. Klemmensen, A., A. Tabor, M.L. Østerdal, et al. "Intake of Vitamin C and E in Pregnancy and Risk of Pre-eclampsia: Prospective Study among 57,346 Women." *BJOG* 116(7) (Jun 2009): 964–74.

160. Kiondo, P., G. Wamuyu-Maina, G.S. Bimenya, et al. "Risk Factors for Pre-eclampsia in Mulago Hospital, Kampala, Uganda." *Trop Med Int Health* 17(4) (Apr 2012): 480–7.

161. Rumbold, A., L. Duley, C. Crowther, et al. "Antioxidants for Preventing Pre-eclampsia." *Cochrane Database Syst Rev* (4) (Oct 2005): CD004227.

162. Ibid.

163. Vadillo-Ortega, F., O. Perichart-Perera, S. Espino, et al. "Effect of Supplementation during Pregnancy with L-Arginine and Antioxidant Vitamins in Medical Food on Pre-eclampsia in High Risk Population: Randomised Controlled Trial." *BMJ* 342 (May 2011) 342.

164. Ibid.

165. Villar, J., M. Purwar, M. Merialdi, et al. "World Health Organisation Multicentre Randomised Trial of Supplementation with Vitamins C and E among Pregnant Women at High Risk for Pre-eclampsia in Populations of Low Nutritional Status from Developing Countries." *BJOG* 116(6) (May 2009): 780–8.

166. Ibid.

167. Levy, T.E. *Stop America's #1 Killer!* Henderson, NV: Livon Books, 2006.

168. Orthomolecular Medicine News Service "No Deaths from Vitamins. America's Largest Database Confirms Supplement Safety." (Dec 28, 2011): www.orthomolecular.org/resources/omns/v07n16.shtml (accessed Nov 2014)

169. Baeten, J.M., E.A. Bukusi, M. Lambe. "Pregnancy Complications and Outcomes among Overweight and Obese Nulliparous Women." *Am J Public Health* 91(3) (Mar 2001): 436–40. Cedergren, M.I. "Maternal Morbid Obesity and the Risk of Adverse Pregnancy Outcome." *Obstet Gynecol.* 103(2):219–24. Sebire, N.J. (2004 Feb), M. Jolly, J.P. Harris, et al. "Maternal Obesity and Pregnancy Outcome: A Study of 287,213 Pregnancies in London." *Int J Obes Relat Metab Disord* 25 (2001): 1175–82.

170. Paiva, L.V., R.M. Nomura, M.C. Dias, et al. "Maternal Obesity in High-Risk Pregnancies and Postpartum Infectious Complications." *Rev Assoc Med Bras* 58(4) (Jul–Aug 2012): 453–8.

171. American College of Obstetricians and Gynecologists.. "Obesity in Pregnancy. Committee Opinion 549" *Obstet Gynecol* 121 (Jan 2013): 213–7. Stothard, K.J., P.W. Tennant, R. Bell, J. Rankin. "Maternal Overweight and Obesity and the Risk of Congenital Anomalies: A Systematic Review and Meta-analysis." *JAMA* 301 (2009): 636–50. Oken, E., E.M. Taveras, K.P. Kleinman, et al. "Gestational Weight Gain and Child Adiposity at Age 3 Years." *Am J Obstet Gynecol* 196 (2007): 322.

172. Hersoug, L.G., A. Linneberg. "The Link between the Epidemics of Obesity and Allergic Diseases: Does Obesity Induce Decreased Immune Tolerance?" *Allergy*;62(10) (Oct 2007): 1205–13.

173. Reichman, N.E., L. Nepomnyaschy. "Maternal Pre-pregnancy Obesity and Diagnosis of Asthma in Offspring at Age 3 Years." *Matern Child Health J* 12(6) (Nov 2008): 725–33. Harpsøe, M.C., S. Basit, P. Bager, et al. "Maternal Obesity, Gestational Weight Gain, and Risk of Asthma and Atopic Disease in Offspring: A Study within the Danish National Birth Cohort." *J Allergy Clin Immunol* 131(4) (Apr 2013): 1033–40.

174. Krakowiak, P., C.K. Walker, A.A. Bremer, et al. "Maternal Metabolic Conditions and Risk for Autism and Other Neurodevelopmental Disorders." *Pediatrics* 2012 May; 129(5): e1121-e1128.

175. Baeten, J.M., E.A. Bukusi, M. Lambe. "Pregnancy Complications and Outcomes among Overweight and Obese Nulliparous Women." *Am J Public Health* 91(3) (Mar 2001): 436–40. Cedergren, M.I. "Maternal Morbid Obesity and the Risk of Adverse Pregnancy Outcome." *Obstet Gynecol.* 2004 Feb;103(2):219–24. Sebire, N.J., M. Jolly, J.P. Harris, et al. "Maternal Obesity and Pregnancy Outcome: A Study of 287,213 Pregnancies in London." *Int J Obes Relat Metab Disord* 25 (2001): 1175–82.

176. National Institutes of Health. U.S. Department of Health and Human Services. Eunice Kennedy Shriver National Institute of Child Health and Human Development. "Does PCOS Affect Pregnancy?" (Jul 14, 2014): www.nichd.nih.gov/health/topics/PCOS/conditioninfo/Pages/pregnancy.aspx (accessed Nov 2014).

177. Lucidi, S., A. Thyer, C. Easton, et al. "Effect of Chromium Supplementation on Insulin Resistance and Ovarian and Menstrual Cyclicity in Women with Polycystic Ovary Syndrome." *Fertil Steril* 84(6) (Dec 2005):1755–7.

178. Werbach, M.R., J. Moss. *Textbook of Nutritional Medicine.* Tarzana, CA: Third Line Press, 1999.

179. Ibid.

180. Tara, F., M.P. Rayman, H. Boskabadi, et al. "Selenium Supplementation and Premature (Pre-Labour) Rupture of Membranes: A Randomised Double-Blind Placebo-Controlled Trial." *J Obstet Gynaecol.* 30(1) (Jan 2010): 30–4.

181. Hoffer, A., A.W. Saul. *Orthomolecular Medicine for Everyone: Megavitamin Therapeutics for Families and Physicians.* Laguna Beach, CA: Basic Health Publications, 2008.

182. Dean, C. *Hormone Balance.* Avon, MA: Adams Media, 2005.

183. Saul, A.W. *Doctor Yourself: Natural Healing That Works.* Laguna Beach, CA: Basic Health Publications, 2003.

184. Klenner, F.R. "Observations on the Dose and Administration of Ascorbic Acid When Employed Beyond the Range of a Vitamin in Human Pathology." *J Applied Nutr* 23(3 & 4) (Winter 1971): 61–88.

185. Hickey, S., A.W. Saul. *Vitamin C: The Real Story: The Remarkable and Controversial Healing Factor* Laguna Beach, CA: Basic Health Publications, 2008.

186. McCormick, W.J. "The Striae of Pregnancy: A New Etiological Concept." *Med Record* (August 1948).

187. Hickey, S., A.W. Saul. *Vitamin C: The Real Story: The Remarkable and Controversial Healing Factor* Laguna Beach, CA: Basic Health Publications, 2008.

188. Balch, J.F., P.A. Balch. *Prescription for Nutritional Healing.* Garden City Park, NY: Avery Publishing Group, Inc., 1990.

189. Balch, J.F., P.A. Balch. *Prescription for Nutritional Healing.* Garden City Park, NY: Avery Publishing Group, Inc., 1990.

190. Holford, P., S. Lawson. *Optimum Nutrition before during and after Pregnancy: Everything You Need to Achieve Optimum Well-Being.* UK: Hachette, 2004.

191. Ibid.

192. Prevention Health Books. *Prevention's Best Vitamin Cures: The Ultimate Compendium of Vitamin and Mineral Cures with More Than 500 Remedies for Whatever Ails You!* New York: Rodale; St. Martin's Paperbacks, 2000.

193. Cassone, A., F. De Barnardis, G. Santoni. "Anticandidal Immunity and Vaginitis: Novel Opportunities for Immune Intervention." *Infect Immun* 75(10) (Oct 2007):4675–86. Hilton, E., H.D. Isenberg, P. Alperstein, et al. "Ingestion of Yogurt Containing Lactobacillus Acidophilus as Prophylaxis for Candidal Vaginitis." *Ann Internal Med* 116(5) (Mar 1, 1992):353–7.

194. Holford, P., S. Lawson. *Optimum Nutrition before during and after Pregnancy: Everything You Need to Achieve Optimum Well-Being.* UK: Hachette, 2004.

195. Cass, H., K. Barnes. *8 Weeks to Vibrant Health.* New York, NY: McGraw Hill. 2004.

196. Fidel, P.L., J. Cutright, C. Steele. "Effects of Reproductive Hormones on Experimental Vaginal Candidiasis." *Infect Immun* 68(2) (Feb 2000):651–7. Dean, C. *Hormone Balance: A Women's Guide to Restoring Health and Vitality.* Avon, MA: Adams Media, 2005.

197. Xu, J., J.D. Sobel. "Candida Vulvovaginitis in Pregnancy." *Curr Infect Dis Rep* 6(6) (Dec 2004): 445–9.

198. Kalkanci, A., A.B. Güzel, I.I. Khalil, et al. "Yeast Vaginitis during Pregnancy: Susceptibility Testing of 13 Antifungal Drugs and Boric Acid and the Detection of Four Virulence Factors." *Med Mycol* 50(6) (Aug 2012): 585–93.

199. Ibid.

200. Lynch, M.E., J.D. Sobel, P.L. Fidel, Jr. "Role of Antifungal Drug Resistance in the Pathogenesis of Recurrent Vulvovaginal Candidiasis." *J Med Vet Mycol* 34(5) (1996): 337–9.

201. Cass, H., K. Barnes. *8 Weeks to Vibrant Health*. New York, NY: McGraw Hill. 2004.

202. Calton, J. and M. Calton. *Rich Food Poor Food*. Malibu, CA: Primal Blueprint Publishing, 2013.

203. Ibid.

204. Cassone, A., F. De Barnardis, G. Santoni. "Anticandidal Immunity and Vaginitis: Novel Opportunities for Immune Intervention." *Infect Immun* 75(10) (Oct 2007):4675–86. Purkh, K., S. Khalsa. "Candida's Curse." *Herb Quarterly* (Summer 1996):18–23.

205. Cass, Hyla, and K. Barnes. 8 Weeks to Better Health. New York, NY: McGraw Hill. 2005.

206. Elias, J., P. Bozzo, A. Einarson, et al. "Are Probiotics Safe for Use during Pregnancy and Lactation?" *Can Fam Physician* 57(3) (Mar 2011): 299–301.

207. Elazab, N., A. Mendy, J. Gasana, J., et al. "Probiotic Administration in Early Life, Atopy, and Asthma: A Meta-analysis of Clinical Trials." Pediatrics. Published online August 19, 2013 (*doi: 10.1542/peds.2013–0246*)

208. Horowitz, B.J., S.W. Edelstein, L. Lippman. "Sugar Chromatography Studies in Recurrent Candida Vulvovaginitis." *J Reprod Med* 29(7) (Jul 1984): 441–3.

209. Purkh, K., S. Khalsa. "Candida's Curse." *Herb Quarterly* (Summer 1996): 18–23.

210. Cassone, A., F. De Barnardis, G. Santoni. "Anticandidal Immunity and Vaginitis: Novel Opportunities for Immune Intervention." *Infect Immun* 75(10) (Oct 2007):4675–86. Hilton, E., H.D. Isenberg, P. Alperstein, et al. "Ingestion of Yogurt Containing Lactobacillus Acidophilus as Prophylaxis for Candidal Vaginitis." *Ann Internal Med* 116(5) (Mar 1, 1992):353–7.

CHAPTER 10. POSTPARTUM PROBLEMS

1. Werbach, M.R., J. Moss. *Textbook of Nutritional Medicine*, 1999.

2. Pauling, L. *Vitamin C and the Common Cold*. San Francisco, CA: W.H. Freeman and Company, 1970.

3. Ibid.

4. Levy, T.E. *Vitamin C, Infectious Diseases, and Toxins: Curing the Incurable*. Philadelphia, PA: Xlibris Corporation, 2002.

5. Levy, T.E. *Vitamin C, Infectious Diseases, and Toxins: Curing the Incurable*. Philadel-

phia, PA: Xlibris Corporation, 2002. Werbach, M.R., J. Moss. *Textbook of Nutritional Medicine*, 1999.

6. Werbach, M.R., J. Moss. *Textbook of Nutritional Medicine*, 1999. Pauling, L. *Vitamin C and the Common Cold*. San Francisco, CA: W.H. Freeman and Company, 1970. Levy, T.E. *Vitamin C, Infectious Diseases, and Toxins: Curing the Incurable*. Philadelphia, PA: Xlibris Corporation, 2002.

7. BabyCenter Medical Advisory Board. "How Breastfeeding Benefits You and Your Baby." www.babycenter.com/0_how-breastfeeding-benefits-you-and-your-baby_8910 .bc?page=1 (accessed Nov 2014).

8. Dermer, A. "A Well-Kept Secret Breastfeeding's Benefits to Mothers." *New Beginnings* 18(4) (Jul–Aug 2001): 124–7.

9. Walters, S. "Dealing with a Plugged Duct or Mastits." *New Beginnings* 24(2) (Mar-Apr 2007): 76–7. Available online at: www.llli.org/nb/nbmarapr07p76.html (accessed Nov 2014).

10. Tilson, B. "Mastitis—Plugged Ducts and Breast Infections." *Leaven* 29(2) (Mar-Apr 1993): 19–21, 26. Available online at: www.lalecheleague.org/llleaderweb/lv/lvmarapr93p19.html (accessed Nov 2014).

11. Walters, S. "Dealing with a Plugged Duct or Mastits." *New Beginnings* 24(2) (Mar-Apr 2007): 76–7. Available online at: www.llli.org/nb/nbmarapr07p76.html (accessed Nov 2014).

12. Ibid.

13. Tilson, B. "Mastitis—Plugged Ducts and Breast Infections." *Leaven* 29(2) (Mar-Apr 1993): 19–21, 26. Available online at: www.lalecheleague.org/llleaderweb/lv/lvmarapr93p19.html (accessed Nov 2014).

14. Cathcart, R.F. "The Third Face of Vitamin C." *J Orthomolecular Med* 7:4 (1993):197–200. Levy, T.E. *Vitamin C, Infectious Diseases, and Toxins: Curing the Incurable*. Philadelphia, PA: Xlibris Corporation, 2002. Werbach, M.R., J. Moss. *Textbook of Nutritional Medicine*. Tarzana, CA: Third Line Press, 1999.

15. Cathcart, R.F. "The Third Face of Vitamin C." *J Orthomolecular Med* 7:4 (1993):197–200.

16. Richards, J.P. "Postnatal Depression: A Review of Recent Literature." *Br J Gen Pract* 40(340) (Nov 1990): 472–6.

17. Centers for Disease Control (CDC). "Prevalence of Self-Reported Postpartum Depressive Symptoms—17 States, 2004–2005." (Apr 11, 2008): 361–6. Available online at: www.cdc.gov/Mmwr/preview/mmwrhtml/mm5714a1.htm (accessed Nov 2014). Richards, J.P. "Postnatal Depression: A Review of Recent Literature." *Br J Gen Pract* 40(340) (Nov 1990): 472–6.

18. Harvard Health Publications. Harvard Medical School. "Exercise and Depression." www.health.harvard.edu/newsweek/Exercise-and-Depression-report-excerpt.htm (accessed Nov 2014).

19. Chatzi, L., V. Melaki, K. Sarri, et al. "Dietary Patterns during Pregnancy and the Risk of Postpartum Depression: The Mother-Child 'Rhea' Cohort in Crete, Greece." *Public Health Nutr* 14(9) (Sep 2011): 1663–70.

20. Jonsson, B.H., A.W. Saul. *The Vitamin Cure for Depression.* Laguna Beach, CA: Basic Health Publications, 2012.

21. Borra, C., M. Iacovou, A. Sevilla. "New Evidence on Breastfeeding and Postpartum Depression: The Importance of Understanding Women's Intentions." *Matern Child Health J* (Aug 21, 2014.) Available online at: http://link.springer.com/article/10.1007%2Fs10995-014-1591-z#page-1 (accessed Nov 2014).

22. Jonsson, B.H., A.W. Saul. *The Vitamin Cure for Depression.* Laguna Beach, CA: Basic Health Publications, 2012.

23. Brody, S. "High-Dose Ascorbic Acid Increases Intercourse Frequency and Improves Mood: A Randomized Controlled Clinical Trial." *Biol Psychiatry* 52(4) (Aug 15, 2002): 371-4.

24. Alpert, J.E., D. Mischoulon, A A. Nierenberg, et al. "Nutrition and Depression: Focus on Folate." *Nutrition* (Jul–Aug 2000) 16(7–8): 544–6. Morris, M.S., M. Fava, P.F. Jacques, et al. "Depression and Folate Status in the US Population." *Psychother Psychosom* 72(2) (Mar-Apr 2003): 80–7.

25. Abou-Saleh, M.T., A. Coppen. "The Biology of Folate in Depression: Implications for Nutritional Hypotheses of the Psychoses." *J Psychiatr Res* 20(2) (1986): 91–101.

26. Coppen, A., J. Bailey. "Enhancement of the Antidepressant Action of Fluoxetine by Folic Acid: A Randomised, Placebo Controlled Trial." *J Affect Disord* 60(2) (Nov 2000): 121–30. Bell, I.R., J. Edman, F.D. Morrow, et al. "Vitamin B1, B2, and B6 Augmentation of Tricyclic Antidepressant Treatment in Geriatric Depression with Cognitive Dysfunction." *J Am Coll Nutr* 11(2) (Apr 1992):159–63.

27. Fava, M., J.S. Borus, J.E. Alpert, et al. "Folate, Vitamin B12, and Homocysteine in Major Depressive Disorder." *Am J Psychiatry* 154(3) (Mar 1997):426–8.

28. Jonsson, B.H., A.W. Saul. *The Vitamin Cure for Depression.* Laguna Beach, CA: Basic Health Publications, 2012.

29. Hollis, B.W., C.L. Wagner. "Vitamin D Requirements during Lactation: High-Dose Maternal Supplementation as Therapy to Prevent Hypovitaminosis D for Both the Mother and the Nursing Infant." *Am J Clin Nutr* 80(6 Suppl) (Dec 2004): 1752S–8S. Hollis, B.W. "Circulating 25-Hydroxyvitamin D Levels Indicative of Vitamin D Sufficiency: Implications for Establishing a New Effective Dietary Intake Recommendation for Vitamin D" *J. Nutr* 135(2) (Feb 2005): 317. Hollis, B.W., D. Johnson, T.C. Hulsey, et al. "Vitamin D Supplementation during Pregnancy: Double-Blind, Randomized Clinical Trial of Safety and Effectiveness." *J Bone Miner Res* 26(10) (Oct 2011): 2341–57.

30. Docherty, J.P., D.A. Sack, M. Roffman, et al. "A Double-Blind, Placebo-Controlled, Exploratory Trial of Chromium Picolinate in Atypical Depression: Effect on Carbohydrate Craving." *J Psychiatr Pract* 11(5) (Sep 2005): 302–14.

31. Challem, J. *The Food Mood Solution.* Hoboken, NJ: John Wiley & Sons, 2007

32. Saul, A.W. *Doctor Yourself: Natural Healing That Works.* Laguna Beach, CA: Basic Health Publications, 2003. Anderson, R., A. Kozlovsky. "Chromium Intake, Absorption, and Excretion of Subjects Consuming Self-Selected Diets," *Am J Clin Nutr* 41(6) (Jun 1985):1177–83. Saul, A.W. *Fire Your Doctor: How to Be Independently Healthy.* Laguna Beach, CA: Basic Health Publications, 2005.

33. McLeod, M.N. *Lifting Depression: The Chromium Connection.* Laguna Beach, CA: Basic Health Publications, 2005.

34. Crayton, J.W., W.J. Walsh. "Elevated Serum Copper Levels in Women with a History of Postpartum Depression." *J Trace Elem Med Biol* 21(1) (2007): 17–21.

35. Jonsson, B.H., A.W. Saul. *The Vitamin Cure for Depression.* Laguna Beach, CA: Basic Health Publications, 2012.

36. American Pregnancy Association. "Omega-3 Fish Oil and Pregnancy." http://americanpregnancy.org/pregnancyhealth/omega3fishoil.html (accessed Nov 2014).

37. Ibid.

38. Su, K.P., S.Y. Huang, T.H. Chiu, et al. "Omega-3 Fatty Acids for Major Depressive Disorder during Pregnancy: Results from a Randomized, Double-Blind, Placebo-Controlled Trial." *J Clin Psychiatry* 69(4) (Apr 2008):644–51.

39. Greenberg, J.A., S.J Bell, W. Van Ausdal. "Omega-3 Fatty Acid Supplementation during Pregnancy." *Rev Obstet Gynecol* 1(4) (Fall 2008): 162–9.

40. Holford, P., S. Lawson. *Optimum Nutrition before during and after Pregnancy: Everything You Need to Achieve Optimum Well-Being.* UK: Hachette, 2004.

CHAPTER 11. HEALTHY BABIES AND HEALTHY KIDS

1. Campbell, R., A.W. Saul. *The Vitamin Cure for Children's Health Problems.* Laguna Beach, CA: Basic Health Publications, 2011.

2. Chen, S., Y. Yang, X. Yan, et al. "Influence of Vitamin A Status on the Antiviral Immunity of Children with Hand, Foot and Mouth Disease." *Clin Nutr* 31(4) (Aug 2012): 543–8.

3. Nilsson, T.K., A. Yngve, A.K. Böttiger, et al. "High Folate Intake Is Related to Better Academic Achievement in Swedish Adolescents." *Pediatrics* 128(2) (Aug 2011): doi10.1542/peds.2010–1481

4. Rao, M., A. Afshin, G. Singh, et al. "Do Healthier Foods and Diet Patterns Cost More Than Less Healthy Options? A Systematic Review and Meta-Analysis." *BMJ Open* 3(2) (Dec 5, 2013): e004277 doi:10.1136/bmjopen-2013–004277.

5. Merenstein, D., M. Murphy, A. Fokar, et al. "Use of a Fermented Dairy Probiotic Drink Containing *Lactobacillus casei* (DN-114 001) to Decrease the Rate of Illness in Kids: The DRINK Study. A Patient-Oriented, Double-Blind, Cluster-Randomized, Placebo-Controlled, Clinical Trial." *Eur J Clin Nutr* 64(7) (Jul 2010): 669–77.

6. Bronchiolitis. Mayo clinic staff. Accessed May 2013 at www.mayoclinic.com/health/bronchiolitis/DS00481

7. American Academy of Pediatrics. Subcommittee on Diagnosis and Management of Bronchiolitis. "Diagnosis and Management of Bronchiolitis." *Pediatrics* 118(4) (Oct 1, 2006): 1774–93. Available online at: http://pediatrics.aappublications.org/content/118/4/1774.full (accessed Nov 2014).

8. Belderbos, M.E., M.L. Houben, B. Wilbrink, et al. "Cord Blood Vitamin D Deficiency Is Associated with Respiratory Syncytial Virus Bronchiolitis." *Pediatrics* 127(6) (Jun 2011): e1513–20. doi: 10.1542/peds.2010–3054.

9. Challem, J. "Low Vitamin D Raises Infection Risk in Infants." *The Nutrition Reporter* 22(3) (Mar 2011).

10. Gadomski, A.M., M. Brower. "Bronchodilators for Bronchiolitis for Infants and Young Children." Published Online: December 8, 2010. http://summaries.cochrane.org/

CD001266/bronchodilators-for-bronchiolitis-for-infants-and-young-children (No longer available on the www).

11. Ibid.

12. Campbell, R., A.W. Saul. *The Vitamin Cure for Children's Health Problems*. Laguna Beach, CA: Basic Health Publications, 2011.

13. Orthomolecular Medicine News Service. "Antibiotics Put 142,000 into Emergency Rooms Each Year. U.S. Centers for Disease Control Waits 60 Years to Study the Problem." (Oct 13, 2008.): www.orthomolecular.org/resources/omns/v04n14.shtml (accessed Nov 2014). Saul, A.W. "Notes On Orthomolecular (Megavitamin) Use of Vitamin C." www.doctoryourself.com/ortho_c.html (accessed Nov 2014).

14. HRSA Health Resources and Services Administration. U.S. Department of Health and Human Services. "National Vaccine Injury Compensation Program." www.hrsa.gov/vaccinecompensation/index.html (accessed Nov 2014).

15. Mercola, J. "Vaccine Makers Profit from Government-Granted Immunity." (Mar 12, 2009): http://articles.mercola.com/sites/articles/archive/2009/03/12/Vaccine-Makers-Profit-from-Government-Granted-Immunity.aspx (accessed Nov 2014).

16. Ibid.

17. U.S. Department of Health and Human Services. Health Resources and Services Administration. National Vaccine Injury Compensation Program. "Data and Statistics." www.hrsa.gov/vaccinecompensation/data.html (accessed Nov 2014).

18. Mercola, J. "Vaccine Makers Profit from Government-Granted Immunity." (Mar 12, 2009): http://articles.mercola.com/sites/articles/archive/2009/03/12/Vaccine-Makers-Profit-from-Government-Granted-Immunity.aspx (accessed Nov 2014).

19. Ibid.

20. Mercola, J. "The Latest in Atrocious Supreme Court Decisions—Only 2 Justices Stand Up for Your Rights . . ." http://articles.mercola.com/sites/articles/archive/2011/03/22/betrayal-of-consumers-by-us-supreme-court-gives-total-liability-shield-to-big-pharma.aspx (accessed Nov 2014).

21. Shaw, W. "Evidence that Increased Acetaminophen use in Genetically Vulnerable Children Appears to Be a Major Cause of the Epidemics of Autism, Attention Deficit with Hyperactivity, and Asthma." *J Restorative Med* 2(1) (Oct 2013): 14–29. Liew, Z., B. Ritz, C. Rebordosa, et al. "Acetaminophen Use during Pregnancy, Behavioral Problems, and Hyperkinetic Disorders." *JAMA Pediatr* 168(4) (Apr 2014): 313–20.

22. Harris, G. "F.D.A. Plans New Limits on Painkillers." *The New York Times* (Jan 13, 2011): www.nytimes.com/2011/01/14/health/policy/14fda.html?_r=0 (accessed Nov 2014).

23. Levy, T.E. "Vitamin C Prevents Vaccination Side Effects; Increases Effectiveness." *Orthomolecular Med News Service* (Feb 14, 2012): http://orthomolecular.org/resources/omns/v08n07.shtml (accessed Nov 2014).

24. Ibid.

25. Ibid.

26. Ibid.

27. Ibid.

28. Fluoride Action Network. "Infant Exposure." FluorideAlert.org. http://fluoridealert.org/issues/infant-exposure/ (accessed Nov 2014).

29. Ibid.

30. Ibid.

31. Ibid.

32. Ibid.

33. Centers for Disease Control and Prevention (CDC). "Recommendations for Using Fluoride to Prevent and Control Dental Caries in the United States." (Aug 17, 2001): www.cdc.gov/mmwr/preview/mmwrhtml/rr5014a1.htm (accessed Nov 2014).

34. Levy, T.E. *Vitamin C, Infectious Diseases, and Toxins: Curing the Incurable.* Philadelphia, PA: Xlibris Corporation, 2002.

35. Gupta, S.K., R.C. Gupta, A.K. Seth, et al. "Reversal of Fluorosis in Children." *Acta Paediatr Jpn* 38(5) (Oct 1996): 513–9.

36. Levy, T.E. *Vitamin C, Infectious Diseases, and Toxins: Curing the Incurable.* Philadelphia, PA: Xlibris Corporation, 2002.

Index

About the Author

Mrs. Case is the author of *The Vitamin Cure for Women's Health Problems* and coauthor of *Vegetable Juicing for Everyone*. She has also published in the *Journal of Orthomolecular Medicine* and the *Orthomolecular Medicine News Service*. She is the daughter of Andrew W. Saul, star of the movie *Food Matters* and author of many popular books including *Doctor Yourself*. She currently lives with her husband and children in western New York.

CPSIA information can be obtained
at www.ICGtesting.com
Printed in the USA
BVHW061401031218
534640BV00030B/1476/P

9 781591 203131